# THE
# PERIODONTIC
# SYLLABUS

## FIFTH EDITION

FIFTH EDITION

# THE PERIODONTIC SYLLABUS

**Arthur R. Vernino, DDS**
Adjunct Clinical Professor, Department of Periodontics
University of Florida College of Dentistry
Gainesville, FL
Professor Emeritus, University of Oklahoma

**Jonathan Gray, DDS**
Clinical Associate Professor
Indiana University School of Dentistry
Indianapolis, IN

**Elizabeth Hughes, RDH, BS, MS**
Associate Professor
Dental Hygiene Division
Department of Periodontics and Allied Dental Programs
Indiana University School of Dentistry
Indianapolis, IN

Wolters Kluwer | Lippincott Williams & Wilkins
Health
Philadelphia · Baltimore · New York · London
Buenos Aires · Hong Kong · Sydney · Tokyo

*Acquisitions Editor:* John Goucher
*Managing Editor:* Kevin C. Dietz
*Marketing Manager:* Hilary Henderson
*Production Editor:* Paula C. Williams
*Designer:* Stephen Druding
*Compositor:* International Typesetting and Composition
*Printer:* Data Reproductions Corporation

351 West Camden Street
Baltimore, MD 21201

530 Walnut Street
Philadelphia, PA 19106

*Printed in the United States of America*

First Edition, 1985
Second Edition, 1989
Third Edition, 1995
Fourth Edition, 2000

**Library of Congress Cataloging-in-Publication Data is available: (ISBN-10: 0-7817-7972-3)**
**(ISBN-13: 978-0-7817-7972-3)**

To purchase additional copies of this book, call our customer service department at **(800) 638-3030** or fax orders to **(301) 223-2320.** International customers should call **(301) 223-2300.**

***Visit Lippincott Williams & Wilkins on the Internet: http://www.LWW.com.*** Lippincott Williams & Wilkins customer service representatives are available from 8:30 am to 6:00 pm, EST.

06 07 08 09 10
1 2 3 4 5 6 7 8 9 10

# Preface

This fifth edition of *The Periodontic Syllabus* is dedicated to the memory of Dr. Peter F. Fedi, who was our mentor and close friend. Dr. Fedi was a leading force in initiating the publication of the book.

This book was originally a publication of the United States Navy. It was intended to accompany a one-week course in periodontics taught at the Naval Dental School, Bethesda, MD. The principle contributors were Drs. Fedi, Gerald Bowers, Joseph Lawrence, and John Williams. Dr. Fedi was largely responsible for the transition to the current publication.

The editors and contributors of *The Periodontic Syllabus* are aware that the ever-expanding information base in periodontics makes it very difficult to "keep up to date." The practice of periodontics is dynamic and continually changing to reflect the changing approaches to therapy. It is no wonder that the practicing dentist and dental hygienist find difficulty remaining current.

The fifth edition, as does its predecessors, attempts to focus attention on the biologic approach to treatment modalities. We strive to continue the basic approach for easy access to various methods for treating diseases of the periodontium and replacement of missing components of the dental arches. This syllabus is not a complete and detailed textbook, but should complement other textbooks on the subject. Our objective is to present a concise, current syllabus.

We originally targeted the dental student and general practitioners as the primary readers. As more and more periodontal therapy is provided in general practice, the role of the dental hygienist has become increasingly important in the treatment of new periodontal diseases. Consequently, there is a greater emphasis placed on including material that would be useful to the dental hygienist and the dental hygiene student.

We welcome suggestions and critiques. This is how we continue to provide you, the user of the syllabus, what you want and need. References have replaced the "Suggested Reading" of previous editions. We hope that the continuing student, who desires greater depth on each subject, will find these lists helpful. Questions for self-assessment have also been included at the end of each chapter.

Additionally, we want to thank all of our contributors, past and present, without whom these five editions could not have been written.

# Contributors

Jane Amme, RDH
Clinical Associate Professor
Department of Periodontics
University of Oklahoma College of Dentistry
Oklahoma City, OK

Stephen Blanchard, DDS, MS
Assistant Professor and Director of Graduate Periodontics
Department of Periodontics and Allied Dental Programs
Indiana University School of Dentistry
Indianapolis, IN

Lorraine Brockman, RDH, MSHE
Assistant Professor
Department of Periodontics
UMKC School of Dentistry
Kansas City, MO

Cheryl Burns, RDH, MS
Clinical Associate Professor
Department of Periodontics
UMKC School of Dentistry
Kansas City, MO

Donald Callan, DDS, MS
Private Practice in Periodontics
Little Rock, AR 72205

Henry Greenwell, DMD, MSD
Professor, Chair, and Director of Graduate Periodontics
Dept of Periodontics, Endodontics, and Dental Hygiene
Graduate Periodontics
Louisville, KY

William Hallmon, DMD, MS
Professor and Chair
Periodontics Department
Baylor College of Dentistry
The Texas A&M University System Health Science
    Center
Dallas, TX

Stephen Harrell, DDS
Clinical Associate Professor
Periodontics Department
Baylor College of Dentistry
The Texas A&M University System Health Science
    Center
Dallas, TX

Gregory Horning, DDS, MS
Associate Professor and Director of Graduate
    Periodontics
Periodontics Department
University of Florida College of Dentistry
Gainesville, FL

Elizabeth Hughes, RDH, BS, MS
Associate Professor
Dental Hygiene Division
Department of Periodontics and Allied Dental
    Programs
Indiana University School of Dentistry
Indianapolis, IN

Vanchit John, DDS, MSD
Associate Professor
Department of Periodontics and Allied Dental
    Programs
Indiana University School of Dentistry
Indianapolis, IN

Donald Newell, DDS, MS
Professor
Department of Periodontics and Allied Dental
    Programs
Indiana University School of Dentistry
Indianapolis, IN

John Rapley, DDS, MS
Professor, Chair, and Director of Advanced Education
    in Periodontics
Department of Periodontics
UMKC School of Dentistry
Kansas City, MO

Terry Rees, DDS, MS
Professor
Periodontics Department
Baylor College of Dentistry
The Texas A&M University System Health Science
    Center
Dallas, TX

Raymond A. Yukna, DDS, MS
Professor, Department of Periodontics
Coordinator of Postdoctoral Periodontics
School of Dentistry Louisiana State University
New Orleans, LA

# Contents

# The Periodontium

Gregory M. Horning

## THE PERIODONTIUM

The main functions of the periodontium are to attach teeth to the bone of the jaws and to maintain the surface integrity of the oral cavity. Other functions include the development of the teeth themselves and their associated tissues, and the repair, regeneration, and maintenance of each tissue throughout the various changes and stresses of life.[1] A healthy periodontium is important in maintaining a functional barrier against the physical and microbial challenges of the gastrointestinal tract, and it is a vital part of good facial esthetics. The periodontium is composed of the gingiva, periodontal ligament, cementum, and alveolar bone.

## GINGIVA

### Terminology

The following terminology is used in describing the gingiva (Fig. 1-1):

### 1. Marginal (Free) Gingiva

That portion of the gingiva surrounding the neck of the tooth, not directly attached to the tooth, and forming the soft tissue wall of the gingival sulcus. It extends from the gingival margin to the gingival groove. The free gingival margin itself is located 1.5 to 2 mm coronal to the cementoenamel junction after tooth eruption,[1] and is about 1 mm thick.[2]

### 2. Gingival Groove

A shallow line or depression on the surface of the gingiva, dividing the free gingiva from the attached gingiva. Present about 50% of the time,[3] the gingival groove often corresponds to the location of the bottom of the gingival sulcus.

### 3. Keratinized Gingiva

The band of keratinized gingiva extending from the gingival margin to the mucogingival junction (Fig. 1-2). The apicocoronal width of the keratinized gingiva varies from less than 1 to 9 mm, and is generally widest in the anterior maxilla and posterior lingual mandible.[4] Certain teeth frequently have a narrow zone of keratinized gingiva. These teeth include mandibular canines and premolars, prominent teeth, and teeth associated with abnormal frenum or muscle attachments. Teeth with less than 1 mm of attached gingiva may be maintained in health. However, when tugging of the lip or cheek results in movement of the free gingival margin or papilla (positive tug test), an increased susceptibility to tissue breakdown may be present. An adequate width of attached gingiva may then be defined as the amount of keratinized tissue necessary to help maintain a noninflamed, stable gingival margin.

### 4. Attached Gingiva

That portion of the gingiva that extends apically from the area of the free gingival groove to the mucogingival junction. In the absence of inflammation the facial attached gingiva is clearly defined. In the hard palate, however, there is no clinical demarcation between the attached gingiva and the remaining masticatory mucosa. Attached gingiva is normally covered by keratinized or parakeratinized epithelium with marked rete ridges. This tissue is designed to withstand the rigors of mastication, tooth brushing, and other functional stresses, and it is tightly bound down to the underlying tooth and bone.

### 5. Mucogingival Junction

The scalloped line dividing the keratinized gingiva from the flexible alveolar mucosa (Fig. 1-1). The mucogingival junction is histologically a transition

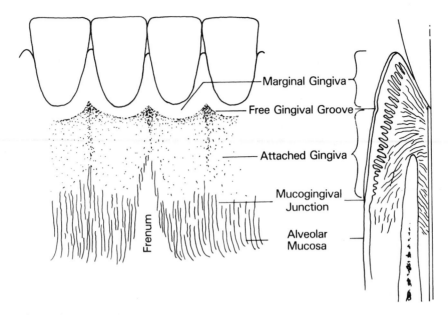

*Figure 1.1* ●

zone,[5] not an abrupt demarcation, which is important to consider in gingival grafting.

## 6. Interdental Groove

The vertical groove, parallel to the long axes of adjacent teeth, found in the interdental area of the attached gingiva.

## 7. Interdental Papilla

The portion of the gingiva that fills the interproximal space between adjacent teeth. The tip of the interdental is concave faciolingually, forming a saddlelike depression called the col (Fig.1-3).

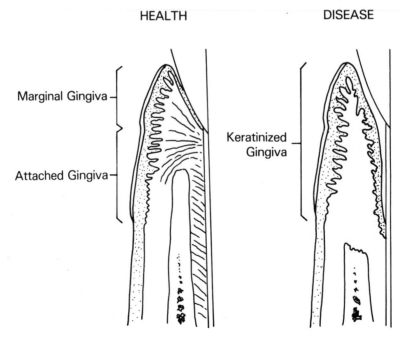

*Figure 1.2* ●

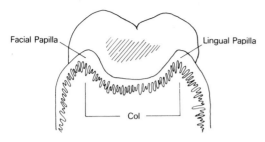

Facial Papilla

Lingual Papilla

Col

**Figure 1.3** ●

### 8. Gingival Sulcus (Crevice)

The space bounded by the tooth and the free gingiva, and having the junctional epithelium as its base. When diseased, it is called a **"pocket."**

## Blood, Lymphatic, and Nerve Supply of the Gingiva

Gingival tissue has a rich vascular supply formed by a plexus of arterioles, capillaries, and small veins that extend from the sulcular epithelium to the outer surface of the gingiva. The blood supply of the gingiva is derived mainly from suprape-

riosteal branches of the internal maxillary arteries. Vessels from both the alveolar bone and the periodontal ligament merge with the supraperiosteal vessels to form the gingival plexus (Fig. 1-4). Peri-implant gingival tissue lacks the periodontal ligament vasculature, and receives its blood supply solely from supraperiosteal vessels.[6]

Lymphatic drainage of the gingiva begins in the connective tissue and progresses into a network that lies external to the periosteum of the alveolar process. Lymphatic vessels drain to regional lymph nodes, particularly the submaxillary group. In addition, lymphatics beneath the epithelium extend into the periodontal ligament and accompany the blood vessels. Innervation of the gingiva comes from labial, buccal, and palatal nerves and from fibers in the periodontal ligament.

## COMPONENTS OF GINGIVA
### Oral and Crevicular Epithelium

Gingival oral epithelium is of the stratified squamous type, and may be parakeratinized or orthokeratinized. It is continuous with the nonkeratinized epithelium lining the gingival sulcus, which at its apical extent forms the epithelial

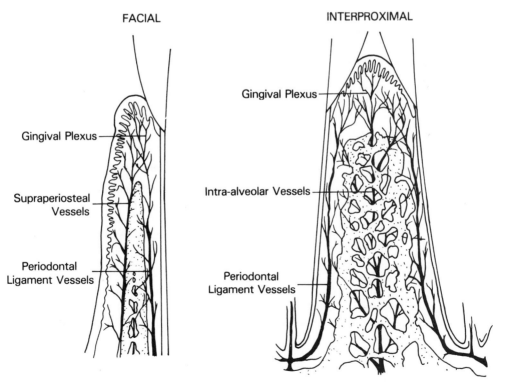

FACIAL

INTERPROXIMAL

Gingival Plexus

Gingival Plexus

Intra-alveolar Vessels

Supraperiosteal Vessels

Periodontal Ligament Vessels

Periodontal Ligament Vessels

**Figure 1.4** ●

DENTOGINGIVAL JUNCTION

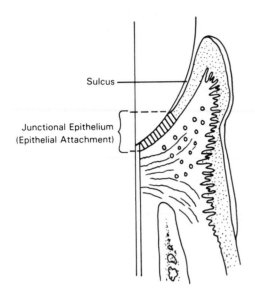

**Figure 1.5** ●

attachment to the tooth (Fig. 1-5). The crevicular epithelium acts like a semipermeable membrane: although crevicular bacteria, toxins, or other injurious products may infiltrate the tissue, the constant seepage of gingival crevicular fluid tends to flush out or dilute these elements. A discrete cuff of inflammatory cells (monocytes/macrophages, lymphocytes, and neutrophils) is generally seen immediately subjacent to the crevicular epithelium in health, although perhaps not in pristine gingiva.[1]

## Dentogingival Junction

The dentogingival junction consists of the epithelial attachment (junctional epithelium) and the gingival fiber apparatus (connective tissue attachment).

## Junctional Epithelium

This term refers to the collar or band of nonkeratinized basal and stratum spinosum-type cells that actually attach to the tooth. It varies in thickness from 15 to 20 cells coronally to 1 to 2 cells apically. The cells of the junctional epithelium have relatively wider intercellular spaces and fewer desmosomes when compared with the gingival epithelium. Its location on the tooth depends on the stage of tooth eruption, but in the adult it is normally considered to be at or near the cementoenamel junction. Migration of the junctional

epithelium apical to this junction is no longer considered to be a physiologic process of aging, but rather a pathologic process.

The ultramicroscopic attachment of the sulcular epithelium to the tooth is comparable to the epithelial connective tissue attachment found in skin or other body surfaces. There is a basal lamina (basement membrane) that consists of two layers: the lamina densa (adjacent to the tooth surface) and the lamina lucida, to which hemidesmosomes (attachment plaques) are attached. A sticky coating (proline or hydroxyproline and mucopolysaccharide), which is secreted by the epithelial cells, also binds the junctional epithelium to enamel or cementum.

## Lamina Propria

This term is used to describe the connective tissue component of the gingiva. The character of the connective tissue determines the differentiation of the overlying epithelium in postsurgical healing: lamina propria signals for the development of keratinized epithelium, whereas submucosal connective tissue codes for the nonkeratinized epithelium seen in oral mucosa.[7] This is an important principle of gingival grafting (see Chapter 16). Like other connective tissues, the lamina propria consists of cells (fibroblasts, mesenchymal cells, mast cells, and macrophages), formed elements (collagenous fibers), a matrix (ground substance) largely consisting of proteoglycans and glycoproteins, and a neurovascular network. The collagenous connective tissue fibers are oriented into the coarse bundles of the connective tissue attachment to the tooth. These are grouped according to location and direction, and are sometimes referred to as the gingival fiber apparatus.

## Gingival Fiber Apparatus

The gingival fiber apparatus serves the important functions of maintaining the gingival margin in close approximation to the tooth and bracing it against the various stresses of mastication. It consists of three groups:

### 1. Gingival Group

These fibers extend from the cementum in three groups (termed a, b, and c) and represent the bulk of the lamina propria facially and lingually (Fig. 1-6).

### 2. Circular Group

Circular fibers encompass the teeth from the margin of the gingiva to the alveolar crest (Fig. 1-7).

GINGIVAL GROUP

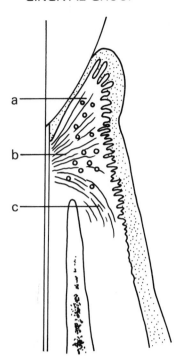

**Figure 1.6** ●

## 3. Transseptal Group

These fibers extend interdentally from the cementum of one tooth to that of the adjacent tooth. Some authors classify this fiber group with the principal fibers of the periodontal ligament rather than with the gingival fiber apparatus (Fig. 1-8).

## Biologic Width

First described by Gargiulo et al. (1961), this term initially referred to the epithelial attachment plus the connective tissue attachment above the crest of alveolar bone, approximately 2 mm.[8] The average crevice depth of 1 mm has been popularly added, making a dimension of 3 mm that the body will tend to reestablish in such cases as caries, tooth fracture, or restoration[9] (also see Chapter 15.) The dimension varies with individuals, and is larger in a thick biotype person.

## Periodontal Biotype

Also known as periodontal phenotype (Fig. 1-9), this refers to the common classification of hereditary thickness of the periodontal tissues as either normal or thin (75% of all patients; Fig. 1-9a) or thick (25%; Fig. 1-9b).[10] A thick biotype displays thick and wide gingiva, wider teeth, and thicker bone. It is less likely to experience gingival recession, more likely to have exostoses, and more likely to have infrabony defects develop during periodontal attachment loss.

## Dimensions and Contours of Therapeutic Importance

The thickness of facial attached gingiva averages a little less than 1.5 mm.[11] The thickness of palatal masticatory mucosa is thicker, averaging 2 to 4 mm.[12] The epithelial portion of palatal mucosa may average 0.34 mm or more in thickness,[13] which has therapeutic importance when harvesting

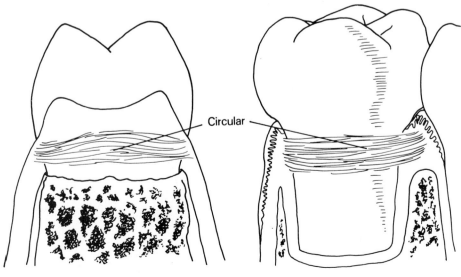

Circular

**Figure 1.7** ●

TRANSSEPTAL GROUP

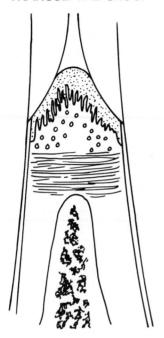

**Figure 1.8** ●

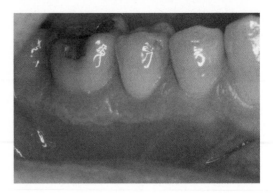

**Figure 1.10** ●

implants, which lack periodontal ligament blood supply and attaching gingival fibers, may only predictably extend 3 mm.[15]

### The Peri-Implant Gingival Attachment

The epithelial attachment (Fig.1-10) to titanium implant surfaces is quite similar to that of teeth, involving junctional or barrier epithelium attaching to the implant surface by a basal lamina and hemidesmosomes.[16] Major differences between the gingival attachment to teeth and to dental implants involve the lack of two major tissues that invest natural teeth: root cementum, and connective tissue of the periodontal ligament and supracrestal fiber groups (a, b, and c). Rather than inserting

gingival connective tissue for periodontal plastic surgical purposes (see Chapter 17). Gingiva may predictably extend 5 mm from the bony crest to the interdental contact about natural teeth, forming the interdental papilla.[14] Gingival tissue about dental

## Periodontal Biotypes

75%
Thin/Normal

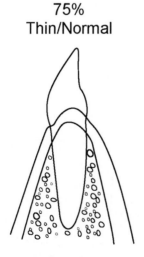

## Periodontal Biotypes

25%
Thick

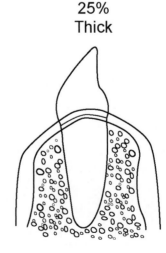

**Figure 1.9a–b** ●

perpendicularly into cementum, connective tissue fibers adjacent to a dental implant run parallel to it.[17] Peri-implant biologic width approximates 3 mm, and consists of about 2 mm of epithelium and 1 to 1.5 mm of connective tissue.[18] The epithelial adhesion to implants may be apparently easily displaced, as gentle probing reveals the connective tissue level in health; in inflamed sites, probing approximates bone level[19] (see Chapters 21–23).

## Clinically Healthy Gingiva

Several terms used in describing the gingival tissues are important. The following terms are used most often to describe normal gingiva:

### 1. Color

Normal gingiva is described as coral pink, but shading varies widely among individuals. Physiologic (melanin) pigmentation is normal in several ethnic groups.

### 2. Size

Inherited biotype determines size; change in size is common in periodontal disease.

### 3. Contour

This term refers primarily to the festooned appearance of the gingiva. It may also refer to such variations in contour as reticular mandibular ridges,[20] which are gingival surface corrugations corresponding to palatal rugae.

### 4. Consistency

The gingiva is firm, resilient, and tightly bound to the underlying bone.

### 5. Surface Texture

A stippled appearance is normal in the attached gingiva; loss of stippling may be a sign of periodontal disease. Stippling is caused by projections of the papillary layer of the lamina propria, which elevate the epithelium into rounded prominences that alternate with indentations of the epithelium.

### 6. Tendency to Bleed on Palpation or Gentle Probing

Clinically healthy gingiva will not bleed when a periodontal probe is gently inserted into the sulcus or when the marginal gingiva is palpated manually.

## ALVEOLAR MUCOSA

The epithelium of the alveolar mucosa is thin, nonkeratinized, and lacks distinct rete ridges. The connective tissue consists of a thin lamina propria and a vascular submucosal layer. The predominant connective tissue fibers are elastic: as a result, the alveolar mucosa is flexible, and is bound loosely to the underlying periosteum of the alveolar process. Clinically, the gingiva and alveolar mucosa are separated by the mucogingival junction. On the facial aspects of the maxillary and mandibular arches, the alveolar mucosa extends to the vestibular fornix. On the lingual aspect of the mandibular arch, the arrangement is similar. In the maxillary arch, the gingiva blends seamlessly with the palatal mucosa, which is dense and firmly attached to the underlying periosteum. It should be emphasized that the alveolar mucosa is not designed to withstand the forces of mastication; therefore, it cannot serve as gingival tissue.

## PERIODONTAL LIGAMENT

The periodontal ligament (Figs. 1-11 and 1-12) is a remarkable connective tissue that coats the root of the tooth and attaches it to the alveolar process. With relatively few elastic fibers, its apparent elasticity is attributable to the wavy configuration of the principal collagen fibers, which permit slight tooth movement downward and about an axis of rotation.

## Functions

The functions of the periodontal ligament include:

1. To physically suspend the tooth within its bony housing via fibrous insertions from the root cementum to the alveolar bone proper.
2. To protect both the tooth and bone from the shock of abnormal occlusal forces. This may be accomplished by a viscoelastic (tissue fluid) mechanism as well as by the toughness of the fibers themselves.

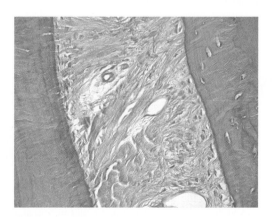

*Figure 1.11* •

PRINCIPAL FIBER GROUPS

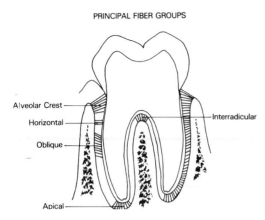

Alveolar Crest
Horizontal
Oblique
Interradicular
Apical

***Figure 1.12*** ●

3. To safely transmit normal external forces from the tooth to the bone, largely converting vertical pressures into tension of the periodontal ligament fibers. This tension in turn is transmitted to the alveolar bone, which may itself flex within physiologic limits, and in time remodel appropriately.
4. To create, regenerate, and remodel alveolar bone and cementum. The periodontal ligament, with its various pluripotential cells, is absolutely required for orthodontic movement and guided tissue regeneration (see Chapter 17), as well as tooth eruption. Its injury or absence can result in inflammatory or replacement root resorption.
5. To supply nutrients and remove waste products via blood and lymph vessels.
6. To detect and transmit tactile pressure and pain sensations by the trigeminal pathway. The sense of localization is imparted through proprioceptive nerve endings.

## Principal Fibers of the Periodontal Ligament

Numerous bundles of collagenous fibers comprise the principal fibers of the periodontal ligament (Fig. 1-12). These fibers are named according to their location and direction of attachment (alveolar crest, horizontal, oblique, and apical). Interradicular fibers are observed on multirooted teeth.

## Width

Width of the periodontal ligament space varies with age, location of the tooth, and the degree of stress to which the tooth was subjected. The mesial side is thinner than the distal side, owing to physiologic mesial drift of teeth. A tooth that is not in function

has a thin periodontal ligament, with loss of orientation of the principal fibers. A tooth under normal use has a thicker periodontal ligament and a normal configuration of the principal fibers. A tooth in functional occlusion has a periodontal ligament space of approximately $0.25 \pm 0.10$ mm.[21] A tooth subjected to abnormal stress has a considerably thicker periodontal ligament space. Periodontal ligament shape is like an hourglass apicocoronally, corresponding to the rotation point of the tooth.

## Blood Supply of the Periodontal Ligament

A particularly rich polyhedral network of periodontal ligament vessels wrap the tooth, derived from three sources:

1. Blood vessels entering the periodontal ligament from the dental artery, itself a branch of the inferior alveolar or palatal arteries.
2. Intraseptal arteries that penetrate the lamina dura (cribriform plate) at all levels of the alveolus.
3. Anastomosing vessels from the gingival plexus.

## Nerve Supply

The nerves are both myelinated and unmyelinated, and have four types of sensory endings. These include pain receptors, two kinds of mechanoreceptors, and spindlelike receptors for pressure and vibration. The nerve bundles follow the course of the blood vessels. Their primary purpose is to transmit proprioceptive sensations via the trigeminal pathways, which give a sense of localization when a tooth is touched.

## CEMENTUM

Cementum is the calcified structure that covers the anatomic roots of teeth. It consists of a calcified matrix with collagenous fibrils. Histologically similar to bone, the inorganic content is approximately 45 to 50%. Cementum is permeable and susceptible to toxins and bacteria if exposed.

## Cementum and Cementoid

When first formed, cementum is uncalcified and is known as cementoid. As new layers are formed, the previously formed matrix is calcified and becomes mature cementum. Microscopically, cementum can be divided into two types, cellular and acellular; functionally, however, there is no difference. Cellular cementum, which often forms during wound healing, contains lacunae with cells called cementocytes. These cells communicate with one another by means of canaliculi. The distribution of cellular and acellular cementum on the roots of teeth varies. Generally, cementum covering the coronal portion of a root is acellular, whereas that covering the apical region is cellular. Cementum is deposited continuously throughout life, and varies in thickness from 1 to 15 μm near the cementoenamel junction to 1,000 μm (1 mm) at the tooth apex.[22] Cementum generally averages 100 μm (0.1 mm) thick in therapeutic areas. Hypercementosis (abnormally thick cementum) may result from occlusal traumatism or from Paget's disease, and cemental tears have been reported in association with localized periodontal defects.

## Functions

Various functions of cementum include:

1. To anchor the connective tissue fibers of the gingiva and periodontal ligament to the tooth.
2. To compensate, by its continuing growth, for the loss of tooth structure through wear.
3. To permit a continual rearrangement of the periodontal ligament fibers.
4. To protect the tooth from apical migration of the junctional epithelium, and protect dentin from resorption when traumatically exposed.

## Cementoenamel Junction

The relationships of the cementum to the enamel at the cementoenamel junction have clinical significance. There are three types of relationships, as demonstrated in Figure 1-13. In 60 to 65% of the cases, the cementum overlaps the enamel. In 30% there is a butt joint. In 5 to 10% of patients, however, the enamel and cementum do not meet, revealing exposed and potentially very sensitive dentin, especially if recession occurs.[23] This defect also enhances accumulation of plaque and calculus. Calculus that forms in this defect defies removal, even when visible.

## Cervical Projection of Enamel

Enamel projections often extend varying distances (grades 1, 2, and 3) from the cementoenamel junction to the mid furcal area (Fig. 1-14). Cervical projections of enamel are covered by an epithelial attachment, potentially weaker than a connective tissue attachment. They may represent a possible pathway for early furcation exposure.

## Palatogingival Groove

A similar developmental defect often associated with advanced periodontal destruction is the palatogingival groove (Fig. 1-15). This groove is most frequently observed on maxillary central and lateral incisors, and it often extends from the cingulum to the apex. The palatogingival groove

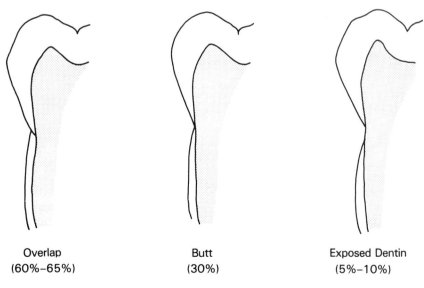

| Overlap | Butt | Exposed Dentin |
| (60%–65%) | (30%) | (5%–10%) |

**Figure 1.13** ●

ENAMEL PROJECTIONS

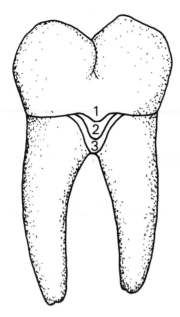

*Figure 1.14* ●

Dentogingival Groove
Maxillary Lateral
(Lingual View)

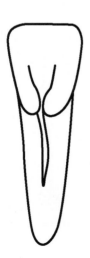

*Figure 1.15* ●

presents a difficult, if not impossible, management problem for the patient and clinician.

## ALVEOLAR PROCESS

The alveolar process is that portion of the maxilla and mandible that forms and supports the sockets (alveoli) of the teeth.

### Divisions

On the basis of function and adaptation, the alveolar process can be divided into two parts:

### 1. Alveolar Bone Proper

The thin layer of compact bone that lines the tooth socket and gives attachment to the periodontal ligament. This bone is also known as the cribriform plate owing to its numerous perforations traversed by blood vessels. Radiographically it is viewed as a narrow but dense opacity about the periodontal ligament space, and is called the lamina dura. Alveolar bone proper contains calcified insertions of bundles of Sharpey's fibers from the periodontal ligament, and may be also called "bundle bone," a term used for other areas of bone in which tendons, ligaments, or muscles insert.

### 2. Supporting Alveolar Bone

The portion of the alveolar process that surrounds the alveolar bone proper and gives support to the sockets. It consists of:

a. **Cortical (compact lamellar) bone** of the exterior aspects of the alveolar process. Cortical plates are typically thick in posterior buccal and palatal areas, but thin in anterior facial areas.

b. **Cancellous bone (spongy bone)** that lies between the alveolar bone proper and the cortical bone. Cancellous bone contains marrow that, in the adult, is mostly of the yellow or fatty type. Foci of red marrow can be found in the maxillary tuberosity and, on occasion, in the maxillary and mandibular molar and premolar areas.

### Blood Supply

The vascular supply of bone is derived from intra-alveolar (intraseptal) arteries, vessels that penetrate the cortical plates (Fig. 1-4). In circumstances in which cortical bone and alveolar bone proper are fused, as on the facial aspect of the anterior teeth, the blood supply is derived chiefly from supraperiosteal vessels. Where the interdental space is less than 0.5 mm (**"kissing roots"**), cancellous bone may again be lacking, and only cortical bone present, with diminished blood supply.[24]

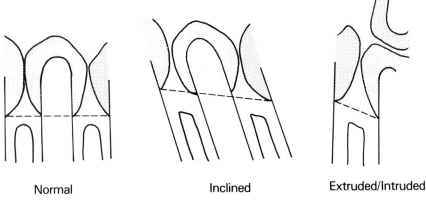

Normal        Inclined        Extruded/Intruded

**Figure 1.16** ●

Once affected by periodontitis, these areas may be difficult to successfully treat.

## Remodeling of Alveolar Bone

The purpose of alveolar bone is to support the teeth in function: when teeth are lost, alveolar bone resorbs. After extraction, 4 mm or more (63%) of bone may be lost horizontally within a 6-month period.[25] Eventually all alveolar bone may resorb, leaving only basal bone of the mandible, and the floors of the sinus and nose in the maxilla, quite inadequate for denture fabrication. Mechanical microstrains have been reported to greatly affect bone remodeling.[26] With minimal loading (less than 0.2% deformation of the mandible), bone atrophy occurs, resulting in fewer and thinner trabeculae and larger medullar spaces. This state is sometimes termed disuse atrophy. With normal loading (0.2 to 0.25% deformation), normal bone turnover and maintenance occurs. With higher loads (0.25 to 0.40% deformation), bone hypertrophy with lamellar bone trabeculae increasing in size occurs, aligned in the path of tensile and compressive stresses. This may be referred to as internal buttressing bone.[27] These findings directly relate to the benefits provided by dental implant therapy in maintaining height and volume of alveolar bone[28] (see Chapter 22). When pathologic loads are imposed (more than 0.40% deformation), woven bone formation occurs. Trauma from occlusion, in which the attachment apparatus can no longer adapt to functional stress, is discussed in Chapter 6.

## Alveolar Bone Contours

In health, the alveolar crest maintains a constant distance from the cementoenamel junction: approximately 1 to 2 mm in health.[29] Teeth that are extruded, intruded, or inclined have an angular interdental crest (Fig. 1-16). This observation is quite important in the radiographic interpretation, where this normal occurrence may be confused with the angular bone defects of periodontitis (see Chapter 2).

The outer contour of the alveolar process conforms to the prominence, size, and position of the roots of the teeth. However, the inherited biotype of the patient greatly affects alveolar bone contours. When the contour of the cementoenamel junction is broad and flat buccolingually (molars and some premolars), the contour of the alveolar process is broad and flat buccolingually. Conversely, the buccolingual contours in the anterior region may be narrow and pointed as a result of the configuration of the cementoenamel junction, just as the gingival contours may be highly scalloped.

Thickness of the labial plate in anterior teeth may be 0.5 mm or less. Overall, the thickness of marginal alveolar bone at 1 mm below its crest averages 1 mm both facially and lingually for anterior teeth and premolars. This thickness is 2 mm for maxillary molars, and 2 to 3 mm for mandibular molars.[30]

## Exostoses, Tori, and Tubercles

Several types of inherited or acquired enlargements in the outer contour of alveolar or palatal bone are commonly seen, and may need to be addressed in periodontal treatment planning (see Chapter 5). These include tori—comprised strictly of cortical bone—palatal tubercles, and buccal alveolar exostoses. There is little evidence these develop in response to heavy occlusal function[30]: they more likely develop as a result of inherited predilection (biotype).

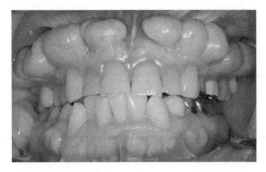

*Figure 1.17* ●

### Palatal Tori:

These occur in approximately 20% of patients, whether dentate or not, and most commonly in white women. Palatal tori may need removal when they interfere with planned prosthodontic treatment.

### Mandibular Tori:

Seen in about 42% of dentate patients, usually bilaterally, mandibular tori may become large enough to impede oral hygiene, and greatly affect periodontal surgery in lingual areas; they may recur after removal.

### Palatal Tubercles:

The most common type of alveolar exostosis, these nodular enlargements are seen in 69% of dentate patients in the maxillary second to third molar area.[31] They generally need removal during crown-lengthening procedures in the posterior

maxilla, and always need to be considered in planning surgical treatment in that area.

### Buccal Exostoses:

(Fig. 1-17) These are seen in about 25% of all teeth, and 77% of all individuals. They may be expressed as alveolar marginal **lipping** (18% of all teeth) or as larger and more globular **buccal exostoses** (7% of all teeth).

### Lingual Exostoses:

These may be seen adjacent to 11% of all teeth, and in 58% of all individuals.[30]

## Dehiscence and Fenestration

**Dehiscence** denotes a cleftlike absence of the alveolar cortical plate, which results in a denuded root surface (Fig 1-18). Although 40% of individuals may have at least one alveolar bone dehiscence, they are present in approximately 4% of all teeth, with most in the mandible, especially in mandibular canines.

**Fenestration** indicates a windowlike defect in the alveolar cortical plate, which similarly exposes the root surface. About 61% of individuals and 9% of all teeth have fenestrations; they are most common in maxillary first molars.[32]

Both of these defects are associated with thin facial bone investing prominent or malaligned teeth. In such cases, there is minimal or no intraalveolar blood supply; the blood supply to the bone is derived chiefly from supraperiosteal vessels and periodontal ligament. Reflecting a

## ALVEOLAR DEFECTS

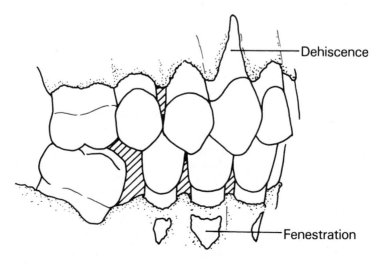

*Figure 1.18* ●

mucoperiosteal flap during periodontal surgery, and so severing the supraperiosteal vessels, may result in the loss of cortical plate or the worsening of a dehiscence or fenestration. If such defects are suspected, every effort should be made to leave connective tissue covering the radicular surface. A partial-thickness flap preserving the supraperiosteal blood supply may be advised.

A similar problem arises if bone contouring is performed adjacent to the thin bone involved with dehiscences or fenestrations: bone resorption during healing may result in extensive osseous dehiscences.

## REFERENCES

1. Lindhe J, Karring T, Lang NP, eds. Clinical Periodontology and Implant Dentistry, 4th ed. Oxford: Blackwell Munksgaard, 2003, pp 1, 3, 198.
2. Alpiste-Illueca F. Dimensions of the dentogingival unit in maxillary anterior teeth: a new exploration technique (parallel profile radiograph). Int J Periodontics Restorative Dent 2004;24:386–396.
3. Ainamo J, Loe H. Anatomical characteristics of gingiva. A clinical and microscopic study of the free and attached gingiva. J Periodontol 1966;37:5–13.
4. Bowers GM. A study of the width of the attached gingiva. J Periodontol 1963;34:210–217.
5. Stanford TW, Levin MP, Payne TF. A comparison of the mucogingival junction in dentulous and edentulous areas. J Periodontol 1976;47:522–524.
6. Berglundh T, Lindhe J, Jonsson K, Ericsson I. The topography of the vascular systems in the periodontal and peri-implant tissues of the dog. J Clin Periodontol 1994;21:189–193.
7. Karring T, Lang NP, Loe HB. The role of gingival connective tissue in determining epithelial differentiation. J Periodont Res 1975;10:1–11.
8. Gargiulo AW, Wentz FM, Orban B. Dimensions and relations of the dentogingival junction in humans. J Periodontol 1961;32:261–267.
9. Nevins M, Cappetta EG. The biologic width: preventing postsurgical recession. In: Nevins M, Mellonig JT, eds. Periodontal Therapy: Clinical Approaches and Evidence of Success, Vol 1. Chicago: Quintessence Publishing, 1998:305–328.
10. Muller HP, Heinecke A, Schaller N, Eger T. Masticatory mucosa in subjects with different periodontal phenotypes. J Clin Periodontol 2000;27:621–626.
11. Goasland GD, Robertson PB, Mahan CJ, Morrison WW, Olson JV. Thickness of facial gingiva. J Periodontol 1977;48:768–771.
12. Wara-aswapati N, Pitiphat W, Chandrapho N, Rattanayatikul C, Karimbux N. Thickness of palatal masticatory mucosa associated with age. J Periodontol 2001;72:1407–1412.
13. Soehren SE, Allen AL, Cutright DE, Seibert JS. Clinical and histologic studies of donor tissues utilized for free grafts of masticatory mucosa. J Periodontol 1973;44:727–741.
14. Tarnow DP, Magner AW, Fletcher P. The effect of the distance from the contact point to the crest of bone on the presence or absence of the interproximal dental papilla. J Periodontol 1992;63:995–996.
15. Gastaldo JF, Cury PR, Sendyk WR. Effect of the vertical and horizontal distances between adjacent implants and between a tooth and an implant on the incidence of interproximal papilla. J Periodontol 2004;75:1242–1246.
16. Gould TR, Westbury L, Brunette DM. Ultrastructural study of the attachment of human gingiva to titanium in vivo. J Prosthet Dent 1984;52:418–420.
17. Listgarten M, Lang N, Schroeder H. Periodontal tissues and their counterparts around endosseous implants. Clin Oral Implants Res 1991;2:1–19.
18. Berglundh T, Lindhe J. Dimension of the periimplant mucosa. Biological width revisited. J Clin Periodontol 1996;23:971–973.
19. Lang NP, Wetzel AC, Stich H, Caffesse RG. Histologic probe penetration in healthy and inflamed peri-implant tissues. Clin Oral Implants Res 1994;5:191–201.
20. Giunta JL. Reticular mandibular ridges. J Periodontol 1986;57:247–250.
21. Coolidge ED. The thickness of the human periodontal membrane. J Am Dent Assoc 1937;24:1260–1270.
22. Newman MG, Takei HH, Carranza FA, eds. Carranza's Clinical Periodontology, 9th ed. Philadelphia: WB Saunders, 2002, pp 15–57.
23. Noyes FB, Schoour I, Noyes HJ. A Textbook of Dental Histology and Embryology, 5th ed. Philadelphia: Lea and Febiger, 19–38.
24. Heins PJ, Wieder SM. A histologic study of the width and nature of inter-radicular spaces in human adult premolars and molars. J Dent Res 1986;65:948–951.
25. Lekovic V, Kenney EB, Weinlaender M, Han T, Klokkevold P, Nedic M, Orsini M. A bone regenerative approach to alveolar ridge maintenance following tooth extraction. Report of 10 cases. J Periodontol 1997;68:563–570.
26. Marx RE, Garg AK. Bone structure, metabolism, and physiology: its impact on dental implantology. Implant Dent 1998;7:267–275.
27. Glickman I, Smulow JB. Buttressing bone formation in the periodontium. J Periodontol 1965;36:365–370.
28. Sennerby L, Carlsson GE, Bergman B, Warfvinge J. Mandibular bone resorption in patients treated with tissue-integrated prostheses and in complete denture-wearers. Acta Odontol Scand 1988;46:135–140.
29. Ritchey B, Orban B. The crests of the interdental alveolar septa. J Periodontol 1953;24:75–87.
30. Horning GM, Cohen ME, Neils TA. Buccal alveolar exostoses: prevalence, characteristics, and evidence for buttressing bone formation. J Periodontol 2000;71:1032–1042.
31. Sonnier KE, Horning GM, Cohen ME. Palatal tubercles, palatal tori, and mandibular tori: prevalence and anatomic features in a U.S. population. J Periodontol 1999;70:329–336.
32. Rupprecht RD, Horning GM, Nicoll BK, Cohen ME. Prevalence of dehiscences and fenestrations in modern American skulls. J Periodontol 2001;72:722–729.

## CHAPTER 1
## REVIEW QUESTIONS

1. An adequate width of attached keratinized gingiva is one that:
   a. Is equal to or greater than 2 mm
   b. Maintains a noninflamed, stable gingival margin
   c. Permits movement of the tip of the interdental papilla on tugging
   d. Extends from the free gingival margin to the gingival groove

2. The periodontal attachment apparatus is comprised of what tissues?
   a. Cementum, epithelium, and enamel
   b. Cementum and epithelium alone
   c. Alveolar bone, epithelium, and cementum
   d. Alveolar bone, periodontal ligament, and cementum
   e. None of the above

3. What is NOT a function of the periodontal ligament?
   a. To regenerate alveolar bone
   b. To supply nutrients to the tooth
   c. To lay down new cementum and protect it from resorption
   d. To suspend the tooth within its bony housing
   e. All of the above are functions

4. Approximately how thick is facial attached gingiva?
   a. 0.25 mm
   b. 1.5 mm
   c. 2 to 4 mm
   d. 5 mm or more

5. After injury, the body soon establishes an epithelial attachment, connective tissue attachment, and crevice of fairly predictable dimensions. This is called the:
   a. Lamina propria
   b. Biologic width
   c. Periodontal biotype
   d. Dimension of Malassez
   e. Dynamic periodontal cuff

6. When interdental spaces or facial alveolar plate are less than 0.5 mm thick:
   a. Alveolar bone proper is lacking
   b. Only cortical bone may be present
   c. Cementum grows thicker to compensate
   d. Intra-alveolar vessels comprise the major blood supply
   e. All of the above

7. What is the most common type of inherited or acquired enlargement in the outer contour of alveolar or palatal bone?
   a. Palatal tori
   b. Mandibular tori
   c. Palatal tubercles
   d. Buccal exostoses
   e. Lingual exostoses

8. A cleftlike absence of the alveolar cortical plate that results in a denuded root surface is termed a:
   a. Dehiscence
   b. Fenestration
   c. Cleft of Serres
   d. Palatogingival groove

9. The differentiation of oral epithelium into either keratinized or nonkeratinized epithelium is dictated by:
   a. The occlusal load of the neighboring tooth
   b. The character of the underlying connective tissue
   c. The amount of function or abrasion the surface is subjected to
   d. Whether the keratinized band is less than or greater than 2 mm
   e. None of the above

10. What major difference is seen between the periodontal gingival attachment and the peri-implant gingival attachment?
    a. Implants have only cellular cementum
    b. The epithelial attachment about implants is longer and stronger
    c. Implants have no root cementum and no supracrestal fiber groups
    d. Teeth have a dynamic epithelial cuff, implants have a passive cuff

# Etiology of Periodontal Disease

Arthur R. Vernino

Periodontal disease may be defined as any pathologic process that affects the periodontium. The vast majority of inflammatory diseases of the periodontium result from bacterial infection. Although other factors may affect this region, the dominating causative agents of periodontal disease are microorganisms that colonize the tooth surface (bacterial plaque and their products).[1–3] Figure 2-1 represents the interaction of etiologic factors that cause periodontal disease. There are a number of systemic disorders that adversely affect the periodontium (see Chapter 3), but no systemic disorder is known to be the initiating cause of periodontitis in the absence of bacterial plaque. In addition, there are other local factors that act in conjunction with bacterial plaque to produce chronic disease of the periodontium. Two factors that may initiate periodontal disease in the absence of bacterial plaque are malignancies and primary occlusal traumatism. The role of each factor in the initiation and progression of periodontal disease is discussed in this chapter.

## TOOTH SURFACE DEPOSITS

To discuss bacterial plaque and its relationship to periodontal disease, it is necessary to define the various materials that accumulate on the tooth surface.[4]

1. Bacterial plaque. There are many types of bacterial plaques, but the ones that are closely allied to periodontal disease can be divided into two major types. The first type consists of a mat of densely packed, colonized, and colonizing microorganisms, which grow on and attach to the tooth. This type may be supragingival or subgingival. The second type is a subgingival plaque that is "free floating" or loosely attached between the soft tissue and the tooth. The attached bacterial plaque is not removed with a forceful water spray, but is readily removed by other mechanical means. The loosely attached plaque consists primarily of anaerobic bacteria.

2. Acquired pellicle. The thin (0.1 to 0.8 μm) primarily protein film that forms on erupted teeth and can be removed by abrasives (e.g., polishing materials). It quickly re-forms after being removed. The source of pellicle is apparently from constituents of saliva. It can form whether or not bacteria are present. Acquired pellicle will stain light pink by erythrosin, a red dye commonly used to stain bacterial plaque. Pellicle is not removed by forceful rinsing, and its role in periodontal disease is unknown.

3. Calculus. Calcified plaque that is usually covered by a soft layer of bacterial plaque.

4. Food debris. Food that is retained in the mouth. Debris, unless impacted between the teeth or within periodontal pockets, is usually removed by action of the oral musculature and saliva, or as a result of rinsing or brushing.

5. Materia alba (literally, white matter). A soft mixture of salivary proteins, some bacteria, many desquamated epithelial cells, and occasional disintegrating leukocytes. This mixture adheres loosely to the surface of the teeth, to plaque, and to gingiva, and can usually be flushed off with a forceful water spray. The toxic potential of materia alba and its role in the formation of bacterial plaque are not known. Table 2-1 summarizes some of the differences between plaque, materia alba, and debris.

6. Stains
   a. Intrinsic:
      (1) Origin: occurs during tooth development and causes changes in the light transmitting of the tooth.[5]

## INTERACTION OF ETIOLOGIC FACTORS

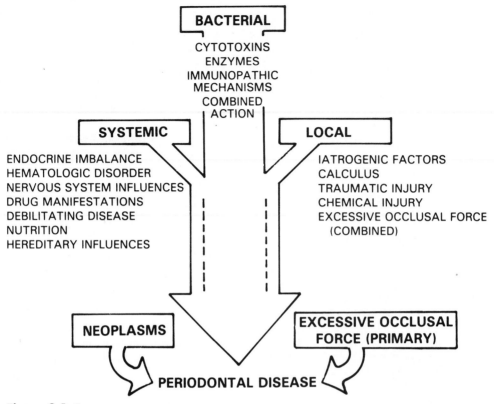

*Figure 2.1* ●

(2) Causes
(a) Metabolic disorders
Examples: alkaptonuria,[6] amelogenesis imperfecta,[7] tetracycline staining,[8] fluorosis.[5]
(b) Systemic disorders
Examples: Ehlers-Danlos syndrome,[9] vitamin D–dependent rickets
b. Extrinsic: discoloration on the tooth surface or in the acquired pellicle[5,10]
(1) Origin: dietary component, beverages, tobacco, mouth rinses, and medications.

(2) Examples: poor oral hygiene, chlorhexidine, Listerine

## BACTERIAL FACTORS IN PERIODONTAL DISEASE

### Morphology of Bacterial Plaque

Studies with light and electron microscopy have yielded evidence to indicate there are distinct morphologic differences between supragingival and subgingival plaque.[9] The morphology of supragingival

## TABLE 2.1

### Some Differences Between Plaque, Material Alba, and Debris

| Characteristic | Plaque | Material Alba | Debris |
|---|---|---|---|
| Adherence | Close | Loose | None |
| Effect of rinsing | None | Dislodged by forceful rinsing | Dislodged readily |
| Structure | Definite | Amorphous | None |

plaque is similar in patients with periodontitis. The bacterial with gingivitis and those with cells appear to be densely packed on the tooth surface and the deposits may be thick (0.5 mm or more). The composition of the microbial deposits includes coccoid and relatively numerous filamentous forms of bacteria. Some of the filamentous bacteria are covered with coccal organisms, which appear as "corncob" formations. Flagellated forms and spirochetes are observed apically and on the outer surface of the supragingival plaque.

Subgingival plaque in periodontitis patients is composed of an inner and an outer layer. The inner layer of tightly adherent bacteria is continuous with, but is thinner and less organized than, supragingival plaque. Outside this tightly adherent layer, and adjacent to the soft tissue of the pocket, is a loosely adherent layer of microorganisms. This layer consists of numerous spirochetes, Gram-negative bacteria, and bacteria grouped into "bottle brush" or "test-tube brush" formations.

## Microorganisms of Plaque

The type of microorganisms found in plaque vary among individuals and sites within the mouth, and with age of the plaque itself. Young plaque (1 to 2 days) consists primarily of Gram-positive and some Gram-negative cocci and rods.[1,2] These organisms normally grow on an amorphous mucopolysaccharide pellicle, less than 1 μm thick, which is attached to the enamel, cementum, or dentin.

From 2 to 4 days of growth, undisturbed plaque changes in the numbers and in the types of organisms present. The number of Gram-negative cocci and rods increases, and fusiform bacilli and filamentous organisms become established.

From 4 to 9 days, this ecologically complex population of microorganisms is further complicated by the presence of increasing numbers of motile bacteria, namely, spirilla and spirochetes.

It was shown recently that there are apparent qualitative differences in the microbial flora associated with periodontal health and disease.[10] Dark-field microscopy has revealed that spirochetes and motile organisms are often associated with disease whereas coccoid forms are usually associated with health. Studies in which plaque bacteria have been cultured show that certain Gram-negative bacteria may be associated with specific types of periodontal disease.[2,3,9] For example, *Porphyromonas gingivalis, Treponema denticola,* and *Tannerella forsythia,* the so-called "red complex," shows a strong association with adult periodontitis; *Prevotella intermedius* has been associated with pregnancy gingivitis. *Haemophilus, Actinobacillus actinomycetemcomitans,* and strains of *Capnocytophaga* are associated with juvenile periodontitis. *Prevotella intermedius, Prevotella nigrescens,* and spirochetes are found in large numbers in necrotizing periodontal diseases.

## Other Constituents of Plaque

Although colonized organisms are the primary constituents of plaque, additional components can be identified by phase-contrast microscopy.

1. Epithelial cells. These are found in almost all samples of bacterial plaque in varying stages of anatomic integrity. They may range from recently desquamated cells with discrete nuclei and clearly defined cell walls to what may be described as "ghosts" of cells swarming with bacteria.
2. White blood cells. Leukocytes, usually polymorphonuclear neutrophils (PMNs), may be found in varying stages of vitality in the several stages of inflammation. It is of interest that vital white cells may be found adjacent to clinically healthy gingiva. Microorganisms are often present within the cytoplasm of the granulocytes. In areas of obvious exudation and purulence, it is often difficult to find any apparently vital cells among the numerous granulocytes present.
3. Erythrocytes. These are readily seen in samples taken from tooth surfaces adjacent to ulcerated gingiva.
4. Protozoa. Certain genera of protozoa, notably *Entamoeba* and *Trichomonas,* can often be seen in plaque taken from surfaces adjacent to acute gingivitis and from within periodontal pockets.
5. Food particles. Occasionally, microscopic shreds of food are seen. Those most readily recognized are muscle fibers, distinguishable by their striations.
6. Miscellaneous components. Nonspecific elements, such as crystalline-appearing particles (which may be fine fragments of cementum, beginning calcification, or unidentified foodstuffs) and what appear to be cell fragments, may also be found in plaque.

## Mechanisms of Bacterial Action

1. Invasion.
Bacterial invasion is not necessary for gingival inflammation to occur. All that is required is that enough bacteria (and possibly specific pathogenic bacteria) be fixed to the tooth, near the gingiva, for a sufficient length of time to

challenge the tissue with their toxic products. No specific organism or group of organisms has been positively or exclusively identified as the cause of periodontal breakdown, but there appears to be a strong association of certain microorganisms with periodontal disease states. There is evidence that bacterial invasion of the connective tissue does occur.[11,12]

2. Cytotoxic agent
   Endotoxins, which are lipopolysaccharide constituents of the cell wall of Gram-negative bacteria, can be a direct cause of tissue necrosis, as well as an initiator of inflammation by triggering an immunologic response and activation of the complement system. Also, endotoxins from certain oral organisms stimulate bone resorption in tissue culture.[13]

3. Enzymes
   a. Collagenase depolymerizes collagen fibers and fibrils, the major formed elements in the gingiva and periodontal ligament. It is of interest that leukocytes are also known to produce collagenase and are present in large numbers in the lesions of the early stages of gingivitis.[10]
   b. Hyaluronidase hydrolyzes hyaluronic acid, an important tissue-cementing polysaccharide, and can act as a "spreading" factor to increase permeability. This enzyme is produced by microorganisms and by the host.
   c. Chondroitinase hydrolyzes chondroitin sulfate, another tissue-cementing polysaccharide.
   d. Proteases, a family of enzymes, contribute to breakdown of noncollagenous proteins and increase capillary permeability.

4. Immunopathologic mechanisms.
   Studies have demonstrated that several plaque antigens induce inflammation in animals by stimulating the immunologic response. Both the humoral and the cell-mediated types of immune response have been observed in patients with periodontitis. The role of the immunologic response in periodontal disease is not completely understood; however, the potential to cause tissue destruction is apparent. The role of the immune response in gingivitis and periodontitis is discussed further in Chapter 5.

5. Combined action.
   It is possible that more than one mechanism may be involved in the initiation and progression of inflammatory periodontal disease. For example, it is conceivable that bacterial enzymes or cytotoxic substances exert a direct effect on the sulcular and subsulcular tissue, as well as initiate an indirect immunopathologic response.[11] The exact mechanism of action of bacterial plaque is

unclear; however, there remains little doubt that bacteria are the primary etiologic agents for inflammatory periodontal disease.

## SYSTEMIC FACTORS AND PERIODONTAL DISEASE

Systemic factors related to periodontal disease are discussed in Chapter 3. However, it should be mentioned that any condition that might reduce the resistance of the periodontium to toxic insult should be expected to contribute to the initiation of inflammation and to influence the rapidity and severity of the disease process.

## LOCAL CONTRIBUTING FACTORS AND PERIODONTAL DISEASE

1. Anatomic factors.[14] These include:
   a. Root morphology (size and shape).[14]
   b. Position of tooth in arch.
   c. Root proximity.
2. Iatrogenic factors. There are a number of procedures, techniques, and materials used in dentistry that indirectly, and on occasion directly, contribute to the initiation or progression of periodontal disease.
   a. Operative procedures. Most injuries to the gingiva that occur during restorative dentistry procedures are of a minor nature and heal readily without loss of form or function of the periodontium. Some precautions, however, should be observed. For example, if a large portion of papilla is destroyed by careless use of a wedge during matrix stabilization, it is likely that the papilla will not regenerate to normal contour. Also, retraction cord, impression tubes, diamond stones, and temporary restorations may result in irreversible damage to the periodontium if either of the following conditions exists.
   (1) Minimal amount of attached gingiva at the operative site. The gingiva can easily become macerated and detached, with ultimate loss of all attached gingiva. Operative procedures performed under such circumstances may result in tissue loss if there is a frenum attachment at the mucogingival junction.
   (2) The gingiva is stripped from a tooth and an overextended temporary restoration is placed, or cementing material is forced between the tooth and the detached tissue and is left in place. In either situation, epithelium will attempt to cover the detached tissue; when the temporary

restoration (or cement) is finally re-moved, a deepened, epithelial-lined pocket will exist. The longer the materials remain interposed between tooth and soft tissue the greater the certainty of perma-nent loss of the gingival attachment.

b. Restorative materials and restorations. Except for plastics, in which excess free monomer is present, no restorative material used in dentistry today has been shown to be, in itself, capable of producing inflammation.

Restorations may play a role similar to that of rough calculus if they have overhanging margins or rough surfaces. Overhanging mar-gins and surface irregularities provide sites for plaque formation and retention.[15] The presence of overhanging margins and rough surfaces makes plaque removal difficult and provides protected areas for microorganisms to multiply and exert their toxic effect.

c. Removable partial dentures. If a prosthesis is so designed as to impinge on the soft tis-sue or to exert torque on the teeth, direct damage to the periodontium can occur. In the presence of bacterial plaque, these in-sults can result in rapid, severe destruction of periodontal structures.

d. Fixed partial dentures. In addition to the necessity for marginal excellence on abut-ments, the design must also be such that the patient can clean all surfaces of the restora-tion. This requirement demands that open interproximal embrasures and generally convex surfaces should be design elements to enhance cleanliness of the prosthesis. These principles are especially critical in pontic design. Failure to instruct patients in the methodology of cleaning fixed partial dentures is the first step toward eventual breakdown of the periodontium.

e. Exodontics. When extractions are performed so that the attachment apparatus of an adja-cent tooth is damaged at or near the den-togingival junction, the damage is frequently irreversible. For example, the soft tissue and bone supporting an adjacent tooth can be destroyed if they are injudiciously used as a fulcrum for a surgical elevator. Poor flap design, as well as poor approximation and fixation of wound edges, can result in tissue contours that are conducive to plaque and food retention. Failure to remove calculus from adjacent tooth surfaces at an extraction site may negate an excellent opportunity for pocket elimination and regeneration of the attachment apparatus around the remaining teeth. This oversight indirectly enhances the progression of periodontal disease.

f. Orthodontics. Fixed appliances (bands and wires) present excellent harbors for bacterial growth and can thus contribute significantly to inflammation. Temporary extracoronal splints, whether composed of welded ortho-dontics bands, wire, or wire and acrylic resin, may also be included in this category. On final analysis, it is evident that poor dentistry of all types may create sites for the accumula-tion of plaque, intensify its production, and prevent its mechanical removal.

3. Calculus formation. Calculus is calcified dental plaque. It should **not** be considered a direct cause of inflammation. Calculus is important in the progression of disease, however, serving as a "coral reef" within which microorganisms can multiply and release their toxic products. The rough surface of calculus makes it difficult, if not impossible, for the patient to remove associated bacterial plaque. There is ample evi-dence that complete removal of calculus is nec-essary for resolution of periodontal pockets.

4. Traumatic factors. Trauma to the periodon-tium can result in the loss of the attachment apparatus and can contribute to the initiation and progression of periodontal disease.

a. Toothbrush abrasion. This can completely destroy a narrow band of attached gingiva and result in extensive recession. In fact, toothbrush abrasion is one of the two most common factors associated with recession, the other being tooth position. Such abra-sion also results in extensive grooving of the root surfaces, which causes cleaning problems for the patient and management problems for the dentist.

b. Factitious disease. Occasionally, patients are encountered who persistently gouge or "scratch" their gingiva with their fingernails (factitious disease).[16] This action usually results in extensive exposure of the root sur-face and localized inflammation. This rare entity is a difficult diagnostic problem. Whenever isolated areas of recession are noted and a thorough evaluation fails to identify the etiology of the condition, facti-tious disease should be considered.

c. Food impaction.[17,18] This is one of the more common local factors that contribute to the initiation and progression of inflammatory periodontal disease. Open contacts, uneven marginal ridges, irregular positions of teeth, and nonphysiologic contours of teeth and restorations can result in the impaction of food on the gingiva and into the gingival sulcus. Some investigators believe that food impaction is an important factor in vertical bone loss. It is not clearly understood what produces the initial breakdown in an area of food impaction or food retention. It is speculated that the forceful wedging of food beneath the gingival tissues can produce inflammation from physical trauma, in addition to tearing of the epithelial attachment. It is just as likely, however, that the initial injury is a result of food degradation and chemical irritation. It is also possible that food impaction and retention afford an excellent breeding ground for bacteria, which initiate the disease process.

5. Chemical injury. Indiscriminate use of topically applied aspirin tablets, strong mouthwashes, and various escharotic drugs may result in ulceration of the gingival tissue. In addition, dentists may inadvertently permit strong bleaches or salts of heavy metals, such as silver nitrate, to come in contact with the tissue. Injuries of this nature are usually transient, but may contribute to the destruction of the periodontium.
6. Excessive occlusal force. See Chapter 6 for a discussion of this type of trauma.

## NEOPLASMS

There are numerous benign and malignant lesions that involve the tissues of the periodontium. It is not within the scope of this book to discuss the various neoplasms of the periodontium, and the reader is referred to a standard text in oral pathology for this information.

## PATHOGENESIS

The pathogenesis of a disease refers to the biologic and histologic events that occur in the tissues during the process of conversion from a healthy state to a diseased state. Understanding the pathogenesis of periodontal disease will allow the clinician to make rational decisions regarding the most predictable methods to prevent or treat this widespread disease.

### Pocket Formation

A pocket is a gingival sulcus pathologically deepened by periodontal disease. It is bordered by the tooth on one side and by ulcerated epithelium on the other, and has the junctional epithelium at its base.[19–21] Deepening of the sulcus can occur in three ways: (1) by movement of the free gingival margin coronally, as observed in gingivitis; (2) by movement of the junctional epithelium apically, with separation of the coronal portion from the tooth; and (3) by a combination of items 1 and 2 (Fig. 2-2).

### Classification of Pockets

Pockets may be classified as follows (Fig. 2-3):

1. Gingival pocket (pseudopocket). Deepening of the gingival sulcus as a result of an increase in the size of the gingiva. There is no apical migration of the junctional epithelium or loss of crestal alveolar bone (Fig. 2-3A).

POCKET FORMATION

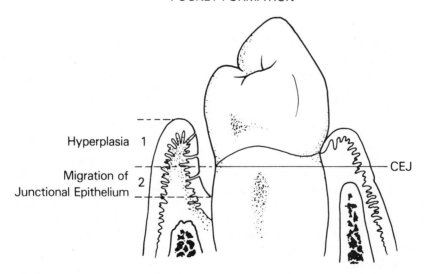

*Figure 2.2* ●

CLASSIFICATION OF POCKETS

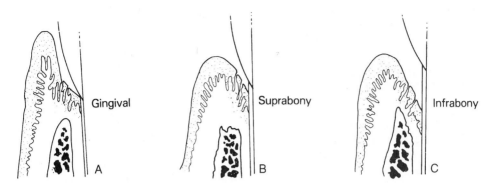

**Figure 2.3** ●

2. Suprabony pocket. Deepening of the gingival sulcus with destruction of the adjacent gingival fibers, periodontal ligament, and crestal alveolar bone associated with apical migration of the junctional epithelium. The bottom of the pocket and the junctional epithelium are coronal to the crest of the alveolar bone (Fig. 2-3B).
3. Infrabony pocket. Deepening of the gingival sulcus to a level at which the bottom of the pocket and the junctional epithelium are apical to the crest of the alveolar bone (Fig. 2-3C). One, two, or three osseous walls, or various combinations thereof, may exist, depending on the amount and pattern of bone loss (see Chapter 17 for classification of osseous defects).

## Horizontal and Vertical Bone Loss

Horizontal bone loss refers to an overall reduction in height of the alveolar crest in which the crestal bone is generally at right angles to the root surface. Vertical bone loss refers to loss of bone at an acute angle to the root surface. Another term for vertical bone loss is angular bone loss. Suprabony pockets are associated with horizontal bone loss (Fig. 2-3B); infrabony pockets are associated with vertical bone loss (Fig. 2-3C).

## Etiology of the Infrabony Pocket

Both suprabony and infrabony pockets are the result of plaque infection; however, there is some difference of opinion as to the factors that influence the formation of the infrabony pocket. Most agree that vertical bone loss and subsequent infrabony pocket formation can occur whenever there is direct extension of inflammation into the periodontal ligament, in the presence of a sufficient thickness of bone. The controversy arises as to what factors alter the pathway of inflammation

from crestal bone to the periodontal ligament space. The etiologic mechanisms that have been proposed are as follows:

1. Large vessels that exit on one side of the alveolus may affect formation of an infrabony pocket.
2. The forceful wedging of food into the interproximal region may result in unilateral destruction of the attachment apparatus and downgrowth of the epithelial attachment.
3. Periodontal traumatism may produce crestal damage of the periodontal ligament (trauma from occlusion) that, in the presence of existing inflammation, can result in the migration of the junctional epithelium into the area of destruction (Fig. 2-4).

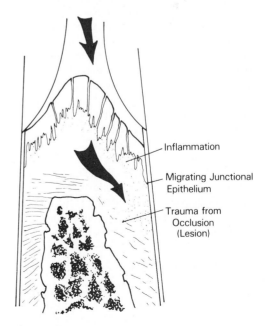

**Figure 2.4** ●

4. Plaque fronts on adjacent teeth advancing at different rates in an apical direction causing the alveolar bone destruction to occur at a more rapid rate on one of the two adjacent teeth, resulting in vertical bone loss.

## PATHOGENESIS OF PLAQUE-RELATED PERIODONTAL DISEASE

Plaque-related periodontal disease is characterized by inflammation. The inflammatory process is activated to limit the spread of the disease process. However, in addition to its beneficial effects, the inflammatory process also has a destructive component. The objective of treatment is to enhance the beneficial aspects of inflammation and to limit or control the destructive potential.

The inflammatory response in plaque-related periodontal disease can be initiated by a variety of factors.[22–24] There is evidence that a number of the lytic enzymes produced by bacteria can cause direct tissue destruction in the periodontium. Other bacterial products (e.g., endotoxin) may activate the complement system, which results in the formation of biologically active proteins that stimulate an increase in vascular permeability with migration of inflammatory cells from the vascular channels, the chemotactic response, cell adherence, and phagocytosis. The end result of complement activation is cell lysis of both host and bacterial cells.

The immunologic response appears to play a significant role in the initiation, and probably the perpetuation, of the inflammatory response.[25–27] The bacteria in plaque contain a multitude of antigens. The antigens can stimulate the B and T lymphocytes of the gingival connective tissues to proliferate, and contribute to both the humoral and cell-mediated immune response, respectively. To support this concept, there is evidence that patients with plaque-related periodontal disease have circulating antibodies to plaque antigens. It also has been shown that cultures of peripheral lymphocytes from patients with plaque-related periodontal disease show a greater cell-mediated immune response to plaque-derived antigens than peripheral lymphocytes from periodontally healthy patients. (See Chapter 5 for a more complete discussion of the role of the immune response).

## HISTOPATHOLOGY

The histologic picture of developing plaque-related periodontal disease has been divided into four stages at the light microscope level (the model proposed by Page and Schroeder).[28]

### The Initial Lesion

The first microscopically observable tissue changes occur after *2 to 4 days* of plaque accumulation. There are small accumulations of polymorphonuclear neutrophils (PMNs) and mononuclear cells subjacent to the junctional epithelium.[29] A decrease of perivascular collagen occurs in this area as well as a decrease of some of the collagen supporting the coronal portion of the junctional epithelium. Gingival fluid can be detected clinically in the gingival sulcus. No more than 5 to 10% of the gingival connective tissue is involved during this stage. Classic vasculitis of vessels subjacent to the junctional epithelium is present.

### The Early Lesion

The early lesion occurs after *4 to 7 days* of plaque accumulation. The changes observed in the initial lesion persist and are more severe at this stage. The major characteristic of the early lesion stage is the formation and maintenance of a dense lymphoid cell infiltrate within the gingival connective tissues. Numerous small and medium-sized lymphocytes accumulate immediately below the junctional epithelium. These cells are the predominant inflammatory cells. The junctional and oral sulcular epithelia begin to form rete ridges (pegs). Numerous injured fibroblasts are observed in close association with lymphoid cells. The collagen content is reduced about 70% in the areas of inflammation.

The events in the sequence of developing plaque-related periodontal disease, thus far, have occurred at the microscopic and biochemical levels. In time, as the inflammatory cells and tissue fluids begin to accumulate, the gingiva will begin to show clinically detectable symptoms, which brings us to the next stage.

### The Established Lesion

The established lesion is a progression of the early lesion and is observed after *2 to 3 weeks* of plaque accumulation. The destructive tissue changes noted in the first two stages persist. The plasma cell is now the predominant inflammatory cell type within the affected connective tissues.

The plasma cells produce immunoglobulins, primarily of the IgG class. The junctional and oral sulcular epithelia continue to proliferate and may now be considered a pocket epithelium. This epithelium varies in thickness and shows areas of ulceration. The inflammatory cells accumulate along vascular channels and between collagen fibers deep in the lesion. The collagen loss persists at the site of active disease, but areas distant from the lesion show foci of collagen formation. The periodontal ligament and alveolar bone show no change at this stage. *Clinical manifestations of the disease can now be observed.*

## The Advanced Lesion

A varying amount of time elapses before the advanced lesion occurs. There are many cases in which the advanced lesion never appears. The area of the lesion enlarges. Strands of pocket epithelium penetrate deep into the connective tissue. There is extensive destruction of the collagen fiber bundles and of the gingiva; however, the transseptal fibers continually regenerate as the lesion moves apically. The plasma cell continues to be the predominant cell type. Many of these cells appear injured, and can be observed deep within the tissue. Crestal alveolar bone resorption occurs, especially in the area of the vascular channels.

## Disease Progression

The initial, early, and established lesions represent varying severities of gingivitis. The advanced lesion can be considered periodontitis. All the events in one stage in the life cycle of plaque-related periodontal disease need not be completed before another stage begins. The stages are a continuum of the disease process, with considerable overlap among stages. Periodontitis must be preceded by gingivitis; however, all untreated gingivitis does not necessarily proceed to periodontitis.

Progression of periodontal disease is now considered by numerous investigators to be a cyclic process. There appear to be extended periods of quiescence with short episodes of disease activity. The attachment loss that occurs during these bursts of disease activity varies from minor loss to relatively extensive tissue loss.

## Spread of Inflammation

Periodontitis usually develops as a sequel to persistent chronic gingivitis. Interdentally, inflammation and bacterial products spread from the gingiva to the alveolar process along the neurovascular bundle of the interdental canal at the crest of the septum (Fig. 2-5A.1). Inflammation spreads along the course of the vascular channels because the loose connective tissue surrounding the neurovascular bundles offers less resistance than the dense fibers of the periodontal ligament.[30] The point at which inflammation enters the bone depends on the location of the vessels. In some instances, large vessels exit at one side of the alveolar crest, permitting direct spread of the inflammation into the marginal portion of the periodontal ligament (Fig. 2-5A.1a). After reaching

## SPREAD OF INFLAMMATION

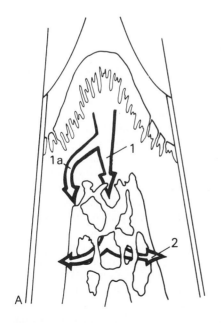
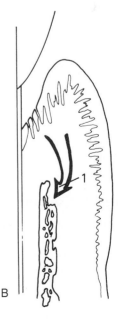

*Figure 2.5* •

the marrow spaces, the destructive process extends laterally into the periodontal ligament via the intra-alveolar opening (Fig. 2-5A.2). On the facial and lingual surfaces, the destructive process spreads along the supraperiosteal vessels and penetrates the marrow space via the channels in the outer cortex (Fig. 2-5B.1).

Extension of the chronic inflammatory process into the alveolar bone is marked by infiltration of the marrow by leukocytes, new blood vessels, and proliferation of fibroblasts. There is marked osteoclastic activity. Progressive extension is accompanied by destruction of the trabeculae and subsequent reduction in the height of the alveolar bone. This destruction is not a continuous process; it is accompanied by osteoblastic activity and new bone formation, even in the presence of inflammation. Likewise, there is constant reformation of the transseptal fibers as the attachment apparatus is destroyed. Alveolar bone loss does not occur until the physiologic equilibrium of bone is disturbed to the point that resorption exceeds formation. The resistance of the individual to disease plays an important role in governing the rate at which bone loss progresses in untreated periodontal disease.

## Genetic Factors in Periodontitis

Familial patterns have been documented for localized juvenile periodontitis (LJP) for decades. Studies of twins have had mixed results. Human leukocyte antigens (HLA) have been associated with various forms of periodontal disease.[27] For example, HLA-A9 increases in the presence of severe adult periodontitis. All such data are premature and inconclusive. Nevertheless, commercial tests for genetic susceptibility for periodontitis are available. There is a great deal of promise in these new tools, but it remains to be seen how they will be applied in clinical practice. It is conceivable that the pathogenesis of periodontitis may differ in these patients and that different treatment modalities may be required.

## Smoking and Periodontitis

Smoking is a major risk factor for periodontitis, and may alter its pathogenesis.[31] One study showed an increased odds ratio of 2.0 to 5.0 using attachment loss as the measurement tool. Smokers appear to have different flora, and do not respond as well to treatment as nonsmokers. When all other factors are eliminated, smoking is as destructive as bacterial plaque.

## Linear vs Burst Theories of Periodontal Disease Activity

Since the 1980s, it has been assumed that periodontal disease occurred in "bursts" of attachment loss at specific sites rather than in a linear fashion.[32] This controversy is being revisited.

At this time there is no answer because our techniques for measuring disease activity—periodontal probing, bleeding on probing, and radiographic changes—are too crude. Much more specific and sensitive tests for disease activity are required to solve this problem.

## Clinical Findings Correlated with Histologic Features

The significance of the clinical findings in periodontitis are more easily understood if they can be correlated with the histologic features of the disease.

## Critical Pathway Theory of Periodontal Disease

It is no longer sufficient to consider periodontal pathogenesis primarily on a cellular level as we have in the past. The model developed by Page and Schroeder that was presented earlier in this chapter is still an excellent way to depict the transition from health to periodontitis, although one must keep in mind that it is occurring at different rates throughout the mouth. To fully understand this subject, one must be able to correlate the biochemical and cellular events. An excellent model, known as the "Critical Pathway Model of Periodontitis," was published in the 1996 World Workshop in Periodontics. There were actually several variations on this model including therapeutic intervention and risk factors such as smoking. We will deal with the basic model.

As the result of poor oral hygiene or exogenous infection, normal flora are converted into pathogenic flora. Inflammation, chemotaxis, antibody production, phagocytosis, activation of the compliment system, and production of prostaglandin $E_2$, leukotrienes, interleukins, and other cytokines occurs. If the body has normal PMNs and antibodies, the invading bacteria will be cleared, and the patient will experience either no disease or limited disease (gingivitis). If, on the other hand, the patient has defective PMNs, the disease process may progress. It may also progress if the bacteria possess virulence factors that enable them to inactivate complement or PMNs, or simply bypass this step by tissue invasion. *Porphyromonas gingivalis*

*(P. gingivalis)* and *Actinobacillus actinomycetem-comitans (A. actinomycetemcomitans)* are examples of bacteria with such capabilities.

Once this has occurred, the predominant cell is the plasma cell, and attachment loss begins. Genetics may predetermine this step involving the monocyte and T-cell response. This causes the release of catabolic cytokines interleukin $1\alpha$, tumor necrosis factor-$\alpha$, and interleukin 6, and the mediator prostaglandin $E_2$. Both host cells and bacteria are stimulated to produce substances that are destructive to the gingiva, such as collagenase and matrix metalloproteins.

Simultaneously, the body is attempting to heal itself. If the balance between catabolism and anabolism shifts in favor of the former, the disease process will continue in a circuitous manner.

## REFERENCES FOR ETIOLOGY

1. Loe H, Theilade E, Jensen SB. Experimental gingivitis in man. J Periodontol 1965;36:177–187.
2. Socransky S, Haffajee A. The bacterial etiology of destructive periodontal disease. J Periodontol 1992; 63:322–331.
3. Slot J, Listgarten MA. *Bacteroides gingivalis, Bacteroides intermedius,* and *Actinobacillus actinomycetemcomitans* in human periodontal diseases. J Clin Periodontol 1988;15:85–93.
4. Schwartz RS, Massler M. Tooth accumulated materials: a review and classification. J Periodontol 1969; 40:407–413.
5. Watts A, Addy M. Tooth discolouration and staining: a review of the literature. Br Dent J 2001;190: 309–316.
6. Link J. Disclorouration of the teeth in alkaptonuria and Parkinsonism. Chron Omaha Dist Dent Soc 1973;36:136.
7. Wright J, Robinson C, Shoe R. Characterization of the enamel ultra structure and mineral content in hypoplastic amelogenesis imperfecta. Oral Surg Oral Med Oral Pathol 1991;126:509–515.
8. van der Bijl P, Pitifoi-Aron G. Tetracycline and calcified tissues. Ann Dent 1995;54:69–72.
9. Tanner A, Maiden MF, Macuch PJ, Murray LL, Kent RL Jr. Microbiota of health, gingivitis, and initial periodontitis. J Clin Periodontol 1998;25:85–98.
10. Sandquist G, Carlsson J, Hanstrom L. Collagenolytic activity of black-pigmented Bacteroides species. J Periodontal Res 1987;22:300–306.
11. Saglie FR, Pertuiset JH, Rezende MT, Sabet MS, Raoufi D, Carranza FA Jr. Bacterial invasion in experimental gingivitis in man. J Periodontol 1987;58: 837–846.
12. Saglie R, Newman MG, Carranza FA, Pattison GL. Bacterial invasion of gingiva in advanced periodontitis in humans. J Periodontol 1982;52:217–222.
13. Daly CG, Seymour GJ, Kieser JB. Bacterial endotoxin: a role in chronic inflammatory periodontal disease. J Oral Pathol 1980;9:1–15.
14. Gher M, Vernino A. Root morphology—clinical significance in pathogenesis and treatment of periodontal disease. J Am Dent Assoc 1980;101:627–633.
15. Lang NP, Kiehl RA, Anderhalden K. Clinical and microbiological effects of subgingival restorations with overhanging or clinically perfect margins. J Clin Periodontol 1983;10:563–578.
16. Stewart G. Minor self-inflicted injuries of the gingiva. J Clin Periodontol 1976;3:128–132.
17. Kepic T, O'Leary T. Role of marginal ridge relationship as an etiologic factor in periodontal disease. J Periodontol 1978;49:570–575.
18. Hirschfeld I. Food impaction. J Am Dent Assoc 1930;17:1504.

## REFERENCES FOR PATHOGENESIS

19. Ritchey B, Orban B. The periodontal pocket. J Periodontol 23: 199–213, 1952.
20. Takata T, Donath K. The mechanism of pocket formation. A light microscopic study on undecalcified material. J Periodontol 1988;59:215–221.
21. Lang NP, Adler R, Joss A, Nyman S. Absence of bleeding on probing. An indicator of periodontal stability. J Clin Periodontol 1990;17:714–721.
22. Consensus report. Periodontal diseases: pathogenesis and microbial factors. Ann Periodontol 1996;1: 926–932.
23. Periodontal diseases: pathogenesis and microbial factors [Review]. J Am Dent Assoc 1998; 129(Suppl):58S–62S.
24. Loe H, Theilade E, Jensen SB. Experimental gingivitis in man. J Periodontol 1965;36:177–187.
25. Offenbacher S. Periodontal diseases: pathogenesis. Ann Periodontol 1996;1:821–878.
26. Landi L, Amar S, Polins AS, Van Dyke TE. Host mechanisms in the pathogenesis of periodontal disease. Curr Opin Periodontol 1997;4:3–10.
27. Male D. Immunology: An Illustrated Outline, 3rd ed. St. Louis: CV Mosby, 1998.
28. Page RC, Schroeder HE. Pathogenesis of inflammatory periodontal disease. A summary of current work. Lab Invest 1976;33:235–249.
29. Crawford JM, Wilton JM, Richardson P. Neutrophils die in the gingival crevice, periodontal pocket, and oral cavity by necrosis and not apoptosis. J Periodontol 2000;71:1121–1129.
30. Weinmann J. Progress of gingival inflammation into the supporting structures of the teeth. J Periodontol 1941;12:71–82.
31. Tonetti MS. Cigarette smoking and periodontal diseases: etiology and management of disease. Ann Periodontol 1998;3:88–101.
32. Theilade E. The non-specific theory in microbial etiology of inflammatory periodontal disease. J Clin Periodontol 1986;13:905–911.

## CHAPTER 2
## REVIEW QUESTIONS

1. Which of the following statements is true?
   a. No systemic disorder is known to be the initiating cause of periodontitis in the absence of bacterial plaque.
   b. Other local factors acting in conjunction with bacterial plaque do not produce chronic disease of the periodontium.
   c. Primary occlusal traumatism will not cause periodontal disease.
   d. Initiation of periodontal disease only occurs in the presence of bacterial plaque.
2. Which of the following is (are) tooth surface deposits?
   a. Bacterial plaque
   b. Acquired pellicle
   c. Calculus
   d. All the above
3. The loosely attached plaque consists primarily of:
   a. Anaerobic bacteria
   b. Supragingival bacteria
   c. Aerobic bacteria
   d. Tightly adherent bacteria
4. Plaque is composed primarily of colonized organisms with additional components such as:
   a. Epithelial cells
   b. White blood cells
   c. Food debris
   d. All the above
5. An enzyme that by definition depolymerizes collagen fibers and fibrils, the major formed elements in the gingiva and periodontal ligament, is:
   a. Collagenase
   b. Hyaluronidase
   c. Protease
   d. Immunase
6. The stage of plaque-related periodontal disease characterized by changes occurring after 2 to 4 days of plaque accumulation is:
   a. Initial lesion
   b. Early lesion
   c. Established lesion
   d. Advanced lesion
7. The stage of plaque-related periodontal disease in which the plasma cell is the predominant inflammatory cell type within the affected connective tissues is:
   a. Initial lesion
   b. Early lesion
   c. Established lesion
   d. Advanced lesion
8. Which of the following statements is true regarding periodontitis?
   a. Periodontitis is preceded by gingivitis.
   b. Untreated gingivitis will proceed to periodontitis.
   c. Occlusal forces can initiate periodontitis.
   d. None of the above
9. Interdentally, inflammation and bacterial products spread from the gingiva to the alveolar process:
   a. Through the base of the sulcus to the periodontal ligament at the crest of the bone
   b. Along the neurovascular bundle of the interdental canal at the crest of the septum
   c. Along the outer aspect of the interdental septal bone
   d. Through the epithelial attachment into the transseptal fibers
10. Examples of bacteria that possess virulence factors that enable them to inactivate complement or PMNs or to simply bypass this step by tissue invasion are:
    a. *Porphyromonas gingivalis (P. gingivalis)* and *Actinobacillus actinomycetemcomitans (A. actinomycetemcomitans)*
    b. *E. coli* and *S. mutans*
    c. Spirochetes
    d. None of the above

# Systemic Contributing Factors

Terry Rees

## INTRODUCTION

It has long been recognized that periodontal diseases are caused by local oral etiologic factors, especially bacterial plaque. It is also well recognized, however, that a significant number of systemic diseases and disorders may reduce or alter host resistance or host response, and predispose individuals to periodontal destruction or to atypical gingival reactions. For example, stress or other systemic disorders may play a role in necrotizing gingivitis, whereas physiologic alterations in steroid hormones during pregnancy can alter gingival response to the presence of plaque. Ingestion of certain medications may lead to gingival overgrowth. The periodontium is made up of bone, tooth structure, connective tissue, and epithelium. Therefore, it is apparent that systemic conditions that affect any body tissues may also have an effect on periodontal tissues. This review will focus on systemic disorders that induce or influence gingivitis or plaque-related periodontitis and the possible role of advanced periodontal disease as a risk factor for systemic disease. The following factors will be discussed:

Aging
Emotional and psychosocial stress
Genetic disorders
Endocrine imbalances
Hematologic disorders
Nutritional deficiencies and metabolic disorders
Drugs and the periodontium
AIDS-related periodontal diseases

## SYSTEMIC CONTRIBUTING FACTORS

### Aging

Epidemiologic studies have established that the incidence of periodontal disease increases with age.

However, although periodontal attachment and alveolar bone loss may increase in the elderly, severe loss is found in only a few sites in a minority of subjects. It is unclear whether these changes represent the cumulative effects of periodontal disease over the course of many years or a reduction in host resistance as a function of the aging process. The increased incidence of systemic diseases and the medicaments used to treat these diseases may also adversely affect host resistance in the elderly. Some authorities consider increasing age as a risk factor for periodontal disease because aging is associated with alterations in the periodontium that, at least in theory, may adversely alter host response. For example, bone density may decrease and healing capacity may be reduced as a result of physiologic slowing of the metabolic processes. **There is also evidence that older individuals with prior attachment loss and inadequate oral hygiene have an increased risk for disease progression. However, the majority of studies indicate that periodontal diseases are not a natural consequence of the aging process and** that periodontal health can be maintained throughout life in the absence of local etiologic factors.[1,2]

### Emotional and Psychosocial Stress

A relationship between emotional or psychosocial stress and oral disease has been proposed for many years. Several studies have indicated an association between severity of periodontal disease and work stresses, life event stresses, and psychological reactions to life events (especially depression). A recent long-term study of nearly 1,500 adults indicated that life event stresses such as financial strain and depression were associated with more severe periodontal disease.[3] It should be noted, however, that the health habits of individuals under stress may decline as reflected by increased smoking, use of alcohol and illicit drugs, sleeplessness, eating disorders, **bruxing,** inadequate oral hygiene, **and failure to seek dental care.** These factors could play an important role in the incidence and severity of periodontal disease. **Several studies, however, have** indicated, that positive coping skills negate the potentially harmful effects of stress on the periodontium. **Necrotizing ulcerative gingivitis is the periodontal disease most often associated with psychosocial stress, but its incidence appears to have markedly diminished among immunocompetent individuals, suggesting that the role of stress as a risk factor for periodontal disease is relatively minor.** Further studies are **needed to determine the degree to which stress alone contributes to periodontal disease.**[2,4,5]

## Genetic Disorders

Currently there is growing evidence that heredity plays an important role in patient susceptibility to plaque-related inflammatory periodontal conditions. For example, studies of identical twins raised in separate environments revealed similar patterns of **periodontitis. Another study, however, has indicated that gingivitis does not have a hereditary component, instead being related to plaque accumulation. It has also been reported that access to routine dental care and proper oral hygiene negate any adverse effect that host genes may have on subgingival plaque in adults.**[6,7] Epidemiologic long-term studies of groups of individuals without access to oral hygiene measures or periodontal treatment suggest that innate host resistance may be the most important factor in determining which individuals experience severe periodontal destruction. More recently an exaggerated monocyte- or macrophage-derived interleukin 1 (IL-1) reaction has been found among individuals susceptible to early onset or severely destructive periodontitis. These individuals appear to possess an IL-1 gene polymorphism that leads to more inflammation and severe periodontal destruction when exposed to dental plaque. Patients found to possess this genotype may require more rigorous preventive and therapeutic periodontal treatment than those who do not possess this risk factor.[8–10]

Several genetic disorders may exert adverse effects on oral and periodontal tissues. These effects are usually the result of deficiencies or dysfunctions of hematologic cells associated with host defense. *Papillon-Lefèvre* syndrome is an autosomal recessive disorder characterized by hyperkeratosis of the palms of the hands and soles of the feet and rapidly progressive periodontitis. The condition is often associated with deficiencies in neutrophil phagocytosis and chemotaxis.[11] Other inherited disorders result in diminished numbers of neutrophils or in faulty neutrophil function. *Down syndrome, chronic idiopathic neutropenia, cyclic neutropenia, Chediak-Higashi syndrome,* and *leukocyte adhesion deficiency (LAD) syndrome* are examples.[12–14]

*Acatalasia* is a rare hereditary condition characterized by a deficiency of the enzyme *catalase,* which leads to accumulation of toxic substances such as hydrogen peroxide in tissues, and induces tissue damage and necrosis. It is associated with precocious destructive periodontitis in infants and children.[15]

The *Ehlers-Danlos* phenomena are a group of eight related hereditary conditions that feature hypermobility of body joints and hyperextensibility and fragility of body tissues, including oral mucosa. Generalized extensive periodontal destruction and delayed wound healing have been reported in some subsyndromes of the condition.[16,17]

*Hypophosphatasia* and *pseudohypophosphatasia* are familial disorders associated with ricketslike bone abnormalities despite normal vitamin D metabolism. The conditions result in a deficiency of alkaline phosphatase in plasma and bone matrix. Susceptibility to periodontal disease and premature loss of primary and secondary dentition may occur as the result of faulty cementum formation, faulty periodontal ligament fibers, abnormal formation of alveolar bone, and defective neutrophil function.[18]

## Endocrine Imbalances

A number of endocrine abnormalities may affect the periodontium directly, or as a result of neutrophil dysfunction or altered wound healing. For example, *hyperparathyroidism* is associated with excessive secretion of parathyroid hormone, which results in imbalanced mobilization of calcium from bone. This may lead to osteoporosis and exaggerated bone loss in the presence of plaque-related periodontitis.[19] A similar response has been noted in individuals who cannot properly utilize vitamin D and among estrogen-deficient women.[20] The resultant osteopenia or osteoporosis may serve as a risk factor for more severe periodontal destruction and tooth loss in the presence of dental plaque. Conversely, estrogen supplementation or the use of bisphonates (estrogen substitutes) may offer a protective effect on the severity of periodontal disease. **It should be noted, however, that injectable bisphonates have recently been reported to occasionally be associated with mandibular osteonecrosis in the presence of dental or periodontal infections. This phenomenon is apparently related to the impact of bisphonates on cellular turnover and replacement in bone.**[21] **Further study is indicated on the role of hormonal factors and osteoporosis in the progression of periodontal disease.** These factors will be of greater importance as the American population ages, with a resultant increase in numbers of postmenopausal women seeking dental treatment.[22]

## Diabetes Mellitus

*Diabetes mellitus* is an abnormality in glucose metabolism characterized by a decrease in insulin production or metabolism. Using the most recent classifications suggested by the American Diabetes Association, type 1 diabetes represents insulin depletion resulting from destruction of the beta cells of the pancreas. Affected individuals require insulin supplementation to achieve metabolic control of their disease. It often develops early in life and is far less common than type 2 diabetes, in which insulin resistance occurs with or without insulin depletion. Type 2 diabetics may be treated with oral hypoglycemic agents or insulin.[23,24] The classic signs and symptoms of uncontrolled diabetes mellitus include excessive thirst, hunger, and urination, as well as fatigue, pruritus (itching), and glycosuria (glucose in urine). Long-term complications may include atherosclerotic cardiovascular, cerebrovascular, or peripheral vascular disease; retinopathy, which often leads to loss of vision; nephropathy; peripheral neuropathy; and periodontal disease. Elevated blood sugar levels (hyperglycemia) may suppress the host's immune response and lead to poor wound healing and recurrent infections. In the oral cavity this may be reflected by multiple or recurrent periodontal abscesses and cellulitis. Patients suffering from undiagnosed or poorly controlled diabetes mellitus are susceptible to gingivitis, gingival hyperplasia, and periodontitis. In part, periodontal destruction is attributable to the factors described above, but the diabetic state is also associated with decreased collagen synthesis and increased collagenase activity. Additionally, altered neutrophil function has been identified in some, but not all, diabetics. Diabetes-induced secondary hyperparathyroidism may predispose the individual to excessive alveolar bone loss in the presence of periodontal infection. The effect of controlled diabetes mellitus on periodontal

disease progression is somewhat controversial. The bulk of evidence suggests, however, that the incidence and severity of gingivitis increases in **poorly controlled** diabetic children, whereas teenage and adult diabetics experience an increased susceptibility to both gingivitis and periodontitis. Recent evidence indicates that meticulous control of the diabetic state is associated with periodontal **health status comparable to that of nondiabetic individuals. However, even nondiabetics may experience increased severity of periodontal disease if they are affected by glucose intolerance.**[25] Conversely, there is strong evidence suggesting that control of infections, including advanced periodontal disease, may be essential to establishment of good metabolic control in diabetics.[26,27] Consequently, the dental practitioner should make the diabetic patient's physician aware if severe periodontal disease **is** present.

Diabetic patients should be treated with caution in dental practice. The dentist must seek medical consultation if there is evidence of poor metabolic control. Patients must be cautioned to take their medication and to follow their usual diet in conjunction with dental appointments, and they must maintain meticulous oral hygiene to assure periodontal health. Patients should be treated in a relaxed, nonstressful environment, and appointments should be short. Decisions regarding use of antibiotics for treatment procedures should be based on the patient's overall health status and the extent of the procedure to be performed. One must always remain alert for evidence of developing insulin shock or diabetic coma.

Several multicenter studies of diabetic patients indicate that strict metabolic control of plasma glucose levels in both type 1 and type 2 patients results in fewer medical complications. These studies also suggest that maintenance of plasma glucose at near normal levels can lead to an increased incidence of hypoglycemia. Some diabetics experience severe hypoglycemia without displaying or sensing the common signs and symptoms. These symptoms may include mood changes, mental confusion, lethargy, bizarre activities, coma, or even death. These symptoms may also be observed in hyperglycemic individuals, although onset of symptoms is more gradual. In most instances it is prudent to treat unexplained reactions in the dental office by diabetic patients as though they are experiencing hypoglycemia. This treatment should include the administration of oral carbohydrates such as soft drinks, candy, orange juice, or Glucola. The unconscious patient can be treated with intravenous administration of dextrose.[28,29]

## Sex Hormones and Pregnancy

Imbalances in sex hormones may have an adverse effect on the gingiva. For example, *gingival inflammatory hyperplasia* has been reported during puberty and pregnancy and as a result of intake of oral contraceptives. Sex hormone–related physiologic changes lead to altered capillary permeability and increased tissue fluids, resulting in an edematous, hemorrhagic, hyperplastic gingivitis in response to dental plaque. **Increased gingival inflammation has also been reported in some women during ovulation and menstruation. These changes appear to be more severe in women with preexisting gingivitis.**[30] Gingival changes have also been reported in males treated with androgenic sex hormones.

Increased susceptibility to gingival inflammation during pregnancy begins in the second month of gestation, peaks in the eighth month, and gradually diminishes in the ninth month and after parturition. These changes closely correlate with progesterone levels during those time periods. There is some evidence to suggest that increases in estrogen and progesterone during pregnancy promote the development of a more anaerobic crevicular microbial flora. *Pyogenic granuloma* (pregnancy tumor) formation sometimes occurs during pregnancy because of the exaggerated tissue response to local irritants induced by altered sex hormone levels.

Periodontal treatment during periods of elevated sex hormone levels is predicated on removal of local irritants and establishment of meticulous oral hygiene. Surgical correction of pregnancy-related gingival hyperplastic changes should be delayed, if possible, until after parturition. Dental treatment can most safely be performed during the second trimester but elective procedures should be deferred when possible.[28]

Characteristics of hormonally deficient women have been discussed above.

## Hematologic Disorders

Gingival inflammation and chronic periodontitis are characterized by histopathologic presence of an inflammatory cell infiltration of polymorphonuclear leukocytes, lymphocytes, macrophages, and plasma cells. Other blood cells (red blood cells, platelets) are intimately involved with periodontal nutrition, hemostasis, and wound healing. For these reasons, systemic hematologic disorders may have a profound effect on the periodontium. Blood dyscrasias such as *polycythemia, thrombocytopenia,* or *clotting factor deficiencies* may result in prolonged hemorrhage after periodontal treatment procedures.[31] Red blood cell disorders such as *aplastic anemia* or *sickle cell anemia* may adversely affect the results of periodontal therapy and induce severe postoperative complications. *Multiple myeloma* is a plasma cell malignancy often associated with gingival bleeding and destruction of alveolar bone. The majority of hematologic disorders associated with periodontal disease, however, are related to white blood cell function or numbers.

*Agranulocytosis* represents depletion of all blood granulocytes whereas *neutropenia* connotes the absence of circulating polymorphonuclear neutrophils. *Cyclic neutropenia* is characterized by cyclic depletion of neutrophil numbers, typically in 3-week cycles. These conditions are associated with severe localized or generalized periodontal destruction.[13,32]

*Leukemia* is a malignant disease characterized by proliferation of white blood cell–forming tissues and increased circulating abnormal leukocytes. Periodontal lesions, including gingival enlargement, are common in patients with leukemia. Gingival changes may be the result of infiltration of leukemic cells into the tissues, hemorrhage into the tissues, and plaque-induced inflammation.[33] Periodontal changes may also occur in patients under treatment for leukemia. Toxicity to chemotherapeutic drugs may directly induce severe gingival erosion and ulceration, whereas bone marrow suppression may lead to neutropenic ulcerations, anemic pallor of the gingiva, bleeding owing to platelet deficiency, and reduced resistance to infection. Meticulous oral hygiene is important in reducing periodontal complications, but close medical-dental coordination is required before performing any periodontal therapy.[12] Functional leukocyte disorders, especially neutrophil dysfunction, are commonly associated with severe periodontal destruction. These disorders were discussed under Genetic Disorders.

## Nutritional Deficiencies and Metabolic Disorders

The relationship of nutritional deficiencies to progression of periodontal disease has been disputed for many years. Tissue-related nutritional deficiencies occur not only as a result of reduced intake of nutritional substances but also because of disruption of proper digestion, absorption, transport, or utilization of the nutritional element. Nutritional disorders have profound effects on all body tissues, including the periodontium. Efforts to correlate periodontal disease progression with nutritional deficiencies have generally been equivocal, and there is no **strong** evidence that nutritional supplementation alone will enhance periodontal health unless a deficiency is present.[34–39]

Severe vitamin C deficiency *(scurvy)* is known to induce dramatic periodontal destruction in humans. Initial changes may manifest as mild-to-moderate gingivitis, followed later by acutely inflamed, edematous, hemorrhagic, gingival enlargement. The oral symptoms are accompanied by significant general physiologic changes, including lassitude, weakness, malaise, sore joints, ecchymosis, and weight loss. If undetected, scurvy will ultimately lead to severe periodontal destruction and spontaneous exfoliation of teeth. Despite these profound effects there is no evidence that vitamin C deficiency will initiate inflammatory periodontal disease in the absence of bacterial plaque. However, individuals who have a minor deficiency in vitamin C intake may be at increased risk for developing periodontitis, especially if they also smoke.[2,39]

*Vitamin D* is a fat-soluble vitamin required for physiologic balance of calcium and phosphorus in the body. Deficiency in vitamin D may lead to the development of osteoporosis, manifesting as rickets in children or osteomalacia in adults.[40] Either condition may be associated with generalized periodontal ligament destruction and alveolar bone resorption as described in the section on Hypophosphatasia.

Severe protein deficiency, such as *Kwashiorkor,* has been associated with necrotizing lesions of the gingiva and other oral tissues and with increased gingival inflammation and periodontal bone loss. These effects may occur as the result of altered immune responses in the presence of plaque-associated periodontitis.

It must be emphasized that mild nutritional deficiencies do not induce periodontal inflammation and destruction. Periodontal changes may be exaggerated, however, when plaque-related infection is present. Nonetheless, it should be obvious that an adequate nutritional status will help assure satisfactory patient response to periodontal therapy.[2]

## Drugs and the Periodontium

Drugs have long been recognized as potential secondary etiologic factors in periodontal disease. For example, drug-induced *xerostomia* may result in increased plaque and calculus accumulation. The ensuing loss of salivary buffering capacity, as well as reduction in salivary immunoglobulins, may alter host resistance to local irritants. Xerostomic potential has been associated with at least 400 drugs, including diuretics, antipsychotics, antihypertensives, and antidepressants. A recent controlled study identified a direct relationship between xerostomia induced by Sjögren's syndrome and established periodontitis.

Various drugs and medicaments may have direct effects on periodontal tissues. Many substances can induce chemical reactions in oral soft tissues, including the gingiva. Reactions range from mild hyperkeratosis to severe burns. Topically applied aspirin, phenolic compounds, volatile oils, anesthetics, fluoride preparations, and astringents are among those agents capable of eliciting such reactions. It may be important to note that chemical burns have been reported with the use of hydrogen peroxide mouth rinses.

Smoking has been recognized for many years as a contributing secondary factor in necrotizing ulcerative gingivitis. More recently it has been identified as a very potent risk factor for periodontal disease and for adversely altering the response to periodontal therapy. Smoking may affect the periodontium by inducing a transient vasoconstriction of the gingival blood vessels and increased levels of cytotoxic substances in gingival crevicular fluid and saliva. Additionally, it is associated with increased tooth surface debris and calculus formation, but the most profound effect appears to be suppression of the host immune system, especially the function of leukocytes and macrophages.

Tobacco products are strongly associated with development of oral leukoplakic lesions with or without epithelial dysplasia or malignant transformation, and the use of smokeless tobacco may induce localized gingivitis, gingival recession, and periodontal attachment loss. Drugs of abuse such as *cannabis* (marijuana) and cocaine can induce gingival leukoplakia and erythema, and heavy intraoral use of cocaine may result in ulcerative gingivitis and alveolar bone destruction.[41]

Drug-induced *agranulocytosis* may result in severe gingival necrosis resembling generalized *acute necrotizing ulcerative gingivitis* (ANUG). Drugs implicated in causing agranulocytosis include the phenothiazines, sulfur derivatives, indomethacin, and some antibiotics.

Hypersensitivity reactions to various drugs, dental materials, flavoring agents, and food products may induce inflammatory, contact lesions of the gingiva and other oral tissues. Erythema multiforme, fixed drug eruptions, and lichenoid drug reactions may also significantly affect gingiva and alveolar mucosa in response to drug ingestion.[42,43]

Drug-induced gingival enlargements have been reported since the 1930s. Phenytoin (Dilantin) was the first agent associated with this phenomenon.

Gingival overgrowth occurs in approximately 50% of patients receiving phenytoin, and the anterior facial gingiva is most often involved. The overgrowth usually becomes evident within 3 to 12 months after initiation of phenytoin therapy, and there is a strong correlation between inadequate plaque control and the tissue changes. Today, other antiepileptic drugs are increasingly being used, and the overall incidence of phenytoin-induced reactions may be decreasing. Some other antiepileptic agents (other hydantoins, barbiturates, and valproic acid), however, have occasionally been associated with gingival overgrowth.

Therapeutic intake of sex hormones such as *estrogen, progesterone,* and *androgens* has been occasionally reported to be associated with gingival enlargement, and most recently, gingival overgrowth has been identified in association with the drug cyclosporin and a family of drugs, the calcium-channel blockers. Nifedipine is the calcium-channel blocking agent that most commonly induces this reaction. Gingival changes are very similar to those described with phenytoin, and reported incidence is believed to be between 10 and 20% of those taking the drug. Incidence is less with the other calcium-channel blocking agents, and isradipine and amlodipine have been identified as rarely if ever causing gingival enlargement.[44]

It is of interest that gingival enlargement has occasionally been reported in response to heavy use of *cannabis* (marijuana). Overall, approximately 20 drugs have been identified as capable of inducing this reaction in the presence of plaque accumulation.[43,44]

## AIDS-Related Periodontal Diseases

*Acquired immunodeficiency syndrome* (AIDS) is characterized by profound impairment of the immune system of affected individuals. A detailed discussion of this condition is beyond the scope of this text. It should be noted, however, that evidence of infection with the causative *human immunodeficiency virus* (HIV) may often manifest in the oral cavity as severe or recurrent *candidiasis, oral hairy leukoplakia, Kaposi's sarcoma,* or as atypical periodontal diseases. The dental health-care provider must be alert for these and other manifestations of immune deficiency and be prepared to assist the patient in management of HIV-associated oral lesions. The terminology used for HIV-related periodontal diseases has been revised, and there is evidence to indicate that the incidence of such diseases may increase with increasing immune deficiency. However, the majority of individuals with AIDS manifest with periodontal health or

conventional forms of gingivitis or periodontitis. Unusual periodontal lesions may occur more frequently in individuals whose immune system is compromised for any reason, and all types of periodontal diseases associated with HIV infection have been reported in HIV-negative patients.[2,45–47]

*Linear gingival erythema* (LGE) is a localized, persistent, erythematous gingivitis that may or may not serve as a precursor to a rapidly progressive *necrotizing ulcerative gingivitis* (NUG) *or periodontitis* (NUP). The inflammation is often limited to marginal gingiva but may extend into attached gingiva as a punctate or diffuse erythema. Linear gingival erythema is often unresponsive to corrective therapy, yet the lesions may disappear spontaneously. Treatment is similar to that recommended for other marginal gingivitis.

An increased incidence of *necrotizing ulcerative gingivitis* (NUG) has been suggested among HIV-infected patients, but the relationship has not been fully substantiated. When found in an HIV-positive patient, the condition should be treated as described elsewhere in this text.

A necrotizing, ulcerative, rapidly progressive form of periodontitis (necrotizing ulcerative periodontitis [NUP]) does occur more frequently among HIV-positive individuals than the general population. Lesions of this type were, however, described long before the onset of the AIDS epidemic in 1981. Necrotizing, ulcerative periodontitis features soft tissue necrosis and rapid periodontal destruction. Lesions may occur anywhere in the dental arches, and they are usually localized. The condition is painful, and bone may be spontaneously exposed. Some evidence suggests an increased incidence of NUP among individuals with severe immune depression. Treatment consists of gentle debridement and scaling and root planing. Meticulous oral hygiene must be established, including home and office use of antimicrobial mouth rinses such as chlorhexidine gluconate. Metronidazole is the drug of choice if systemic antibiotic therapy is indicated.

*Necrotizing ulcerative stomatitis* (NUS) represents an extension of NUP to involve mucosal tissue and bone. It occurs in only a relatively small number of HIV-positive individuals, and it probably represents noma or cancrum oris, which was described many years ago. As mentioned earlier, most HIV-infected patients experience periodontal disease of the same nature and severity as the general population. With proper home care and appropriate periodontal therapy, these individuals can maintain good periodontal health throughout the course of their disease. In AIDS treatment centers there is a clinical impression that the incidence of

AIDS-related periodontal diseases has diminished since newer antiviral agents and drug combination therapies have been introduced.[22,48]

# PERIODONTAL INFECTIONS AND SYSTEMIC DISEASES

Although the potential for systemic conditions to contribute to plaque-induced periodontitis is well documented, a growing body of evidence suggests that the presence of generalized, severe periodontitis may also contribute to certain systemic disorders or adversely influence their control. An association has been identified between infections, including advanced periodontitis, and premature births or delivery of low birth-weight infants, and recent interventional studies suggest that periodontal treatment may reduce the risk for these birth complications The adverse events are believed to occur because accumulations of Gram-negative microorganisms such as those found in periodontitis results in increased release of prostaglandins and cytokines, which may act on distant sites such as the placenta.[49–52]

A similar relationship has been suggested between acute systemic infections and the occurrence of cardiovascular disease to include myocardial infarction and stroke. This may indicate that excessive accumulations of Gram-negative organisms contribute to atherosclerosis. The mechanism of action is not clearly defined, although animal and some human studies indicate that Gram-negative bacteremias may induce platelet aggregation, creating hypercoagulation and increased blood viscosity, all of which appear to be important features of atheroma formation.[53–67]

Available evidence indicates that periodontitis is a potential risk factor for poor glycemic control in individuals with diabetes mellitus. Diabetic individuals with severe periodontitis have been demonstrated to experience a worsening of glycemic control with time when compared with individuals in good periodontal health.[28] Additionally, some studies indicate that periodontal therapy in diabetic patients with periodontal disease may improve the degree of glycemic control.[68]

Severe periodontitis has also been associated **with** both upper and lower respiratory diseases such as hospital-acquired pneumonia. This type of pneumonia is usually associated with microorganisms rarely found in the oral cavity of healthy individuals but that are harbored in plaque of hospitalized individuals with periodontal disease. Conversely, periodontal disease does not appear to represent a risk factor for community-acquired pneumonia.

The relationship between periodontitis and systemic disorders is an area of intense interest at present, and several studies are underway to evaluate this relationship. To date, ample evidence exists to encourage the dentist to advise medical colleagues of the relationship and to encourage periodontal health as an important component in the management of some systemic diseases.[26,53–55,59,61,63,65,66,69]

# REFERENCES

1. Centers for Disease Control and Prevention (CDC). Public health and aging: retention of natural teeth among older adults—United States, 2003. MMWR Morb Mortal Wkly Rep 2003;52:1226–1229.
2. Stanford TW, Rees TD. Acquired immune suppression and other risk factors/indicators for periodontal disease progression. Periodontol 2000 2003;32:118–135.
3. Genco RJ, Ho AW, Kopman J, Grossi SG, Dunford RG, Tedesco LA. Models to evaluate the role of stress in periodontal disease. Ann Periodontol 1998;3:288–302.
4. Firestone JM. Stress and periodontitis. J Am Dent Assoc 2003;134:1591–1596.
5. Solis AC, Lotufo RF, Pannuti CM, BGrunheiro EC, Margues AH, Lotufo-Neto F. Association of periodontal disease to anxiety and depression symptoms, and psychosocial stress factors. J Clin Periodontol 2003;31:633–538.
6. Michalowicz BS, Diehl SR, Gunsolley JC, Sparks BS, Brooks CN, Koertge TE, Califano JV, Burmeister JA, Schenkein HA. Evidence of a substantial genetic basis for risk of adult periodontitis. J Periodontol 2000;71:1699–1707.
7. Michalowicz BS, Wolff LF, Klump D, Hinrichs JE, Aeppli DM, Bouchard TJ Jr, Pihlstrom BL. Periodontal bacteria in adult twins. J Periodontol 1999;70:263–273.
8. Kim JS, Park JY, Chung WY, Choi MA, Cho KS, Park KK. Polymorphisms in genes coding for enzymes metabolizing smoking-derived substances and the risk of periodontitis. J Clin Periodontol 2004;31:959–964.
9. Nares S. The genetic relationship to periodontal disease. Periodontol 2000 2003;32:36–49.
10. Suzuki A, Ji G, Numabe Y, Ishii K, Muramatsu M, Kamoi K. Large-scale investigation of genomic markers for severe periodontitis. Odontology 2003;92:43–47.
11. Lundgren T, Renvert S. Periodontal treatment of patients with Papillon-Lefevre syndrome: a 3-year follow-up. J Clin Periodontol 2004;31:933–938.
12. Deas DE, Mackey SA, McDonnell HT. Systemic disease and periodontitis: manifestations of neutrophil dysfunction. Periodontol 2000 2003;32:82–104.
13. Myoken Y, Sugata T, Fujita Y, Asaoku H, Fujihara M, Mikami Y. Fatal necrotizing stomatitis due to

*Trichoderma longibrachiatum* in a neutropenic patient with malignant lymphoma: a case report. Int J Oral Maxillofac Surg 2002;31:688–691.

14. Waldrop TC, Anderson DC, Hallmon WW, Schmalsteig FC, Jacobs RL. Periodontal manifestations of heritable Mac1, LFA1 deficiency syndrome. Clinical, histopathologic and molecular characteristics. J Periodontol 1987;58:401–416.

15. Goth L, Pay A. Genetic heterogeneity in acatalasemia. Electrophoresis 1996;17:1302–1303.

16. Fridrich KL, Kempf KK, Moline DO. Dental implications in Ehlers-Danlos syndrome. Oral Surg Oral Med Oral Pathol 1990;69:431–435.

17. Rahman N, Dunstan M, Teare MD, Hanks S, Douglas J, Coleman K, Bottomly WE, Campbell ME, Berglund B, Nordenskjold M, Forssell BN, Burrows N, Lunt P, Young I, Williams N, Bignell GR, Futreal PA, Pope FM. Ehlers-Danlos syndrome with severe early-onset periodontal disease (EDS-VIII) is a distinct, heterogeneous disorder with one predisposition gene at chromosome 12p12. Am J Hum Genet 2003;73:19–204.

18. Oh TJ, Eber R, Wang HL. Periodontal diseases in the child and adolescent. J Clin Periodontol 2002; 29:400–410.

19. Franenthal S, Nakhoul F, Machtei EE, Green J, Ardekian L, Laufer D, Peled M. The effect of secondary hyperparathyroidism and hemodialysis therapy on alveolar bone and periodontium. J Clin Periodontol 2002;29:479–483.

20. Murayama T, Iwatsubo R, Akiyama S, Amano A, Morisaki I. Familial hypophosphatemic vitamin D-resistant rickets: dental findings and histologic study of teeth. Oral Surg Oral Med Oral Pathol Oral Radiol Endod 2000;90:310–316.

21. Bagan JV, Murillo J, Jimenez Y, Poveda R, Milian MA, Sanchis JM, Silvrstre FFJ, Scully C. Avascular jaw osteonecrosis in association with cancer chemotherapy: series of 10 cases. J Oral Pathol Med 2005;34:120–123.

22. Mealey BL, Rees TD, Rose LF, Grossi SG. Systemic factors impacting the periodontium. In: Rose LF, Mealey BL, Genco RJ, Cohen DW, eds. Periodontics Medicine, Surgery, and Implants. St. Louis: Elsevier Mosby, 2004, pp 790–845.

23. American Diabetes Association. Expert Committee on the Diagnosis and Classification of Diabetes. Committee report. Diabetes Care 1997;20:1183–1197.

24. Muzyka BC. Diabetes mellitus: a clinical update of terminology, prevalence, and economics. Pract Proced Aesthet Dent 2004;16:522.

25. Saito T, Shimazaki Y, Kiyohara Y, Kato I, Kubo M, Iida M, Koga T. The severity of periodontal disease is associated with the development of glucose intolerance in non-diabetics: the Hisayama study. J Dent Res 2004;83:485–490.

26. Renvert S. Destructive periodontal disease in relations to diabetes mellitus, cardiovascular diseases, osteoporosis and respiratory diseases. Oral Health Prev Dent 2003;1(Suppl 1):341–357.

27. Saremi A, Nelson RG, Tulloch-Reid M, Hanson RL, Sievers ML, Taylor GW, Shlossman M, Bennett PH, Genco R, Knowler WC. Periodontal disease and mortality in type 2 diabetes. Diabetes Care 2005; 28:27–32.

28. Mealey BL, Moritz AJ. Hormonal influences: effects of diabetes mellitus and endogenous female sex steroid hormones of the periodontium. Periodontol 2000 2003;32:59–81.

29. Rees TD. Periodontal management of the patient with diabetes mellitus. Periodontol 2000 2000;23: 63–72.

30. Diaz-Guzman LM, Castellanos-Suarez JL. Lesions of the oral mucosa and periodontal disease behavior in pregnant patients. Med Oral Patol Oral Cir Bucal 2004;9:434–437, 430–433.

31. Owais Z, Dane J, Cumming CG. Unprovoked periodontal hemorrhage, life-threatening anemia and idiopathic thrombocytopenia purpura: an unusual case report. Spec Care Dentist 2003;23:58–62.

32. Nakai Y, Kshihara C, Ogata S, Shimoto T. Oral manifestations of cyclic neutropenia in a Japanese child: case report with a 5-year follow-up. Pediatr Dent 2003;25:383–388.

33. Pereira CM, Gasparetto PF, Coracin FL, Marques JF, Lima CS, Correa ME. Severe gingival bleeding in a myelodysplastic patient: management and outcome. J Periodontol 2004;75:483–486.

34. Boyd LD, Madden TE. Nutrition, infection, and periodontal disease. Dent Clin North Am 2003;47: 337–354.

35. Bsoul SA, Terezhalmy GT. Vitamin C in health and disease. J Contemp Dent Pract 2003;15:1–13.

36. Enwonwu CO, Phillips RS, Ibrahim, CD, Danfillo IS. Nutrition and oral health in Africa. Int Dent J 2004;54(Suppl 1):a344–351.

37. Leggott PJ, Robertson PB, Rothman DL, Murray PA, Jacob RA. The effect of controlled ascorbic acid depletion and supplementation on periodontal health. J Periodontol 1986;57:472–479.

38. Munoz CA, Kiger RD, Stephens JA, Kim J, Wilson AC. Effects of a nutritional supplement on periodontal status. Comp Cont Educ Dent 2001;22:425–428, 430, 432 passim.

39. Nishida M, Grossi SG, Dunford RG, Ho AW, Trevisan M, Genco RJ. Dietary vitamin C and the risk for periodontal disease. J Periodontol 2000;71: 1057–1066.

40. Zambrano M, Nikitakis NG, Sanchez-Quevedo MC, Sauk JJ, Sedano H, Rivera H. Oral and dental manifestations of vitamin D-dependent rickets type I: report of a pediatric case. Oral Surg Oral Med Oral Pathol Oral Radiol Endod 2003;95:705–709.

41. Yukna RA. Cocaine periodontitis. Int J Periodont Restor Dent 1992;11:73–79.

42. Ciancio SG. Medications' impact on oral heatlh. J Am Dent Assoc 2004;135:1440–1448.

43. Rees TD. Drugs and oral disorders. Periodont 2000 1998;18:21–36.

44. Seymour RA. Dentistry and the medically compromised patient. Surgeon 2003;1:207–214.

45. Barasch A, Gordon S, Geist RY, Geist JR. Necrotizing stomatitis: report of 3 *Pseudomonas aeruginosa*-positive patients. Oral Surg Oral Med Oral Pathol Oral Radiol Endod 2003;96:136–140.

46. EC Clearinghouse on Oral Problems Related to HIV Infection and WHO Collaborating Center on Oral Manifestations of the Immunodeficiency Virus. Classification and diagnostic criteria for oral lesions in HIV infection. J Oral Pathol Med 1993;22: 289–291.

47. Lausten LL, Ferguson BL, Barker BF, Cobb CM. Oral Kaposi sarcoma associated with severe alveolar bone loss: case report and review of the literature. J Periodontol 2003;74:1668–1675.

48. Rees TD. Aids and the periodontium. In: Carranza FA Jr, Newman MG, eds. Clinical Periodontology, 9th ed. Philadelphia: WB Saunders, 2005, in press.

49. Canakei V, Canakei CF, Canakci H, Canakci E, Cicek Y, Ingee M, Ozgo M, Demir T, Dilsiz A, Yagiz H. Periodontal disease as a risk factor for pre-eclampsia: A case control study. Aust NZ J Obstet Gynaecol 2004;44:568–573.

50. Goepfert AR, Jeffrcoat MK, Andrews WW, Faye-Petersen O, Cliver SP, Goldenberg RL, Hauth JC. Periodontal disease and upper genital tract inflammation in early spontaneous preterm birth. Obstet Gynecol 2004;104:777–783.

51. Moore S, Ide M, Coward PY, Randhawa M, Borkowska E, Baylis R, Wilson RF. A prospective study to investigate the relationship between periodontal disease and adverse pregnancy outcome. Br Dent J 2003;197:251–258.

52. Sanchez AR, Kupp LI, Sheridan PJ, Sanchez DR. Maternal chronic infection as a risk factor in preterm low birth weight infants: the link with periodontal infection. J Int Acad Periodontol 2004;6: 89–94.

53. Chun YH, Chun KR, Olguin D, Wang HL. Biological foundation for periodontitis as a potential risk factor for atherosclerosis. J Periodontal Res 2005;40:87–95.

54. Dave S, Batista EL JR, Van Dyke TE. Cardiovascular disease and periodontal diseases; commonality and causation. Compend Contin Educ Dent 2004;25(Suppl 1):26–37.

55. Deliargyris EN, Madianos PN, Kadoma W, Marron I, Smith SC Jr, Beel JD, Offenbacher S. Periodontal disease in patients with acute myocardial infarction-prevalence and contribution to elevated C-reactive protein level. Am Heart J 2004;147:1005–1009.

56. Desvarieux M, Demmer RT, Rundek T, Boden-Albala B, Jacobs DR Jr, Papapanou RN, Sacco RL; Oral Infections and Vascular Disease Epidemiology Study (INVEST). Stroke 2003;34:2150–2155.

57. Dorfer CE, Bevcher H, Ziegler CM, Kaiser C, Lutz R, Jorss D, Lichy C, Buggle F, Bultmann S, Preusch M, Grau AJ. The association of gingivitis and periodontitis with ischemic stroke. J Clin Periodontol 2004;31:396–401.

58. Elter JR, Offenbacher S, Toole JF, Beck JD. Relationship of periodontal disease and edentulism to stroke/TIA. J Dent Res 2003;82:998–1001.

59. Geerts SO, Legrand V, Charpentier J, Albert A, Rompen EH. Further evidence of the association between periodontal conditions and coronary artery disease. J Periodontol 2004;75:1274–1280.

60. Grau AJ, Becher H, Ziegler CM, Lichy C, Buggle F, Kaiser C, Lutz R, Bultmann S, Preusch M, Dorfer CE. Periodontal disease as a risk factor for ischemic stroke. Stroke 2004;35:496–501.

61. Hung HC, Joshipura KJ, Colditz G, Manson JE, Rimm EB, Speizer FE, Willett WC. The association between tooth loss and coronary heart disease in men and women. J Public Helath Dent 2004;64: 209–215.

62. Janket SJ, Baird AE, Chuang SK, Jones JA. Meta-analysis of periodontal disease and risk of coronary heart disease and stroke. Evid Based Dent 2004; 5:69.

63. Meurman JH, Sanz M, Janket SJ. Oral health, atherosclerosis, and cardiovascular disease. Crit Rev Oral Biol Med 2003;1:403–413.

64. Muhlestein JF, Anderson JL. Chronic infection and coronary artery disease. Cardiol Clin 2003;21: 333–362.

65. Nakib SA, Pankow JS, Beck JD, Offenbacher S, Evans GW, Desvarieux M, Folsom AR. Periodontitis and coronary artery calcification: the Atherosclerosis Risk in Communities (ARIC) study. J Periodontol 3004;75:505–510.

66. Paquett DW. The periodontal-cardiovascular link. Compend Contin Educ Dent 2004;25:681–682, 685–692.

67. Scannapioco RA, Bush RB, Paju S. Associations between periodontal disease and risk for atherosclerosis, cardiovascular disease, and stroke. A systematic review. Ann Periodontol 2003;8:38–53.

68. Grossi SG. Treatment of periodontal disease and control of diabetes: an assessment of the evidence and need for future research. Ann Periodontol 2001;6:138–145.

69. Terpenning MS. The relationship between infections and chronic respiratory diseases: an overview. Ann Periodontol 2001;6:66–70.

## CHAPTER 3
## REVIEW QUESTIONS

1. Which of the following is true regarding the relationship of aging to periodontal health?
   a. Periodontal health can be maintained for life in the absence of local etiologic factors.
   b. Advanced age should be considered a major risk factor for periodontal disease.
   c. The incidence of periodontal disease does not increase with age.
   d. Loss of bone density usually results in an increase in periodontal disease with advancing age.

2. Emotional or psychosocial stress:
   a. Has no effect on periodontal disease risk
   b. May result in a decline of oral health habits
   c. Affects periodontal health despite positive coping skills
   d. Should be considered a major risk factor for periodontal disease

3. Genetic susceptibility factors:
   a. Have no effect on periodontal health
   b. May profoundly affect risk of severe periodontal disease
   c. Will cause increased periodontal disease despite adherence to proper oral hygiene and regular dental visits
   d. May result in enhanced neutrophil function and more periodontal disease

4. Type 1 diabetes:
   a. Results from an increase in insulin production
   b. Is more common than type 2 diabetes
   c. Is not associated with increased periodontal disease risk
   d. May be more easily controlled in patients with excellent periodontal health

5. During pregnancy, susceptibility to increased gingival inflammation tends to peak in the:
   a. Second month
   b. Sixth month
   c. Eighth month
   d. Ninth month

6. Which of the following is associated with severe generalized or localized periodontitis?
   a. Neutropenia
   b. Anemia
   c. Increased red blood cells (polycythemia)
   d. Decreased platelets (thrombocytopenia)

7. Which of the following drug groups have **all** been associated with gingival enlargement?
   a. Phenytoin, cyclosporine, acetaminophen
   b. Phenytoin, cyclosporine, angiotensin-converting enzyme inhibitors
   c. Phenytoin, calcium-channel blockers, angiotensin-converting enzyme inhibitors
   d. Phenytoin, cyclosporine, calcium-channel blockers

8. Oral use of which drug is most likely to be associated with ulcerative gingivitis and alveolar bone destruction?
   a. Marijuana
   b. Methamphetamine
   c. Alcohol
   d. Cocaine

9. Soft tissue necrosis and rapid periodontal destruction in an individual with AIDS is best described as:
   a. Necrotizing ulcerative gingivitis
   b. Necrotizing ulcerative periodontitis
   c. Linear gingival erythema
   d. Aggressive periodontitis

10. Which of the following statements is **true**?
    a. Periodontal disease has been clearly identified as a major risk factor for several systemic diseases.
    b. Interventional studies indicate that periodontal therapy in pregnant women may reduce risk of premature births.
    c. There is no evidence of an interrelationship between periodontal disease and stroke.
    d. There is no evidence that periodontal therapy will benefit diabetic control in affected individuals.

# Host Defenses in Periodontal Disease

Vanchit John

Inflammatory periodontal disease, which is primarily chronic in nature, usually results from the presence of bacterial plaque. However, the presence of bacterial plaque does not sufficiently account for all periodontal destruction. The host response plays a major role in the disease process. Therefore, severity and progression of periodontal disease and the resulting tissue destruction are highly dependent on the host response to the presence of infecting bacteria. The human body has a complex array of interdependent defense mechanisms to eliminate infecting microorganisms, to heal, and thus to maintain health. These systems are referred to as the inflammatory response and the immune system. Paradoxically, these systems that are intended to protect and heal the body have been shown to be responsible for some of the destruction in periodontal disease. Periodontal disease progression has been described as the *initial, early, and established lesions* with regard to gingivitis and as the *advanced lesion* describing periodontitis.[1,2] However, clinical observation of periodontal disease and its progression has indicated differing levels of susceptibility among patients. This, combined with a more sophisticated understanding of the immune response, has led to a more prominent role for the host response in periodontal disease.

Immunology is an extraordinarily complex subject. Furthermore, separating inflammation and immunity into distinct entities is difficult because there are many situations in which their activities overlap. This chapter presents an overview of the workings of the inflammatory response and the immune system, and discusses their role in periodontal healing and destruction.

## THE ROLE OF INNATE IMMUNITY AND RESISTANCE TO THE PROGRESSION OF PERIODONTAL DISEASE

The body's natural resistance to infectious agents present in the environment is referred to as *innate immunity.* Innate immunity refers to antigen-nonspecific defense mechanisms that a host uses immediately or within several hours after exposure to almost any infectious agent. Commonly encountered infectious agents include bacteria, viruses, fungi, and a variety of different parasitic organisms. In health most of these infectious agents are dealt with as a result of the presence of an intrinsic innate immunity. Innate immunity, which functions as the first line of defense, results from the presence of soluble factors and cells. Soluble factors may include those that are part of the complement system along with the more recently described acute-phase proteins and interferons.

A challenge to the host usually results in *inflammation* as the first response (Fig. 4-1). Periodontitis, which is an infectious disease process, leads to inflammation of the small blood vessel plexus present deep to the junctional epithelium. The process of inflammation is designed to protect the host from infections as well as to limit the damage that results to the host. Inflammation is an orderly sequence of events that occurs in response to any injury or infection; therefore, it is considered to be nonspecific in nature. Inflammation is the initial response, occurring before activation of the immune system. It occurs in three stages:

1. Increased vascular supply
2. Increased vascular permeability

# THE INFLAMMATORY RESPONSE

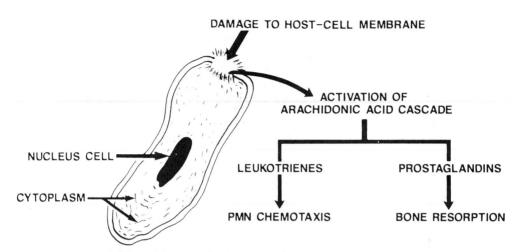

DAMAGE TO CERTAIN CELL MEMBRANES CAN RESULT IN THE FORMATION AND LIBERATION OF FACTORS THAT ARE RESPONSIBLE FOR THE CLINICAL SIGNS OF INFLAMMATION: ERYTHEMA, EDEMA, PAIN, AND TEMPERATURE ELEVATION. IN ADDITION, SOME OF THESE FACTORS ARE NOW KNOWN TO CAUSE BONE RESORPTION.

*Figure 4.1* ●

3. Active migration of phagocytic cells into the affected area

The primary cells responsible for inflammation are the leukocytes (polymorphonuclear cells [PMNs]), which are formed in the bone marrow from the same stem cell that forms monocytes. Specific cell surface markers determine which promyelocytes will become PMNs and which will become macrophages.

These markers are lost after cell differentiation. In the periodontium, the presence of a few PMNs in the junctional epithelium in health is considered to be normal. An increase in their number indicates the initiation of host defenses.

The macrophage is the next cell involved in inflammation. It is derived from the circulating monocyte and arrives at the site of inflammation after the PMN. It is a large cell with phagocytic capabilities similar to the PMN. It also plays a critical role in the immune response.

Lymphocytes arrive late at the site of inflammation and are associated with chronic inflammation.

Other cells involved include the mast cells, which are similar to the circulating basophil. They release histamine, platelet-activating factor (PAF), prostaglandin $E_2$ ($PGE_2$), and leukotrienes $B_4$ ($LTB_4$) and $D_4$ ($LTD_4$), all of which have profound inflammatory effects. In addition, the platelets release serotonin, an important inflammatory mediator. Other important soluble factors are those of the complement system.

## Serum Complement System

The *serum complement system* is composed of more than 20 serum proteins that, when activated, have potent biologic activity. These proteins function mainly to control the inflammatory response. This is done through the activation of immune cells and enhancing the immune response.

There are two major pathways by which proteins of the complement system are activated. The first, the *classic pathway (specific activation),* follows binding of antibody to bacterial cell wall surfaces. The second pathway, the *alternate pathway (nonspecific activation),* can be activated directly by constituents of cell walls of certain Gram-negative bacteria. These constituents are called endotoxins. The following are some of the many effects of complement activation by both pathways:

1. Substances form that enhance the ingestion of microbial cells and microbial products by white blood cells (phagocytes). These substances are called opsonins. When activated, serum complement generates potent opsonic factors.
2. Activated serum complement induces mast cells to release substances such as histamine. These factors cause blood vessels to dilate and to become permeable, resulting in an influx of

serum and serum factors into the local tissue spaces. Among the serum factors are antibodies and additional complement components.

3. A very powerful chemoattractant (for phagocytes) is generated when serum complement is activated. This chemoattractant, or chemotactic factor, causes neutrophils and macrophages to migrate toward a specific area in tissue.

4. Activated serum complement can result in factors that destroy microbial cell walls and cell membranes. This feature is important in killing certain bacteria. In the periodontal area, the large numbers of microbial cells and associated high levels of their metabolic products require that host responses consistently and efficiently control their concentrations and potential for invasion if serious infection is to be avoided.

The biologically active factors generated from serum complement probably play an important role in defense against microbial assault in periodontal tissues by directly destroying bacteria and by augmenting other host defense responses in controlling local concentrations of the microbial population. The complement system appears to be downregulated in patients with periodontal disease. As with all host responses, potential for periodontal tissue injury exists when complement activation occurs.

In addition to complement, other soluble factors that have been elucidated more recently include acute-phase proteins such as α-2 macroglobulin and the C-reactive proteins (CRPs), among several others. The role of CRPs has received much attention of late because of its increased level with increased periodontal disease activity or in the presence of untreated periodontal disease. Increased CRP levels have been proposed to be a risk factor for atherosclerosis, which can lead to cardiovascular and cerebrovascular disease.

## Molecular Components of Inflammation

Histamine is a potent agent that increases vascular permeability, thus permitting inflammatory cells easier access to the affected site. It is released from mast cells and basophils. Serotonin (5-hydroxytryptamine) also increases vascular permeability. Basophils, neutrophils, and macrophages release PAF. PAF increases the release of serotonin from platelets. Neutrophil chemotactic factor (NCF) is released from mast cells and is chemotactic for PMNs.

Chemokines are released from leukocytes. They constitute a large collection of cytokines, which cause mast cell degranulation and chemotaxis of PMNs. (The terminology can be very confusing. All molecules that affect or control the immune or inflammatory responses are referred to as cytokines. Accordingly, all chemokines are cytokines, but there are many other cytokines that are not chemokines.)

Activated compliment C3a causes mast cell degranulation. Activated compliment C5a causes mast cell degranulation, phagocyte chemotaxis, activation of PMNs, and increased capillary permeability (Fig. 4-2).

## COMPLEMENT

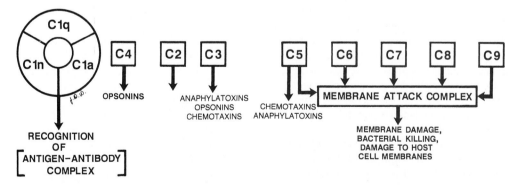

THE ELEVEN PROTEINS OF THE CLASSIC COMPLEMENT SYSTEM ARE INDICATED AT THE TOP OF THE FIGURE.

THE ACTIVATION CASCADE PROCEEDS IN SEQUENCE FROM LEFT TO RIGHT. SOME OF THE BIOLOGIC EFFECTS OF THE ACTIVATION OF VARIOUS COMPONENTS ARE DESIGNATED BY ARROWS.

*Figure 4.2* ●

Bradykinin from the kinin system causes vasodilation and increased vascular permeability. Fibrinopeptides are byproducts of the clotting mechanism, and are chemotactic for PMNs and macrophages.

$PGE_2$ is a product of the cyclooxygenase pathway and causes vasodilation while potentiating vascular permeability caused by histamine and bradykinin.

$LTB_4$ has its origins in the lipoxygenase pathway. It stimulates PMN chemotaxis and is synergistic with $PGE_2$ in increasing vascular permeability.

$LTD_4$, which is also produced through the lipoxygenase pathway, aids in vascular permeability.

NCF is released from basophils.

Selectins are a group of three molecules responsible for assisting with migration of PMNs and macrophages across vessel walls. E selectins and P selectins are specific for PMNs, and L selectins are selective for macrophages. They help slow the cells down before adhesion to the endothelial wall. There are at least 12 other molecules from three different families that perform similar functions, including a group known as intracellular adhesion molecules (ICAMs).

## THE ROLE OF ADAPTIVE IMMUNITY AND RESISTANCE TO THE PROGRESSION OF PERIODONTAL DISEASE

Adaptive (acquired) immunity refers to antigen-specific defense mechanisms that take several days to become protective and are designed to react with and remove a specific antigen. There are two major branches of the adaptive immune responses: humoral immunity and cell-mediated immunity. Humoral immunity involves the production of antibody molecules in response to an antigen and is mediated by B lymphocytes. Cell-mediated immunity involves the production of cytotoxic T lymphocytes, activated macrophages, activated natural killer (NK) cells, and cytokines in response to an antigen and is mediated by T lymphocytes.

Although these designations are still useful, immunologists now tend to characterize the immune system into those components that recognize cell-associated antigens and those that recognize free antigens.

### Cellular Elements of the Immune System

1. *B cells* (B lymphocytes) are produced in the bone marrow in humans and carry surface immunoglobulin (antibody), which reacts to antigens. Some B cells mature into plasma cells.

2. Plasma cells or *antibody-forming cells* (AFCs) are terminally differentiated B cells. They produce antibodies to specific antigens (invaders), and are divided into two groups, B-1 and B-2 cells.
   a. B-1 cells develop early in response to common bacteria.
   b. B-2 cells comprise the majority of all B cells and produce a greater variety of antibodies.

3. Produced in the thymus gland, *T cells* are responsible for the production of cytokines known as lymphokines. These cells play a dual role. First, they are tasked with killing virally infected cells and tumor cells. T cells also play a significant role in the modulation and amplification of the immune response. They are divided into two major subsets based on their cell surface markers, CD4 and CD8.
   a. T helper cells have $CD4^+$ and $CD8^-$ cell surface markers. They are referred to generically as Th0 cells with two subsets, Th1 and Th2. The antigen is presented to them by the appropriate cell listed in the following, and cytokines necessary for continuation of the immune process are released: (1) Th1 cells interact with mononuclear phagocytes such as activated macrophages, and (2) Th2 cells release cytokines that are required for differentiation of B cells into plasma cells.
   b. T cytotoxic cells are $CD8^+$ and are most effective against virally infected cells and tumors.
   c. T suppressor cells (Ts) have no unique cell surface marker. They are capable of increasing or decreasing the immune response in response to appropriate cytokines.
   d. Memory cells are populations of long-lived T cells and B cells that remain after exposure to an antigen. They provide a rapid response if that antigen is encountered in the future.

4. *Killer cells* are mononuclear cells that are capable of killing target cells, such as a tumor cell, sensitized with antibody.

5. *Natural killer (NK) cells* have the same ability as killer cells, except that the target cell need not be sensitized. These cells possess innate surface receptors to identify target cells.

6. *Monocytes* are circulating cells that can migrate into the tissues, becoming macrophages. They have phagocytic capability, produce cytokines, and "present" antigens to B cells and Th1 cells for further processing. The B cells then produce antibody specific for that antigen, and the Th1

# THE PHAGOCYTE (PMN)

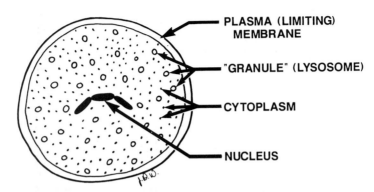

THE "GRANULE" IS ALSO CALLED THE LYSOSOME, ALSO
REFERRED TO AS "SUICIDE PACKETS." THE ENZYMES
THAT DAMAGE BACTERIAL CELL WALLS AND HOST CELL
MEMBRANES ARE CONTAINED IN THE LYSOSOMES. THE
CYTOPLASM CONTAINS THE CYTOSKELETAL ELEMENTS.
WHEN STIMULATED THESE ELEMENTS BECOME
ORGANIZED AND ARE RESPONSIBLE FOR THE CELLULAR
MOVEMENT DURING CHEMOTAXIS.

***Figure 4.3*** ●

cells render the antigen for phagocytosis by macrophages.

7. *PMNs* are cells that phagocytize antigens coated with antibody (Fig. 4-3).

## Cytokines and Other Molecular Components

Cytokines are non-antibody molecules that influence a wide range of activity in the immune and inflammatory systems as well as complement, clotting, bradykinin, and arachidonic acid pathways. The most important cytokines are as follows:

1. *Interleukins* are a diverse group of cytokines. Most are produced by and act on other cells in the immune or inflammatory response and have intertwining biologic activity.
   a. Lymphocytes, fibroblasts, and macrophages produce IL-1. It has the following functions: (1) stimulation of the production of endothelial adhesion molecules such as selectins to begin the inflammatory process; (2) production of prostaglandins by fibroblasts and osteoclasts; (3) activation of phagocytes that makes T-cell surfaces more receptive to antigens; and (4) stimulation of the release of IL-2 by T cells, B cells, and NK cells.
   b. IL-1 stimulates prostaglandin synthesis.
   c. IL-2 enhances T cell and NK cell growth and activation.
   d. IL-4 causes B cells to activate and divide. It promotes immunoglobulin and is also a growth factor for mast cells.
   e. IL-6 is produced by macrophages and CD4+ T cells and stimulates the production of B cells and mast cells.
   f. IL-8 is an important cytokine. It is produced by fibroblasts, endothelial cells, and monocytes and stimulates activation and chemotaxis by macrophages, PMNs, and T cells.
   g. IL-10 is produced by CD4+ T cells and inhibits the production of cytokines by CD8+ T cells.

2. *Interferons* are cytokines usually associated with antiviral activity. Interferon-γ plays an important role in periodontal disease. It is released by the CD4+ T cells and enhances phagocytosis via a number of pathways.

3. *Migration inhibitory factor* (MIF) is produced by activated T cells and prevents the migration of macrophages from an area of inflammation or infection, thereby increasing the population of macrophages in that area.

4. *Tumor necrosis factor* (TNF) aids in the formation of selectins and intracellular adhesion molecules on endothelial walls, thus aiding in migration of leukocytes.

5. *Lymphotoxin* (LT) is produced by activated T cells. It works together with IFN-γ to activate leukocytes.
6. *Transforming growth factor-β* (TGF-β) is a group of cytokines produced by macrophages and platelets. Its primary role appears to be the inhibition of the immune system.
7. *Prostaglandins* and *leukotrienes* were discussed earlier in this chapter.
8. *Matrix metalloproteinases* (MMPs) are a group of enzymes that degrade collagen, the ground substance, and other structures. The nine that have been identified have been classified into four groups based on the substrates on which they act.
9. *Elastase, glucuronidase,* and *hyaluronidase* are lysosomal enzymes produced by the destruction of PMNs and fibroblasts.
10. *Colony-stimulating factors* (CSFs) exist for granulocytes, lymphocytes, and macrophages. They are cytokines derived from T cells that control hematopoiesis.

## Immunoglobulins (Antibodies)

1. IgM is the first antibody on the scene. It initiates the complement cascade and is the main antibody in response to T-cell–independent antigens.

2. IgG is the next antibody to arrive; it remains the longest. Having several subclasses, IgG is also the most predominant antibody. It coats antigens (opsonization) for destruction by phagocytes, prepares other antigens for destruction by killer cells, and also activates the complement cascade.
3. IgA is found in the saliva (secretory IgA) and other areas where there are mucous membranes.
4. IgD is a trace antibody on differentiating B cells. It disappears after differentiation.
5. IgE binds to mast cells and basophils, stimulating the release of vasoactive substances such as histamine, prostaglandins, and leukotrienes (Fig. 4-4).

## Acute Inflammatory Process in Periodontal Disease

Although acute inflammation may result when the host is presented with a bacterial challenge, in some patients the presence of periodontal pathogens does not initiate an acute inflammatory response. The presence of an intact gingival sulcular epithelium and junctional epithelium can serve as a barrier against penetration by the bacterial products and components. However, as bacterial plaque continues to accumulate in the gingival sulcus, the following events may occur:

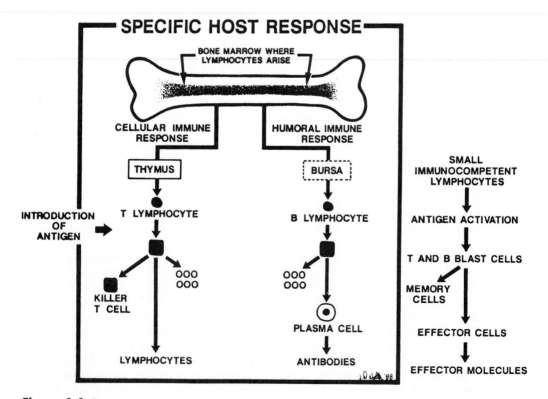

**Figure 4.4** ●

A widening of the spaces results between the cells of the junctional epithelium, which allows for diffusion of bacterial products. This is followed by a migration of a large number of leukocytes as well as Langerhans cells along with other HLA-DR-positive antigen-presenting cells. The vascular supply is increased by vasodilation in the affected area. Mediators such as histamine and $PGE_2$ are responsible for this process. Serotonin, C5a, bradykinin, fibrinopeptides, $PGE_2$, $LTB_4$, and $LTD_4$ cause increased vascular permeability and retraction of the endothelial cells. Selectins and ICAMS slow the PMNs, permitting them to migrate into the connective tissue. Migration and phagocytosis of PMNs are mediated by chemotactic factors such as NCF and chemokines, and C5a, fibrinopeptides, and $LTB_4$ enhance phagocytosis and neutrophil chemotaxis. The principal phagocytic cells involved in the host response to infectious microorganisms are the polymorphonuclear neutrophils and the macrophages. Killing of microorganisms by these cells usually, but not always, occurs after the microorganisms have been taken up or ingested by the cells.

## PHAGOCYTIC SYSTEM

### Non–Oxygen-Dependent Phagocytosis

This consists of a battery of degenerative substances contained in organelles located in the cytoplasm of the phagocytes. These organelles are referred to as granules or lysosomes.

The degenerative activities of enzymes carry out the granular contents and other factors broadly classified as cationic proteins, neutral proteases, acid hydrolases, and other constituents such as lactoferrin.

The usual mode of killing by these enzymes occurs after the bacteria have been ingested. However, during the process of phagocytosis, these enzymes "leak out" of the phagocyte and enter the external environment of the cells. Possibly, this phenomenon is important in the sulcular, or pocket, fluid where bacterial killing, without prior ingestion, could be important to the defense of periodontal tissues. Furthermore, lysosomal enzymes may be important in neutralizing the actions of destructive enzymes and toxins synthesized and released by bacteria—whether or not the enzymes and toxins were first ingested into phagocytic cells.

### Oxygen-Dependent Phagocytosis

This system kills microorganisms inside the cell in an organelle called the phagolysosome. In this system, toxic oxidants and hydrogen peroxide are generated from oxygen radicals and a lysosomal enzyme, myeloperoxidase. The result of formation of these factors is extensive and lethal damage to bacterial cell walls.

The relationship of the PMN to periodontal health and disease has been the subject of numerous studies. When humans or animals have defective neutrophils, as in agranulocytosis or leukocyte adherence deficiency, periodontal disorders are common and severe. Animals depleted of or congenitally lacking PMNs undergo rapid periodontal destruction and tooth exfoliation (or loss). Extensive studies of humans with defects in PMN function have shown these individuals to demonstrate high susceptibility for periodontal tissue destruction. In the 1996 World Workshop in Periodontics, Offenbacker proposed that individuals with normal PMN function would have either gingivitis or periodontal health regardless of the bacterial challenge. Conversely, those with PMN deficiency or malfunction are much more likely to experience attachment loss. Conclusions from these studies indicate that the PMN is essential for the maintenance of periodontal health but can also be responsible for periodontal destruction.

### Destruction of Host Tissues

It is well known that the body is responsible for much of the destruction that occurs during periodontal disease. This destruction can be viewed as an overreaction to a chronic infection. The following substances have the capability of destroying periodontal tissues during the process of defending against invading bacteria and their byproducts:

1. CSFs
2. IFN-$\gamma$
3. IL-1
4. IL-6
5. Lymphotoxin
6. Matrix metalloproteinases
7. $PGE_2$
8. TGF-$\beta$
9. TNF

These will be discussed in greater detail later in this chapter.

### Immune Response in Periodontal Disease

If bacterial plaque is permitted to collect in the gingival sulcus, a lag period of several days occurs, during which there is no detectable antibody. After several days, the body responds to the presence of the bacteria and their byproducts.

Fibroblasts, macrophages, and lymphocytes release IL-1, IL-2, IL-6, and IL-8. Selectins and ICAMs are activated, beginning the process of PMN diapedesis (movement through the vessel wall), migration, and chemotaxis. The process of diapedesis is enhanced, and the PMNs are followed by macrophages. Both are activated and enhanced by cytokines. This produces the initial redness of gingivitis.

Antigens are "presented" to B cells and monocytes with the aid of T helper cells. The latter release cytokines that cause the production of B cells, which produce antibody specific for the antigen. The antigens are opsonized and phagocytized, and, in the process, substances that are harmful to collagen and the ground substance are released. C3a and C5a cause mast cells to release histamine, which increases vasodilation and allows more protective cells to migrate into the area. Eventually, the sulcular epithelium becomes ulcerated, permitting more rapid ingress of the bacterial antigens. At this point, the gingiva is swollen and bleeding, and may be slightly painful.

Cytokines produced by fibroblasts, PMNs, and other host cells are both helpful and harmful in the protective process. The area becomes infiltrated with lymphocytes and finally by plasma cells. If treatment is not provided, or if the host defenses are insufficient, attachment loss will occur both as a result of the bacteria and the body's response to the bacteria.

## Summary

Periodontitis is an infectious disease that is caused primarily by a bacterial challenge; however, the role of the host defense helps determine in a majority the extent of the disease process. Bacteria and host defense mechanisms are in balance in health. In disease, an imbalance exists, in which both the bacteria and the body's attempts to kill the bacteria and heal itself actually contribute to the destruction of periodontal tissue. This imbalance may be a result of bacterial virulence factors, altered host defenses, or external modifying factors such as tobacco smoke.

## REFERENCES

1. Page RC, Schroeder HE. Pathogenesis of inflammatory periodontal disease. A summary of current work. Lab Invest 1976;34:235–249.
2. Payne WA, Page RC, Ogilvie AL, Hall WB. Histopathologic features of the initial and early stages of experimental gingivitis in man. J Periodontal Res 1975;10:51–64.

## CHAPTER 4
## REVIEW QUESTIONS

1. The cell that is considered to be the first cell of the immune system that responds to a bacterial challenge is:
   a. The peripheral mononuclear leukocyte
   b. The macrophage
   c. The basophil
   d. The leukocyte
2. The sole cause of inflammatory periodontal disease is bacterial plaque.
   a. True
   b. False
3. Innate immunity refers to antigen-nonspecific defense mechanisms that a host uses immediately or within several hours after exposure to almost any infectious agent.
   a. True
   b. False
4. Chronic inflammatory periodontal disease can be considered:
   a. An infectious disease process
   b. An inflammatory disease process
   c. An infectious disease process with the presence of inflammation
   d. All the above
   e. None of the above
5. The complement system appears to be down-regulated in patients with periodontal disease.
   a. True
   b. False
6. Adaptive (acquired) immunity refers to antigen-specific defense mechanisms that take several days to become protective and are designed to react with and remove a specific antigen.
   a. True
   b. False
7. Cytokines are non-antibody molecules that influence a wide range of activity in the immune and inflammatory systems.
   a. True
   b. False
8. Interferons are cytokines usually associated with antiviral activity.
   a. True
   b. False
9. Substances that have the capability of destroying periodontal tissues during a process of defending against invading bacteria and their byproducts include:
   a. CSFs
   b. IFN-γ
   c. IL-1
   d. All the above
   e. None of the above
10. The host defense response, while protective in nature, is also responsible for some of the destruction that is seen in periodontal disease.
    a. True
    b. False

# Diagnosis, Prognosis, and Treatment Planning

Jonathan L. Gray

The successful management of periodontal disease depends on the systematic conversion of examination data into a comprehensive, written treatment plan. This is a step-by-step process that requires discipline and attention to detail. The process is as follows. One first evaluates the data gathered during the examination; this must not be restricted to periodontal findings, because other considerations, such as restorative dentistry or endodontics, may be critical elements of the final treatment plan; likewise, the patient's medical history and age may prove consequential. Next, the gathered data are used to arrive at a diagnosis(es)—some patients may have multiple diagnoses. A list of etiologic factors is then compiled for each diagnosis, and evaluated to determine which factors are reversible and which are beyond the control of the clinician and the patient. The prognosis for individual teeth, and the entire dentition, is established using aforementioned information, and finally a treatment plan can be prepared. Failure to follow all these steps in sequence may result in inappropriate or unsuccessful treatment. A major failing of some practitioners is to proceed directly from the examination to the treatment plan, disregarding the critical intermediate steps of the process. This chapter serves as a guide for the gathering of information and discusses its use in the formation of a prognosis and treatment plan.[1]

## DIAGNOSIS

### Periodontal Chart

The practitioner's approach to periodontal diseases will be more productive and less frustrating if information is recorded on a form that serves as a fact-gathering guide, allows brief shorthand notations, and provides space in which to formulate the treatment plan.

The basic means of gathering data that precedes periodontal therapy may be considered as a series of surveys. As these surveys are completed, it is helpful to estimate the comparative influence of each survey area on the patient's condition. The survey areas are:

1. Health survey
2. General dental survey
3. Periodontal survey
4. Occlusal survey
5. Radiographic survey
6. Deposits survey

Virtually all periodontal disease is a very complex interaction between host factors, environmental factors, and bacterial plaque. Every single factor surveyed simply modifies the influence of either the disease agent or the host resistance.

### Health Survey

The health survey includes a medical and a dental history.

#### Medical History

A medical history should be obtained first by a written questionnaire. Once the written questionnaire is completed, it should be reviewed with the patient so that a thorough explanation of any areas of concern may be provided. This is the appropriate time to refer patients for a medical consultation if any condition exists that might affect the progression of the periodontal disease or the management of the patient. A written consultation report from the physician, rather than a telephone report, is essential.

The medical history is vital for three major reasons:

1. To detect oral manifestations of certain systemic conditions. These may include leukemia, diabetes mellitus, hormonal disturbance, and so forth. An alert diagnostician, in addition to ensuring good management for the patient, may detect conditions having important health implications. The interaction between periodontal health and general health is the subject of increasing interest and has potentially far-reaching implications for patients' health. It is discussed in detail in Chapter 4.
2. To ascertain systemic conditions, such as pregnancy, diabetes mellitus, blood dyscrasias, nutritional deficiencies, and hypertensive cardiovascular diseases that may alter the response of the host to the bacterial insult.
3. To determine certain systemic conditions that require modification, of both primary and supportive periodontal therapy. These include allergic conditions, rheumatic fever syndrome, diabetes mellitus, endocrine disorders, cardiovascular diseases and valvular prostheses, drug therapy (endocrine, corticosteroid, anticoagulant), psychological problems, and use of tobacco products. Patients at risk for subacute bacterial endocarditis, or those who have received prosthetic joint replacements, must be premedicated in accordance with the appropriate guidelines.[2,3]

## Dental History

Before the intraoral examination, a complete dental history should be obtained. By obtaining this history, the practitioner is afforded the opportunity to assay the patient's attitude, establish rapport, and learn of past dental disease and response to treatment. It is also important to determine what methods of home care the patient is presently using, and the patient's general dental I.Q.

## General Dental Survey

The overall impression gained by this survey will begin to establish the magnitude of the problem. The following points should be observed and noted:

1. *Soft tissue survey.* This is the oral cancer search. Other lesions must be noted also, but few have consequences as severe, especially if not detected early or if completely overlooked.
2. *Positioning.* Arch alignment, morphologic malocclusion, and migration of teeth.
3. *Caries.* Location, type, and extent.

4. *Restorative dentistry.* Adequacy of restorations and prostheses. These must be viewed in relation to plaque retention, prevention of plaque removal, traumatogenic occlusion, and excessive leverage from torquing forces.
5. *Habits.* Examples include smoking, tongue thrusting, bruxism, and clenching, and factitious disease.
6. *Pulpal status of teeth, especially those with advanced bone loss* (particularly when associated with teeth that have deep restorations or furcation involvement). The relationships between pulpal status and periodontal disease have become increasingly important and may alter treatment planning.
7. *Mobility of teeth.* This is a critical diagnostic and prognostic consideration. Some mobility is normal and may vary during the day, according to diet and stress. Pathologic mobility has several principal causes:
   a. Gingival and periodontal inflammation.
   b. Parafunctional occlusal habits.
   c. Occlusal prematurities.
   d. Loss of supporting bone.
   e. Traumatic torquing forces applied to clasped teeth by removable partial dentures.
   f. Periodontal therapy, endodontic therapy, and trauma may cause transient mobility.

Tooth movement is measured by applying force buccolingually between two dental instrument handles. Mobility is usually graded as 1, 2, or 3 (Fig. 5-1), as follows:

*Grade 1* represents the first distinguishable sign of movement greater than normal.
*Grade 2* is recorded if there is a total movement of about 1 mm.

### GRADES OF MOBILITY

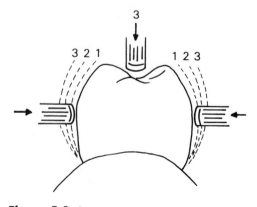

**Figure 5.1** ●

*Grade 3* is recorded if the tooth moves more than 1 mm in any direction or is depressible.

Reduction or control of pathologic tooth mobility may be achieved through removal or modification of the causative factors (see Chapter 6).

## Periodontal Survey

This survey (Fig. 5-2) is a critical part of the diagnostic process. A calibrated periodontal probe, a furcation explorer, a front reflective surface examining mirror, adequate light, palpation, and air

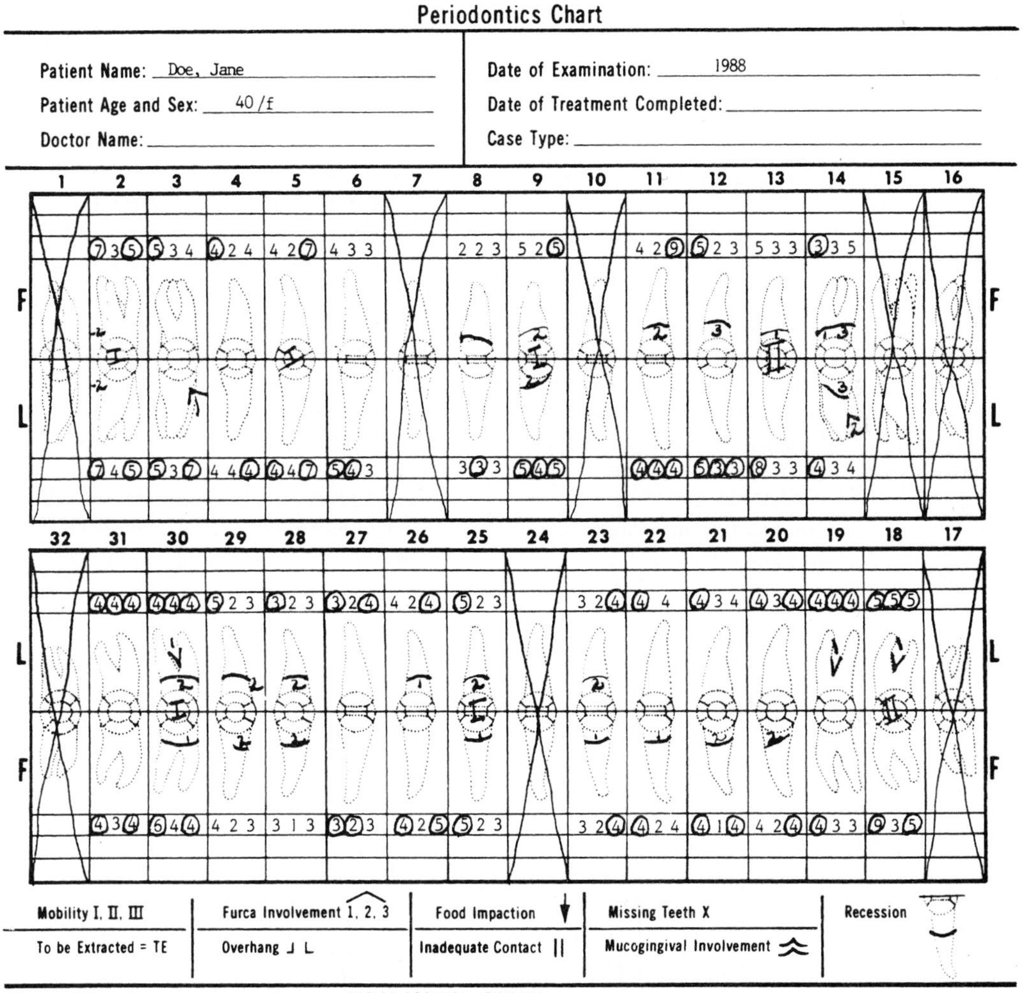

### Periodontics Chart

Patient Name: Doe, Jane  
Patient Age and Sex: 40/f  
Doctor Name: _____

Date of Examination: 1988  
Date of Treatment Completed: _____  
Case Type: _____

| Legend | | | | |
|---|---|---|---|---|
| Mobility I, II, III | Furca Involvement 1, 2, 3 | Food Impaction ↓ | Missing Teeth X | Recession |
| To be Extracted = TE | Overhang ⌐ L | Inadequate Contact \|\| | Mucogingival Involvement ≈ | |

#### INITIAL OCCLUSAL FINDINGS

| | | | | | | | | | | | | | | | | | |
|---|---|---|---|---|---|---|---|---|---|---|---|---|---|---|---|---|---|
| CENTRIC RELATION OCCLUSION | 1 | (2) | 3 | 4 | 5 | 6 | 7 | 8 | 9 | 10 | 11 | 12 | (13) | 14 | 15 | 16 | |
| | 32 | (31) | 30 | 29 | 28 | 27 | 26 | 25 | 24 | 23 | 22 | 21 | (20) | 19 | 18 | 17 | |
| RIGHT LATERAL | 1 | 2 | 3 | 4 | (5) | 6 | 7 | 8 | 9 | 10 | 11 | 12 | (13) | (14) | 15 | 16 | CR = CO |
| | 32 | 31 | 30 | 29 | 28 | 27 | 26 | 25 | 24 | 23 | 22 | 21 | (20) | (19) | 18 | 17 | Hor. Vert. |
| LEFT LATERAL | 1 | (2) | (3) | 4 | 5 | 6 | 7 | 8 | 9 | 10 | (11) | (12) | (13) | 14 | 15 | 16 | |
| | 32 | (31) | (30) | 29 | 28 | 27 | 26 | 25 | 24 | 23 | 22 | 21 | 20 | 19 | 18 | 17 | |
| PROTRUSIVE | 1 | 2 | 3 | 4 | 5 | 6 | 7 | (8) | (9) | 10 | 11 | 12 | 13 | 14 | 15 | 16 | |
| | 32 | 31 | 30 | 29 | 28 | 27 | 26 | (25) | 24 | (23) | 22 | 21 | 20 | 19 | 18 | 17 | |

Occlusal Treatment Plan _____

**Figure 5.2** ●

blast must all be used to supplement visual examination of the periodontal tissues. There are endless variations of periodontal charts for recording the results of the periodontal survey, including electronic and computer-generated forms. Some charts include space for repeat measurements at subsequent appointments; others must be completed in full. Electronic storage and retrieval of charting information is the most efficient means of tracking these data, and in some cases, permits assessment of changes from one appointment to another.

1. *Gingival color, form, and consistency.* These should be observed and recorded.
2. *Bleeding and purulent exudation.* These are clinical indicators of disease activity and should be noted. Exudation may be spontaneous or may be evident only on probing or palpation. Bleeding and suppuration are not necessarily indicators of the severity of the disease, but may signify ulceration of the epithelial wall of the pocket. Bleeding scores have many false positives and false negatives. For example, smokers bleed less than nonsmokers despite the fact that they often have more periodontal disease.

3. *Pocket (probing) depth.* Measurement is taken from the gingival margin on all teeth with the aid of a calibrated probe. The instrument is held as close to the tooth surface as possible and is gently inserted into the sulcus or pocket until resistance is met. Any bleeding or suppuration is noted and recorded. The probe is walked along the tooth surface, keeping it parallel to the long axis of the tooth. Three measurements are recorded on both the facial and lingual surfaces: distal, midfacial/midlingual, and mesial (Fig. 5-3). When there is heavy calculus formation, it is often impossible to measure pocket depth accurately, because calculus will impede the insertion of the probe. It may then be necessary to perform a gross debridement before pocket measurement is taken. The measurements are then recorded.[4]
4. *Relationship of gingival margin to cementoenamel junction (recession).* This information is recorded as a continuous line on a chart. If this step is neglected, pocket measurements are meaningless. A 3-mm pocket, for example, on a tooth with 5 mm of gingival recession would signify greater destruction of the attachment apparatus than a 5-mm pocket on a tooth with hyperplastic gingiva (Fig. 5-4).

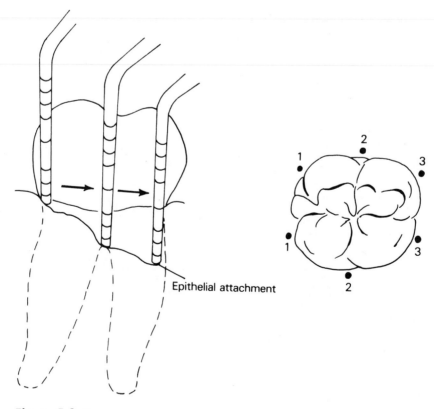

Epithelial attachment

**Figure 5.3** ●

RECESSION HYPERPLASIA

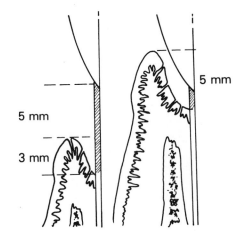

5 mm

5 mm

3 mm

**Figure 5.4** ●

5. *Relationship of cementoenamel junction (CEJ) to the bottom of the pocket (attachment level).* This measurement should be recorded. The location of the base of the pocket in relation to the CEJ affects the prognosis of an individual tooth more than the pocket depth. For example, a tooth with 3-mm probing depth and 5 mm of recession has an attachment level loss of 8 mm, whereas a tooth with a 5-mm probing depth and no recession would have an attachment level loss of only 5 mm. This measurement is especially important when comparing with attachment levels at subsequent visits for reevaluation or maintenance. Attachment level loss may be an indication of disease activity.

6. *General width of keratinized gingiva, relationship of probing depth to mucogingival junction, and influence of various frenal and muscle attachments on the gingival margin.* These should all be observed and recorded.

7. *Pathologic invasion of furcation areas.* Careful probing with a curved furcation probe (e.g., a Nabors furcation probe) will help make this determination. The complicated anatomy of these regions presents diagnostic and therapeutic challenges, but one's ability to determine the extent of furcation invasions will improve with experience. There are several classification systems for furcation invasions. Two of the most common systems are described below:

   a. Glickman classification
      i. Grade I—incipient
      ii. Grade II—cul-de-sac

      iii. Grade III—through-and-through
      iv. Grade IV—same as grade III; however, no gingiva covers the furcation
   b. Nyman classification
      i. Degree 1—≥1/3 the width of the tooth
      ii. Degree 2—≤1/3 the width of the tooth, but not through-and-through
      iii. Degree 3—through-and-through

## Occlusal Survey

Occlusal trauma has been implicated in progression of periodontal destruction, although not without controversy. A thorough examination of the occlusion is an essential component of all periodontal examinations.[5] Please refer to Chapter 6 for a comprehensive discussion of the occlusal analysis.

## Radiographic Survey

Radiographs are indispensable aids in the diagnosis of periodontal disease, but they alone are not diagnostic. Radiographic interpretation should be considered along with clinical data to establish a final, accurate diagnosis. Each diagnostic regimen serves to monitor the accuracy of the other.

There are certain general requirements of a complete radiographic survey:

1. These film series should be included.
   a. Full-mouth periapical series
   b. Four-film periodontal bitewing series
   c. Panoramic radiographs as an adjunct
2. High-quality radiographs. Films should be technically adequate in density, contrast, and angulation, and should include all pertinent anatomic detail.

Radiography will demonstrate the following information (Fig. 5-5 depicts many of the features):

1. Root length and morphology
2. Clinical crown-root ratio
3. Approximate amount of bone destruction
4. Relationship of maxillary sinus to the periodontal deformity
5. Condition of interproximal bony crests; horizontal and vertical resorption. It should be noted that the height of normal interseptal bone is usually parallel and 1 to 2 mm apical to a line connecting the CEJs of adjacent teeth. When these landmarks are not on the same horizontal plane, the resulting angular appearance of a normal alveolar crest may resemble a pathologic infrabony defect. The astute diagnostician must be aware of these CEJ relationships, as well as of the dense appearance of

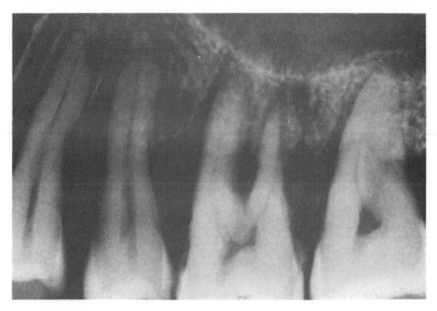

**Figure 5.5** ●

healthy crestal lamina dura, to avoid unnecessary periodontal osseous surgery.

6. Widening of periodontal ligament space on the mesial and distal aspects of the root
7. Advanced furcation involvement
8. Periapical pathosis
9. Calculus
10. Overhanging restoration
11. Root fractures
12. Caries
13. Root resorption

Radiography will not demonstrate the following information (radiographs will not show disease activity, but the effects of the disease):

1. Presence or absence of pockets
2. Exact morphology of bone deformities, especially tortuous defects, dehiscences, and fenestrations
3. Tooth mobility
4. Position and condition of the alveolar process on the facial and lingual surfaces
5. Early furcation involvement
6. Level of connective tissue attachment and the junctional epithelium

## Deposits Survey

A survey of the existing plaque and calculus is extremely important. To determine accurately the prevalence and distribution of plaque, it is necessary, even to the trained eye, to use disclosing solutions. For optimal usefulness in monitoring

therapeutic progress, these accumulations should be measured and recorded repeatedly by using a plaque index. The deposits survey is conducted last because the disclosing media used in this examination mask other important clinical signs, such as changes in gingival coloring. Some clinicians prefer to question patients regarding their current tooth-cleansing procedures at this time rather than during the dental history survey. The timing is unimportant, so long as the information that permits the clinician to correlate technique with effectiveness is obtained.

## DIAGNOSIS

### Classification of Periodontal Diseases

To diagnose periodontal disease, one must have a classification system with which to work. In the past 15 years, several systems for the classification of periodontal disease have been proposed.[6–8] Disagreement over the current periodontal disease classification remains, and without doubt, other classifications will be developed in the future. The situation is very fluid because the very nature of "periodontal diseases" requires further investigation and definition.[9] The classification system presented below is the result of the *1999 International Workshop for a Classification of Periodontal Diseases and Conditions.*[10] The report of this workshop discusses the classification, the characteristics of the diseases and conditions, and the rationale for this particular taxonomy.

1. Gingival disease
   a. Dental plaque-induced gingival disease
      i. Gingival disease modified by systemic factors
      ii. Gingival disease modified by medications
      iii. Gingival disease modified by malnutrition
   b. Non–plaque-induced gingival lesions
      i. Gingival disease of specific bacterial origin
      ii. Gingival diseases of viral origin
      iii. Gingival diseases of fungal origin
      iv. Gingival lesions of genetic origin
      v. Traumatic lesions
      vi. Foreign body reactions
2. Chronic periodontitis
   a. Localized
   b. Generalized
3. Aggressive periodontitis
   a. Localized
   b. Generalized
4. Periodontitis as a manifestation of systemic diseases
   a. Associated with hematologic disorders
      i. Neutropenia
      ii. Leukemias
      iii. Other
   b. Associated with genetic disorders
      i. Familial and cyclic neutropenia
      ii. Down syndrome
      iii. Leukocyte adhesion deficiency syndrome
      iv. Papillon-Lefèvre syndrome
      v. Chediak-Higashi syndrome
      vi. Histiocytosis syndrome
      vii. Glycogen storage disease
      viii. Infantile genetic agranulocytosis
      ix. Cohen syndrome
      x. Ehlers-Danlos syndrome (types IV and VII)
      xi. Hypophosphatasia
      xii. Other
5. Necrotizing periodontal diseases
   a. Necrotizing ulcerative gingivitis
   b. Necrotizing ulcerative periodontitis
6. Abscesses of the periodontium
   a. Gingival abscesses
   b. Periodontal abscesses
   c. Pericoronal abscesses
7. Periodontitis associated with endodontic lesions
   a. Combined periodontic-endodontic lesions
8. Developmental or acquired deformities and conditions
   a. Localized tooth-related factors
      i. Tooth anatomic factors
      ii. Dental restorations or appliances
      iii. Root fractures
      iv. Cervical root resorption and cemental tears
   b. Mucogingival deformities and conditions around teeth
      i. Gingival tissue recession
      ii. Lack of keratinized gingiva
      iii. Decreased vestibular depth
   c. Mucogingival deformities and conditions on edentulous ridges
      i. Vertical or horizontal ridge deficiency
      ii. Lack of gingival or keratinized tissue
      iii. Gingival or soft tissue enlargement
      iv. Aberrant frenum or muscle position
      v. Decreased vestibular depth
      vi. Abnormal color
   d. Occlusal trauma
      i. Primary occlusal trauma
      ii. Secondary occlusal trauma

## Plaque-Induced Gingivitis

Plaque-induced gingivitis is inflammation of the gingiva associated with bacteria. Epidemiologic studies have shown that this is the most common periodontal disease. The inflammation is confined to the gingiva and is characterized by swelling, alterations in color, contour, and bleeding, and increased gingival crevicular fluid. As the condition becomes chronic, the gingiva may become more fibrotic and less edematous. Although there may be increased probing depth resulting from coronal migration of the swollen gingival margin, there is no attachment loss or alveolar bone loss. This form of gingivitis is reversible with improved plaque control or professional care.[10]

## Chronic Periodontitis

The term "chronic periodontitis" is a time-honored phrase that was discarded in 1989 in favor of "adult periodontitis." It has been revived under the 1999 International Classification. In its current form, it is much more clearly defined and applicable to a broader group of patients. "Adult periodontitis" is misleading, as it is age limiting. This disease has been demonstrated in both the primary and secondary dentition, in children, adolescents, and adults, thereby rendering the word "adult" inappropriate. The International Workshop also concluded that the diagnosis "rapidly progressive periodontitis" should be discontinued because the criteria for this disease were imprecise.

Chronic periodontitis is defined as "an infectious disease resulting in inflammation within the supporting tissues of the teeth, progressive attachment, and bone loss. It is characterized by pocket formation and/or gingival recession." It is the most common form of periodontitis and is characterized by the following: association with a wide variety of microbes, subgingival calculus, an amount of destruction consistent with the local factors, and progression that is slow to moderate with the potential for periods of rapid destruction. Both prevalence and age are associated with increased destruction. A wide variety of host and environmental risk factors play a major role in the progression of chronic disease. These will be discussed in detail later in this chapter. The term "refractory periodontitis" was discarded because it was deemed too heterogeneous, and because a variety of therapies had been shown to be effective in some of these patients.[10]

## Aggressive Periodontitis

Aggressive periodontitis is a new classification, combining a group of diseases that had been referred to as "early-onset periodontitis." The fact that rapid destruction of the periodontium can occur at any age, rather than younger than age 35—the arbitrary age ceiling for early-onset periodontitis—makes the phrase "early-onset" unsuitable. Aggressive periodontitis has the following characteristics: the patients are in good health, and there is rapid loss of attachment and alveolar bone. This disease seems to have a familial tendency. Other characteristics that may or may not be present are amounts of bacterial plaque not consistent with the amount of attachment loss, elevated numbers of particular bacteria, particularly *Actinobacillus actinomycetemcomitans* and *Porphyromonas gingivalis,* and defects in phagocytosis. A patient need not have all the above characteristics to be assigned a diagnosis of aggressive periodontitis.

Aggressive periodontitis is subdivided into localized and generalized forms, which have differing presentations. The localized form has a circumpubertal onset, and is localized to the first molars and incisors. There must be interproximal attachment loss on at least two permanent teeth; one of these teeth must be a first molar; no more than two teeth other than first molars and incisors can be involved. There is a strong serum antibody response to the associated bacterial plaque.

Generalized aggressive periodontitis usually, but not always, occurs in patients younger than the age of 30. There are noticeable periods of exacerbation and remission of attachment loss and bone loss. The bone loss must affect at least three teeth other than first molars and incisors, distinguishing it from localized aggressive

periodontitis. The serum antibody response to bacterial plaque is poor.[10]

## Periodontitis Modified by Systemic Factors

Systemic factors that modify periodontitis, and qualify for the diagnosis "periodontitis modified by systemic factors," are listed above. It is interesting to note the absence of diabetes mellitus. Although discussed at length in the review paper written for the workshop group who dealt with this diagnosis, diabetes was not included in the final taxonomy, nor was there any explanation for its exclusion.[10]

## Necrotizing Periodontal Diseases

The 1999 Workshop classification combined "necrotizing ulcerative gingivitis (NUG)" and "necrotizing ulcerative periodontitis (NUP)" as "necrotizing periodontal disease." NUG is defined as "an infection characterized by gingival necrosis, presenting as 'punched-out' papillae, with gingival bleeding and pain."[10] There may also be a characteristic halitosis called "fetid" and formation of a grayish pseudomembrane over the surface of the involved areas. NUG is associated with spirochetes and *Prevotella intermedia,* and is believed to be caused by factors that alter host resistance such as smoking, stress, inadequate diet, inadequate sleep, and HIV.

NUP shares the clinical characteristics of NUG, but the infection involves the alveolar bone and periodontal ligament in addition to the gingiva. It is found in individuals with severe malnutrition, HIV, and other forms of immunosuppression.[10]

## Abscesses of the Periodontium

Gingival abscesses are a localized collection of pus surrounded by inflamed and necrotic tissue that is confined to the gingiva. Periodontal abscesses involve the alveolar bone and periodontal ligament. Pericoronal abscesses occur within the tissue surrounding an incompletely erupted tooth.[10]

## Periodontic-Endodontic Lesions

In the past, there have been several complex classification systems for periodontic-endodontic lesions based on the origin of the initial infection, either the pulp or the periodontium. The 1999 International Workshop simplified the classification, recommending only a single category, the "Periodontic-Endodontic Lesion," that did not take into consideration the origin of the initial lesion.[10]

## Tooth-Related Issues

The "tooth-related issues" listed above either enhance the retention and propagation of bacterial plaque or help the bacteria gain entry to the periodontium. Some of these issues result in localized breakdown in a periodontium that is otherwise healthy. This phenomenon can be an important diagnostic aid.[10]

## Mucogingival Deformities

A "mucogingival deformity" is defined as "a departure from the normal dimension and morphology of and/or interrelationship between the gingiva and alveolar mucosa."[10] These deformities are often coupled with a similar defect in the underlying alveolar bone.[10]

## Occlusal Trauma

"Occlusal trauma is an injury resulting in tissue changes within the attachment apparatus as a result of occlusal force(s)."[10] There are two types of occlusal trauma, primary and secondary. Primary occlusal trauma is the result of excessive occlusal force on a tooth with normal bone levels and attachment levels. Secondary occlusal trauma results from normal or excessive occlusal force on a tooth with a reduced periodontium. There was insufficient evidence of proper quality to include the term "combined occlusal trauma."[10] Advocates of that concept should be aware that the lack of evidence does not mean that the theory is invalid; it simply means that scientific evidence that meets current standards does not exist (see Chapter 6).[10]

## PROGNOSIS

Prognosis is a forecast of the probable response to treatment and the long-term outlook for maintaining a functional dentition. Hopeless cases generally present few problems in establishing an accurate prognosis. Likewise, cases of simple gingivitis, which can be expected to respond favorably when local and systemic factors can be controlled, present few problems in defining a prognosis. In borderline cases, however, the forecasting process becomes challenging.

Problems are compounded when the prognosis concerns strategic, severely involved individual teeth on which a large and complex restorative treatment plan often depends. This situation places a heavy burden of responsibility on the diagnostician under any circumstance. No formula can be established for such situations. Rules of proportional

bone loss (such as one-third or one-half of the supporting bone) have been expressed in the literature as condemning a tooth for extraction. In practice, such rules are of little value. If adhered to rigidly, such rules may lead to the sacrifice of teeth that might have been retained in health. The difficulty with any formula or rule is that there are many exceptions. The best way of meeting the problem is to establish certain basic principles, criteria of judgment, and probable behavior patterns of doubtful teeth under the conditions in which they must function.

Researchers have identified several risk factors for periodontal diseases. Some of these risk factors can be modified, thus improving the prognosis, although others cannot, making the prognosis less certain.[11] Below is a list of the most common risk factors:

1. Risk factors that can be modified
   a. Bacterial plaque
   b. Smoking
   c. Diabetes mellitus and some other systemic conditions
   d. Faulty dentistry
   e. Stress
2. Risk factors that cannot be modified
   a. Age
   b. Male gender
   c. History of prior periodontal disease and initial mean bone level
   d. Hereditary factors
   e. Some systemic conditions

The ability of the therapist or the patient to correct risk factors is critical to a successful outcome in periodontal therapy. Bacterial plaque and smoking (cigarettes, pipes, or cigars) are the most critical risk factors. Control of both is essential to a favorable prognosis. Risk factors that can be modified should become part of the treatment plan.

Research has shown that our ability to predict the outcome of periodontal therapy is flawed. In study, only a prognosis of "good" was consistently accurate. Prognoses of "fair," "poor," and "hopeless" were often erroneous.[12] Increased probing depth, more severe furcation involvement, greater mobility, unsatisfactory crown-to-root ratio, malpositioned teeth, and teeth used as fixed abutments are factors that were associated with a decreasing prognosis.[13]

## Overall Prognosis

There are two aspects of prognosis, the overall prognosis and the prognosis of individual teeth. Overall prognosis deals with the dentition as a whole and is the basic determinant of the extent of dental treatment to be provided. It includes consideration of the following factors:

1. *Oral hygiene.* The success of periodontal treatment depends primarily on effective daily plaque control. Without patient cooperation and deep personal commitment and involvement in personal therapy, the prognosis is poor. This fact holds true no matter how skilled the managing practitioner.
2. *Smoking.* Smoking has been identified as a major risk factor for periodontal destruction. The mechanisms by which it affects the periodontium are still unclear, but every effort should be made to encourage patients to cease smoking. Those who are successful have an improved prognosis for periodontal therapy.
3. *Maintenance availability.* It is increasingly evident that overall, long-term prognosis is dependent on the patient's availability and motivation to seek frequent maintenance recall visits, preferably at 3-month intervals. Patients who are unable to participate in a regular maintenance program, for whatever reason, are poor risks for periodontal therapy.
4. *Preexisting periodontal disease.* A history of prior periodontal disease and a reduced level result in a poorer prognosis for most patients.
5. *Systemic background.* The patient's systemic background affects the overall prognosis in several ways. When extensive periodontal destruction cannot be attributed to local factors, it is reasonable to assume a contributing systemic influence. The detection of systemic factors and the resolution of systemic factors may be extremely difficult. For these reasons, the prognosis in such patients is often poor. However, if patients have known systemic disorders that could affect the periodontium (e.g., use of tobacco, diabetes, nutritional deficiency, hyperthyroidism, and hyperparathyroidism), the prognosis improves on correction of the disorder. If periodontal surgery is contraindicated because of the patient's health, the prognosis is uncertain. Incapacitating conditions that prevent adequate plaque control by the patient (such as Parkinson's disease) adversely affect the prognosis.
6. *Genetic factors.* Genetic factors, such as the overproduction of interleukin 1-β, result in a poorer prognosis. As yet, there is no method to alter genetic factors.
7. *Male gender.* This is associated with greater periodontal destruction, and a poorer prognosis. However, this may be attributable to the fact that men seek care less often than women.

8. *Age of patient.* Generally, the younger the patient, the poorer the prognosis. Given two patients with periodontal involvement of the same degree, it is logical to assume that the younger has far less resistance, because equal damage occurred in a shorter period. It follows that in a patient with weak resistance, healing and repair may also be impaired.
9. *Stress and coping.* Some types of emotional stress and inappropriate coping mechanisms have been associated with periodontal diseases. However, the nature and extent of the relationship is still unclear.
10. *Number of remaining teeth.* If the number and the distribution of remaining teeth are inadequate to support a satisfactory prosthesis, the overall prognosis is poor. Periodontal injury from extensive fixed or removable prostheses constructed on an insufficient number of natural teeth may hasten bone loss. Inability to establish a satisfactory functional environment for remaining natural teeth diminishes the likelihood of maintaining periodontal health.
11. *Malocclusion.* Irregular alignment of the teeth, malformation of teeth and jaws, and disturbed occlusal relationships may be important *factors* in the etiology and the progression of periodontal disease. Correction by orthodontic or prosthodontic means is often essential if periodontal treatment is to succeed. The overall prognosis is poor when relevant occlusal deformities are not amenable to correction.
12. *Tooth morphology.* The prognosis is poor in patients whose teeth have short, tapered roots and relatively large crowns. The disproportionate crown-root ratio and the reduced root surface available for periodontal support render the periodontium more susceptible to injury by occlusal forces, and any loss of attachment apparatus has a more significant effect.

## Prognosis of Individual Teeth

The following factors should be considered:

1. *Mobility.* Tooth mobility is caused by one or more of the following factors:
   a. Gingival and periodontal inflammation
   b. Parafunctional habits
   c. Occlusal prematurities
   d. Torquing forces
   e. Loss of supporting bone

   Mobility is usually correctable, unless it results solely from loss of the attachment apparatus; this is not likely to be corrected. The likelihood of restoring tooth stability is inversely related, then, to the extent to which it is caused by loss of the attachment apparatus.

2. *Teeth adjacent to edentulous areas.* Abutment teeth are subjected to increased functional demands. Standards that are more rigid are required in evaluating the prognosis of teeth in such locations.

3. *Location of remaining bone in relation to individual root surfaces.* When extensive bone loss has occurred on only one root surface, the center of rotation of that tooth is more coronal than if all root surfaces were extensively involved (Fig. 5-6). Thus, leverage on the periodontium is more favorably tolerated than would be expected given the extensive bone loss on the one root surface.

4. *Relation to adjacent teeth.* When a tooth has a questionable prognosis, the chances of successful treatment should be weighed against the effects on adjacent teeth if that tooth were extracted. Unsuccessful attempts at treatment frequently jeopardize adjacent teeth. Strategic extraction is often followed by partial restoration of bone, improving support of adjacent teeth (Fig. 5-7; with permission from Dr. Ronald L. Van Swoll). This result is enhanced if the adjacent teeth are scaled and root planed at the time of the extraction.

5. *Attachment level.* The location of the base of the pocket in relation to the CEJ affects the prognosis of an individual tooth more than the pocket depth. For example, a tooth with minimal pocket depth and extensive recession can present a poorer prognosis than a tooth with a deeper pocket and no recession and less bone loss. Additionally, proximity of pockets to frenal attachments and to the mucogingival junction may jeopardize the prognosis unless corrective procedures are included in the treatment plan. When the periodontal pocket has extended to involve the apex, the prognosis is generally poor.

6. *Infrabony pockets.* The likelihood of eliminating infrabony pockets and their associated osseous defects is influenced by the number of remaining bony walls.

7. *Furcation involvement.* Bifurcation or trifurcation involvement does not always indicate a hopeless prognosis. Added support gives multirooted teeth an advantage over single-rooted teeth with comparable bone loss. Several factors

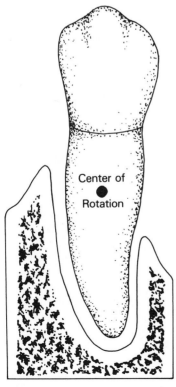
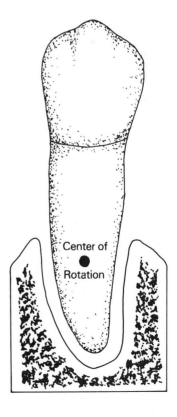

*Figure 5.6* ●

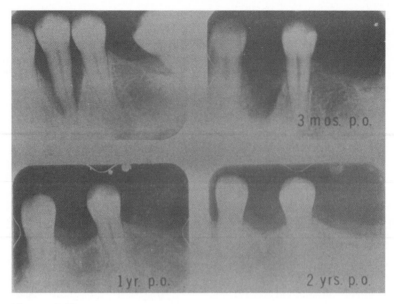

3 mos. p.o.

1 yr. p.o.                    2 yrs. p.o.

*Figure 5.7* ●

influence the prognosis of teeth with attachment loss involving the furcation.
a. Extent of furcation involvement (see Chapter 18).
b. Access to the furca for surgical management. A narrow interradicular space offers a poor prognosis for new attachment procedures or root resection because of the close proximity of the adjacent roots. It also compromises the plaque control efforts of the patient. Generally, the more divergent the roots, the better the prognosis. For example, mandibular second molars have a poorer prognosis than mandibular first molars because their roots are shorter and the interradicular space is more constricted.
c. Access to the furca for plaque control. Generally, mandibular molars with furcation involvement have a better prognosis than maxillary molars with furcation involvement, because patients have better access to the furcas of the mandibular molars. Maxillary premolars with furcation involvement are poor candidates for therapy because of ˙root morphology and poor access for plaque control before and after therapy.
8. *Caries, nonvital teeth, and root resorption.* In teeth mutilated by extensive caries, the feasibility of adequate restoration and endodontic therapy influences periodontal treatment. Extensive idiopathic root resorption jeopardizes tooth stability and adversely affects the response to periodontal treatment. The periodontal

prognosis is not significantly affected in endodontically treated teeth.
9. *Developmental defects.* Developmental defects, such as the palatogingival groove observed on incisor teeth and molars, present a poor prognosis for successful management. Root concavities observed in some teeth, particularly the maxillary first premolar, complicate the prognosis for surgical success as well as for maintenance after surgery.
10. *Faulty dentistry.* Factors such as overhanging margins or poorly contoured crowns are responsible for the accumulation of dental plaque. This may result in periodontal disease in susceptible patients.

## TREATMENT PLANNING

After the diagnosis and prognosis are established, treatment is planned. The treatment plan is the road map for case management. It includes all procedures required for the establishment and maintenance of oral health.

Periodontal treatment requires long-range planning. The value of periodontal treatment to the patient is measured in years of healthful service of the entire dentition, not by the number of teeth retained at the time of treatment. The treatment plan, therefore, is concerned with the entire dentition as well as with the individual teeth. Its principal purpose is to provide a healthy foundation for the future rather than simply to salvage those teeth that were affected in the past. It is directed toward establishing and maintaining an atmosphere of health of the periodontium throughout the mouth, not solely toward spectacular efforts to "tighten" loose teeth.

The welfare of the overall dentition should not be jeopardized by heroic attempts to retain questionable teeth. The clinician should be concerned with practicing periodontics, not "herodontics." The clinician is primarily interested in teeth that can be retained with maximal longevity. Such teeth provide the basis for a constructive total treatment plan. A treatment plan should be developed to achieve these objectives:

1. Patient education directed at the patient's specific problem(s), with emphasis on the need to quit smoking, if appropriate, and the importance of lifelong maintenance.
2. Reduction or removal of all etiologic and risk factors that can be removed.
3. Reestablishment of periodontal health, whether by nonsurgical or surgical therapy.
4. Maintenance of periodontal health through adequate plaque control by the patient and regular visits to the dentist.

If the clinician can successfully attain these objectives, most cases of periodontal disease can be arrested on a long-term basis.

## Order of Treatment

The detailed treatment plan must be based on the patient's dental and medical histories, emotional status, clinical and radiographic examinations, and the other factors that have been mentioned. Treatment plans, therefore, have many variations, but, in general, may consist of four phases: bacterial plaque control, surgical therapy, restorative treatment, and maintenance.

### Bacterial Control

This phase has also been called "initial preparation" or "phase 1 therapy" and usually includes these steps:

1. *Premedication.* Attention must be given to the need for premedication for subacute bacterial endocarditis, heart disease, hypertension, and other systemic conditions, as well as preoperative sedation, when indicated.
2. *Emergency care.* Immediate treatment of periodontal abscesses, necrotizing ulcerative gingivitis (NUG), large carious lesions, tooth pain, and so forth.
3. *Patient instruction and motivation.* The patient learns personal, bacterial plaque control

procedures. *Success depends primarily on the patient's willingness to participate as a serious co-therapist.*

4. *Extraction of teeth.* Teeth with a hopeless prognosis and those whose removal will improve prognosis of adjacent teeth are extracted.
5. *Scaling and root planing.* These should be performed to remove calculus and contaminated cementum. This enables the patient to begin a program of personal plaque control as early as possible.
6. *Antibiotics.* Antibiotics are recommended only after mechanical therapy and improved home care have been completed. If, at 1 to 3 months after these treatments, the condition has not improved, or has worsened, systemic or local antimicrobials can be used.[14] It may be necessary to repeat drug therapy at intervals of about 3 months or more. There is no consensus regarding the value or sequencing of microbial culturing.
7. *Removal of overhanging restorations and other plaque-retentive areas.*
8. *Minor tooth movement.*
9. *Temporary stabilization.* This may be required to facilitate overall treatment or to aid in determining the prognosis of certain teeth.
10. *Preliminary occlusal adjustment and odontoplasty* (if indicated). Obvious gross occlusal abnormalities (plunger cusps, initial prematurities, defective marginal ridges) should be evaluated early in treatment and corrected, if necessary.
11. *Evaluation of results.* Elimination of etiologic factors may produce sufficient improvement to permit modification of the original treatment plan. In this sense, the infection control phase may actually be complete and satisfactory therapy. The patient's attitude toward plaque control responsibility is also evaluated. Additional instruction may be required, even though the patient is making a sincere effort to practice recommended techniques. On the other hand, a patient's failure to cooperate in this critical area should prompt the clinician to modify, limit, or terminate the course of treatment at this point.

### Surgical Therapy (Phase 2 Therapy)

This phase of treatment includes procedures designed to gain access to the root surface for debridement, reduce or eliminate the pocket by resection, the relocation of the gingival margin, or the use of regenerative procedures. This phase may also include surgical procedures for the correction of mucogingival defects.

## Restorative Treatment (Phase 3 Therapy)

The restorative phase usually involves definitive occlusal adjustment, operative dentistry, replacement of missing teeth by fixed or removable prostheses, and permanent splinting, when indicated.

## Maintenance (Phase 4 Therapy)

Patients are carried in the maintenance phase for a lifetime. Most patients who have been treated for moderate to advanced periodontitis require maintenance at least every 3 months. The length of time between recall appointments is dictated by the level of disease control accomplished by patients during the interval between recall visits. This phase of therapy is often downgraded by both the patient and the practitioner, yet it spells the difference between long-term success and failure (see Chapter 23).

## REFERENCES

1. American Academy of Periodontology Position Paper. Diagnosis of periodontal diseases. J Periodontol 2003;74:1237–1247.
2. Dajani AS, Taubert KA, Wilson W, Bolger AF, Bayer A, Ferrieri P, Gewitz MH, Shulman ST, Nouri S, Newburger JW, Hutto C, Pallasch TJ, Gage TW, Levison ME, Peter G, Zuccaro G Jr. Prevention of bacterial endocarditis: recommendations by the American Heart Association. J Am Dent Assoc 1997;128:1142–1151.
3. American Dental Association; American Academy of Orthopedic Surgeons. Antibiotic prophylaxis for dental patients with total joint replacements. J Am Dent Assoc 2003;134:895–899.
4. Listgarten M. Periodontal probing: what does it mean? J Clin Periodontol 1980;7:165. Proceedings of the World Workshop in Clinical Periodontics; July 23–27, 1989, Princeton, NJ.
5. Parameter on occlusal traumatism in patients with chronic periodontitis. American Academy of Periodontology. J Periodontol 2000;71:873–875.
6. Ferris RT, Listgarten MA, Caton JG, Armitage GC, Burmeister JA, Jeffcoat M. Koch RW, Kornman KS, Lamster IB, Lang NP, Loughlin DM, Newman MG, Page RC, Robertson PB, Sugarman MM, Suzuki JB, van Dyke TE. Consensus report. Discussion section. In: Proceedings of the World Workshop in Clinical Periodontics. Princeton: American Academy of Periodontology, 1989;23–32.
7. Attström R, van der Velden U. Consensus report of session 1. In: Lang NP, Karring T, eds. Proceedings of the 1st European Workshop on Periodontology. London: Quintessence, 1994;120–126.
8. Armitage GC. Development of a classification system for periodontal diseases and conditions. Ann Periodontol 1999;4:1–6.
9. Baelum V, Lopez R. Defining and classifying periodontitis: need for a paradigm shift? Eur J Oral Sci 2003;111:2–6.
10. International Workshop for Classification of Periodontal Diseases and Conditions. Ann Periodontol 1999;4:1–112.
11. Fardal O, Johannessen AC, Linden GJ. Tooth loss during maintenance following periodontal treatment in a periodontal practice in Norway. J Clin Periodontol 2004;31:550–555.
12. McGuire MK. Prognosis versus actual outcome: a long-term survey of 100 treated periodontal patients under maintenance care. J Periodontol 1991;62:51–58.
13. McGuire MK, Nunn ME. Prognosis versus actual outcome. II. The effectiveness of clinical parameters in developing an accurate prognosis. J Periodontol 1996;67:658–665.
14. American Academy of Periodontology Position Paper. Systemic antibiotics in periodontics. J Periodontol 2004;75:1553–1565.

## CHAPTER 5
## REVIEW QUESTIONS

1. Which of the following statements is true?
   a. Treatment planning is a systematic stepwise process.
   b. Treatment such as operative dentistry or exodontia is not included in a periodontal treatment plan.
   c. Medical and dental history are inconsequential in a treatment plan.
   d. Treatment planning is done before data gathering.

2. The dental history should be obtained before the intraoral examination.
   a. True
   b. False

3. _____ is not usually considered a grade of mobility.
   a. 1
   b. 2
   c. 3
   d. 4

4. Smokers gingiva bleeds more than nonsmokers.
   a. True
   b. False

5. Measurement of the location of the _____ is necessary to determine attachment loss.
   a. Mucogingival junction
   b. Cementoenamel pearls

c. Cementoenamel junction
d. Incisal edge

6. Which probe is best for probing furcations?
   a. A UNC probe
   b. A Nabors probe
   c. A PSR probe
   d. A Michigan probe

7. The Glickman furcation classification consists of degrees 1–3.
   a. True
   b. False

8. Radiographs show current disease activity.
   a. True
   b. False

9. Abscesses of the periodontium include all of the following except:
   a. Necrotizing ulcerative gingivitis
   b. Gingival abscesses
   c. Periodontal abscesses
   d. Pericoronal abscesses

10. Periodontal trauma consists of each of the following except:
   a. Primary
   b. Secondary
   c. Tertiary

# Occlusion as a Risk Factor for Periodontal Disease

William Hallmon, Stephen Harrel

Occlusion and its effect on the periodontal supporting tissues of the teeth has generated considerable interest and debate through the years. The controversy surrounding this relationship is centered around the difficulty of correlating scientific studies of the effect of occlusion with the perceived negative effect of occlusion that many observe clinically. In the simplest context, one may consider excessive occlusal force(s) as a risk factor for periodontal destruction and its subsequent progress. It has consistently been reported that occlusal trauma alone does not initiate periodontal pocket formation.[1,2] Periodontal disease has been consistently demonstrated to be causally associated with the accumulation and persistence of bacterial plaque.[3] Therefore, it would seem reasonable to conclude that by effectively controlling plaque, the chances of the genesis and progression of disease(s) of the periodontium would be minimized. However, like numerous other chronic inflammatory and degenerative conditions, periodontal destruction is a complex interaction of the initiating agent (i.e., plaque) and multiple host-related risk factors.[4] Occlusal trauma, resulting from excessive forces(s), can be viewed as one of the risk factors that may influence the progression of the periodontal destructive process.

## Definitions

In an attempt to clarify the role of occlusion and its effect on the periodontium, the following terms as defined by the 1999 International Workshop for Classification of Periodontal Diseases and Conditions will be reviewed.[5] Occlusal trauma is defined as an injury within the attachment apparatus of the dentition that results when excessive occlusal force(s) exceeds the adaptive capability of the affected tissues. Two types of occlusal trauma are described, primary and secondary. Primary occlusal trauma refers to injury resulting in (periodontal) tissue changes from excessive occlusal forces applied to a tooth or teeth with normal support. It occurs in the presence of (1) normal bone levels, (2) normal attachment levels, and (3) excessive occlusal force(s). Secondary occlusal trauma describes injury resulting in tissue changes (to the periodontium) from normal or excessive occlusal forces that are applied to a tooth or teeth with reduced support. This condition occurs in the presence of (1) bone loss, (2) attachment loss, and (3) "normal" or excessive occlusal forces (assumes average tooth and root anatomy). The basic injury to the periodontium is the same in both instances; it is only the circumstances surrounding its occurrence that are different (Figs. 6-1 and 6-2).

## Studies Evaluating the Effect of Occlusion on the Periodontium

Our current understanding of the effects of occlusion on the supporting tissues of the periodontium is largely based on animal investigations and human studies.[6–8] Early human data were derived primarily from human necropsy materials and retrospective analysis.[8] More recently, human clinical studies have attempted to assess associations of occlusal effects on the periodontium by site-specific examination of comparative changes in periodontally diseased and healthy dentitions presenting with and without occlusal disharmonies, and treatment with and without occlusal therapy.[9,10] Because of the necessity of following diagnosed but untreated periodontal disease, prospective

Primary Occlusal Traumatism

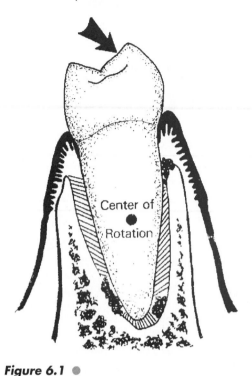

**Figure 6.1** ●

Secondary Occlusal Traumatism

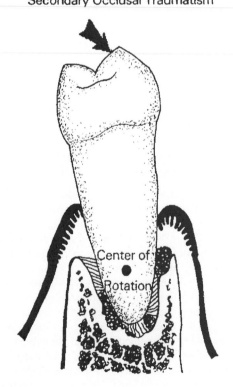

**Figure 6.2** ●

randomized clinical trials of the diverse occlusal variables are deemed unethical. Animal studies have been used to histologically investigate occlusion-related effects and outcomes on the affected periodontium. Extensive animal studies have been conducted using beagle dog and squirrel monkey models using different occlusal force applications.[6,7] These studies have consistently shown that occlusal trauma can cause extensive changes in the bone but does not cause the loss of attachment without the presence of plaque. Although informative, one must be cautious in applying the outcomes of these studies directly to human beings.

Earlier human observations and interpretations by Glickman and associates led to the proposal that excess occlusal force(s) could influence the progression of periodontal destruction in the presence of a superimposed inflammatory lesion affecting the coronal soft tissues of the periodontium.[11] These authors felt that when the plaque-associated inflammatory lesion affecting the soft tissues coronal to the transseptal or dentogingival fibers (zone of irritation), combined with occlusally mediated injury of the supporting tissues apical to the transseptal or dentogingival fibers (zone of codestruction), the affected periodontium was at greater risk for progressive and more advanced periodontal destruction. Although frequently referenced, this hypothesis remains unproven.

More recent human clinical investigations seem to indicate that there is a relationship between occlusal trauma and periodontal disease. In a controlled study by Burgett et al.,[12] it was shown that patients who had their occlusion adjusted responded statistically better to surgical therapy than a similar group of patients that did not have their occlusion adjusted. In addition, retrospective studies by Harrel and Nunn[9,10] have shown that sites (individual teeth) that were undergoing occlusal trauma had a greater increase in pocket probing depths with time than did the sites that did not have occlusal trauma. These same studies also showed that when occlusal adjustments were performed, the increase in pocket probing depths was less than those teeth that had occlusal trauma and did not receive an occlusal adjustment.

At this time, it appears that occlusal trauma is a significant risk factor for the progression of periodontal disease but that occlusal trauma alone does not act as a causative agent for the initiation of periodontal disease. In the clinical treatment of patients, it is imperative that the buildup of plaque be addressed as the primary cause of periodontal disease. However, given the fact that most patients rarely achieve a consistent level of ideal plaque control, the control of other risk factors for progressive periodontal destruction is also an important consideration in the treatment of periodontal disease. In this light, in the patient with established periodontal disease, the control of occlusal trauma should be a routine part of periodontal treatment.[13]

## CLINICAL AND RADIOGRAPHIC INDICATORS OF OCCLUSAL TRAUMA

Because occlusal trauma is defined by histologic injury to the supporting periodontium, the clinician is dependent on identifying clinical and radiographic modifiers (or indicators) that have been associated with the presence of this injury.[5] These clinical and radiographic indicators of occlusal trauma will assist the clinician in diagnosing occlusal trauma during the course of the clinical examination or evaluation. Clinical indicators of occlusal trauma may include fremitus (mobility of the tooth in function), progressive tooth mobility, occlusal prematurities, tooth migration, dull ache, fractured or cracked teeth, sensitivity to thermal change, and wear facets or unusual wear patterns. Radiographic indicators of occlusal trauma may include bone loss, root resorption, widened periodontal ligament (PDL) space(s), alterations in the lamina dura, and hypercementosis. Presence and recognition of these indicators will help the clinician to diagnose and effectively treat occlusal trauma during the course of comprehensive patient management.

## CLINICAL EVALUATION OF THE OCCLUSION

Excessive occlusal forces and occlusal trauma may occur in two ways. If the teeth do not contact equally during routine closure of the mouth or during side to side movements of the mandible, the teeth that contact first (often called a premature contact[14]) will receive more stress than the teeth that contact after the teeth slide to a position of maximum contact. This can be termed occlusal trauma during functional occlusion. A second form of occlusal trauma occurs when patients grind or clench their teeth. This type of movement is termed parafunctional movement[14] or movement "outside" of normal function. Both of these types of occlusal trauma have been shown to be detrimental to periodontal health, and both

types may exist in the same patient. Occlusal trauma, regardless of type, should be addressed during the treatment of the patient with periodontal disease.

## OCCLUSAL TRAUMA DURING FUNCTIONAL MOVEMENTS

To determine whether a patient has a tooth (or teeth) that contact before the rest of their teeth, it is necessary to perform an examination of the occlusal contacts. This can be done in several ways, and the following steps are provided as an acceptable approach to occlusal examination.

Step one in evaluating the patient's occlusion consists of manipulating the mandible into a relaxed or neutral position. This is accomplished by using two hands to exert moderate posterior and upward pressure against the mandible. This procedure is accompanied by gentle controlled up and down movement of the mandible by the operator (Fig. 6-3). The goal of this maneuver is to position the head of the mandibular condyle into the depression of the glenoid fossa.

It needs to be emphasized that only controlled gentle pressure should be used during this procedure. There is some controversy concerning the amount of pressure to be used during this maneuver and what is the ideal location of the mandibular head in the glenoid fossa. The clinician, with experience, will develop a "feel" for when the correct position is obtained. Once the condyles are seated in the fossa, often called centric relation,[14] patients are asked to slowly close until they feel initial contact of their teeth. This point of contact is recorded in the examination chart as the "initial contact in centric relation or CR" (Fig. 6-4). Patients are then requested to carefully continue to close until maximum contact of the teeth is obtained. This position of maximum contact is often called centric occlusion or CO.[14] During the movement from the first contact in centric relation to the maximum

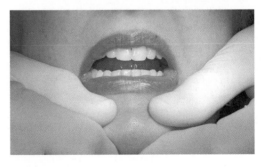

***Figure 6.3*** •

| Centric Prem aturies (CR:CO) | 1 | 2 | 3 | 4 | 5 | 6 | 7 | 8 | 9 | 10 | 11 | 12 | 13 | 14 | 15 | 16 |
|---|---|---|---|---|---|---|---|---|---|---|---|---|---|---|---|---|
| | 32 | 31 | 30 | 29 | 28 | 27 | 26 | 25 | 24 | 23 | 22 | 21 | 20 | 19 | 18 | 17 |
| Right Lateral Excursion (RLE) | 1 | 2 | 3 | 4 | 5 | 6 | 7 | 8 | 9 | 10 | 11 | 12 | 13 | 14 | 15 | 16 |
| | 32 | 31 | 30 | 29 | 28 | 27 | 26 | 25 | 24 | 23 | 22 | 21 | 20 | 19 | 18 | 17 |
| Left Lateral Excursion (LRE) | 1 | 2 | 3 | 4 | 5 | 6 | 7 | 8 | 9 | 10 | 11 | 12 | 13 | 14 | 15 | 16 |
| | 32 | 31 | 30 | 29 | 28 | 27 | 26 | 25 | 24 | 23 | 22 | 21 | 20 | 19 | 18 | 17 |
| Protrusive | 1 | 2 | 3 | 4 | 5 | 6 | 7 | 8 | 9 | 10 | 11 | 12 | 13 | 14 | 15 | 16 |
| | 32 | 31 | 30 | 29 | 28 | 27 | 26 | 25 | 24 | 23 | 22 | 21 | 20 | 19 | 18 | 17 |

**Figure 6.4** ●

contact in centric occlusion, the amount of movement at the cuspid is recorded (in millimeters) in the occlusal examination chart. The distance of this movement is often termed the CR – CO shift.

$$CR - CO\ shift = 2\ mm$$

## Comments

Step two in evaluating the patient's occlusion is to determine how the teeth contact in lateral (side to side) movements. Although this can be observed by starting from centric relation or from centric occlusion position, it is much simpler to record these contacts from the centric occlusion position and that is the method that will be described. Starting with the teeth in a position of maximum contact (CO), patients are instructed to slowly move their mandible to the right (or left) side while maintaining light contact between the teeth. If all of the teeth but the cuspids disengage contact or disclude, this relationship is termed cuspid rise or cuspid protection[14] (Fig. 6-5).

If multiple maxillary and mandibular teeth contact during this lateral excursion, this relationship is termed group function[14] (Fig. 6-6). During this procedure, the teeth should be examined for the associated indicators of occlusal trauma previously described.

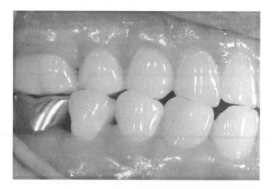

**Figure 6.6** ●

The teeth that contact on the side that the jaw is moving toward (i.e., the right side when the jaw is moving toward the right) are termed working contacts.[14] Teeth that contact on the opposite side during this excursion (i.e., the left side when the jaw is moving toward the right) are termed nonworking or balancing contacts[14] (Fig. 6-7). Findings should be recorded in the occlusal examination chart (Fig. 6-4).

Step three includes evaluating tooth contact(s) during anterior movement of the mandible from the centric occlusion (CO) position. The forward movement of the mandible constitutes protrusive movement. For this evaluation, patients are asked to close their teeth until maximum contact (centric occlusion) is observed, and then slowly advance the mandible anteriorly or to "protrude" their jaw. Ideally, the anterior teeth (i.e., cuspids and incisors) of both jaws will be the only teeth that contact during this movement. This is termed anterior guidance.[14] If any posterior teeth contact during the forward movement of the mandible, they may be experiencing occlusal trauma and the clinician should look for any associative indicators of occlusal trauma previously described.

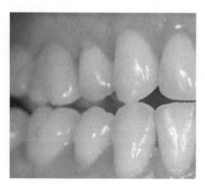

**Figure 6.5** ●

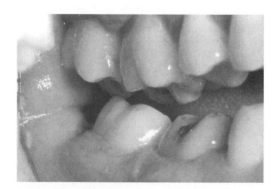

**Figure 6.7** ●

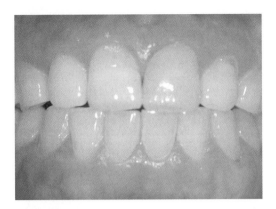

**Figure 6.8** ●

All contacts during protrusive movement are recorded in the occlusal examination chart (Figs. 6-4 and 6-8).

If this evaluation indicates that there is a significant distance between centric relation and centric occlusion (i.e., CR – CO shift > 1 mm) or if the posterior teeth contact during lateral or protrusive movements, the patient is diagnosed as having premature contacts that may be associated with occlusal trauma. In patients with active periodontal disease, these contacts are an indication for adjustment of the occlusion by selective grinding of the occlusal surfaces (Fig. 6-9).

The goal of occlusal adjustment by selective grinding is to eliminate or minimize the premature contacts and, by conservative reshaping of the contacting surfaces, to establish an ideal and harmonious occlusal relationship. The beginning practitioner should approach this procedure with caution to avoid irreversible damage to the teeth. Under these circumstances, when possible, initial occlusal adjustment(s) by the beginning practitioner should be performed with close supervision by an experienced clinician.

## OCCLUSAL TRAUMA DURING PARAFUNCTIONAL MOVEMENTS

The only visible clinical sign that is characteristic of parafunctional movement is the presence of flattened areas of wear on the occlusal surfaces of affected teeth. These characteristic patterns are termed wear facets. Unfortunately, a diagnosis of current parafunctional habits cannot be made solely on the presence of wear facets. Wear facets may be the result of parafunctional habits that were present many years ago but are no longer occurring, or may have been associated with teeth or restorations that are no longer present. Additionally, some wear of the teeth can be expected as the result of years of normal mastication, especially among individuals with a very abrasive diet or who work in an environment with abrasive elements in the air (i.e., dust). Nonetheless, the presence of wear facets on the teeth should be evaluated and an extensive patient dental history review completed (Fig. 6-10).

If parafunctional habits are suspected, the patient should be asked whether they are aware of any grinding or clenching of their teeth. Although some patients with parafunctional habits will

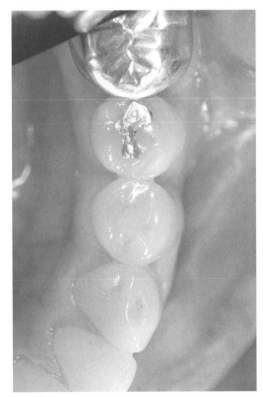

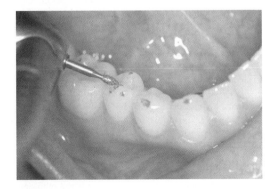

**Figure 6.9** ●

**Figure 6.10** ●

answer affirmative to this question, many patients who have parafunctional habits are often unaware of them. The possibility of parafunctional habits should be discussed in detail with the patient, and they should be given information regarding the signs that may indicate parafunction. The patient should be instructed to watch for the following: waking with their teeth clenched together; presence of "tired" or sore muscles in the morning; and, in more advanced cases, tenderness of the temporomandibular joint or TMJ. If patients have experienced these clinical signs, it is probable that they have parafunctional habits that should be treated.

Most adverse parafunctional habits occur during sleep (night grinding), and these should be treated with a "night guard" or occlusal appliance. These usually consist of a plastic retainer-like device that provides a layer of plastic that covers the occlusal surfaces (Fig. 6-11).

Although patients wearing an occlusal appliance will still tend to grind their teeth, the occlusal appliance will prevent excess pressure (force) on the teeth and will allow wear to occur on the plastic appliance instead of the tooth. Although most parafunctional movements will occur during sleep, such movement is certainly possible during waking hours. Waking parafunctional movement usually occurs during periods of intense concentration or stress. Often, waking parafunctional movements can be minimized by pointing out the damaging effects to the patient and making the patient consciously aware of it and the importance of prevention. Once aware of the problem, many patients will reduce the amount of time they clench or grind their teeth while awake. In severe cases, it may be necessary to recommend an occlusal appliance for daytime use. The 24-hour use of an occlusal appliance should be approached with caution and is not recommended unless the practitioner is experienced in the treatment of occlusal problems.

Although the exact role of occlusion in the progression of periodontal disease remains somewhat unclear, the preponderance of human studies indicate that occlusion should be considered one of the many risk factors associated with this disease progress. As with all risk factors, it is the clinician's responsibility to limit the effect of occlusal trauma as part of the routine treatment of patients with periodontal disease. To ameliorate the effects of this risk factor, the treating dentist needs to make a detailed evaluation of the patient's occlusion during initial periodontal examinations and make a conscience decision whether occlusal treatment is a necessary part of that patient's periodontal therapy.

## REFERENCES

1. Ramfjord SP, Ash MM. Significance of occlusion in the etiology and treatment of early, moderate and advanced periodontitis. J Periodontol 1981;52: 511–517.
2. Svanberg GK, King GJ, Gibbs CH. Occlusal considerations in periodontology. Periodontol 2000 1995; 9:106–117.
3. Loe H, Theilade E, Jensen S. Experimental gingivitis in man. J Periodontol 1965;36:177–187.
4. Nunn M. Understanding the etiology of periodontitis: an overview of periodontal risk factors. Periodontol 2000 2003;32:11–23.
5. Hallmon W. Occlusal trauma: effect and impact on the periodontium. Ann Periodontol 1999;4: 102–108.
6. Ericsson I. The combined effects of plaque and physical stress on periodontal tissues. J Clin Periodontol 1986;13:918–922.
7. Polson A, Heijl LC. Occlusion and periodontal disease. Dent Clin North Am 1980;24:783–795.
8. Glickman I, Smulow JB. Further observations on the effects of trauma from occlusion in humans. J Periodontol 1967;38:280–293.
9. Nunn ME, Harrel SK. The effect of occlusal discrepancies on periodontitis. I. Relationship of initial occlusal discrepancies to initial clinical parameters. J Periodontol 2001;72:485–494.
10. Harrel SK, Nunn ME. The effect of occlusal discrepancies on periodontitis. II. Relationship of occlusal treatment to the progression of periodontal disease. J Periodontol 2001;72:495–505.
11. Glickman I. Inflammation and trauma from occlusion, co-destructive factors in chronic periodontal disease. J Periodontol 1963;34:5–10.
12. Burgett FG. Trauma from occlusion—periodontal concerns. Dent Clin North Am 1995;39:301–311.
13. Harrel SH. Occlusal forces as a risk factor for periodontal disease. Periodontol 2000 2003;32: 111–117.
14. The American Academy of Periodontology. Glossary of Terms, 2001, 4th ed.

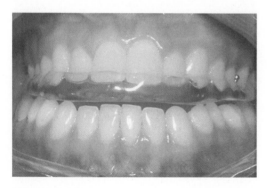

**Figure 6.11** ●

## CHAPTER 6
## REVIEW QUESTIONS

1. Excessive occlusal forces are a risk factor for periodontal destruction.
   a. True
   b. False

2. Occlusal trauma initiates periodontal pocket formation.
   a. True
   b. False

3. Secondary occlusal trauma occurs when _____ forces are applied to a tooth with reduced support.
   a. Normal
   b. Excessive
   c. Normal and excessive
   d. Normal or excessive

4. The basic injury to the periodontium is the same in both primary and secondary occlusal trauma.
   a. True
   b. False

5. _____ is not a clinical indicator of occlusal trauma.
   a. Mobility
   b. Discomfort
   c. Widened periodontal ligament
   d. Fremitus

6. _____ is a radiographic indicator of occlusal trauma.
   a. Cemental tears
   b. Normal periodontal ligament
   c. Caries
   d. Mobility

7. Premature contacts receive more stress than other teeth.
   a. True
   b. False

8. Parafunction includes _____.
   a. Clenching
   b. Grinding
   c. Both
   d. Neither

9. Step two in evaluating the patient's occlusion is assessment of centric occlusion.
   a. True
   b. False

10. Wear patterns associated with occlusal trauma are called facets.
    a. True
    b. False

# Plaque Control

Lorraine Brockman

Bacterial plaque is the primary cause of inflammatory periodontal diseases. Without plaque control, periodontal health can neither be achieved nor be maintained. The success of virtually every aspect of clinical dentistry is dependent on plaque control, from the maintenance of a disease-free mouth to the maintenance of the most complex treatment involving dental implants.

Plaque control may be categorized into professional plaque control and patient plaque control. The clinician is tasked with the responsibility to render a patient as free as possible of plaque and calculus. Once this end is achieved, the patient then assumes the major responsibility in maintenance. Professional visits remain important; however, the patient's daily plaque control routine remains the single most important factor to success.

Informing and educating the patient are our first responsibilities. If the patient does not understand why plaque control is important, it is unlikely the patient will comply. It is surprising, indeed disappointing, the number of adult patients who have never been informed of proper home care and its direct relationship to the health of their teeth and gingiva. Too often, plaque control instruction is accomplished hastily, or not at all. Plaque control instruction is most likely the first component omitted from the appointment in an effort to save time.

Plaque control is an integral part of periodontal disease management. This message should be conveyed to patients. If it is not conveyed, it is doubtful the patient's plaque control will change and, therefore, the cycle of disease will continue.

Plaque control instruction has the potential to be interpreted by the patient as routine and mundane. Unfortunately, too many patients equate plaque control instruction with a nagging, "You need to floss more!" For plaque control to be effective, the patient must be informed, educated, and motivated. Once these criteria are fulfilled, the patient needs good manual dexterity. Absence of even one of these criteria will compromise success.

The most effective means to communicate the presence of disease and the need for improved plaque control is to show your patient the disease in his or her own mouth. Pamphlets, illustrations, and manikins are valuable adjuncts to instruction, but by themselves have only a mild impact. You will gain your patient's attention when you point out the problem areas in their own mouth. For example, show your patient how deep the probe can be inserted subgingivally and how easily the gingiva bleeds. Point out color changes in the gingiva. The patient should be shown the plaque in his or her mouth. Disclosing agents are excellent tools for this purpose.

## DISCLOSING AGENTS

Patients cannot adequately remove plaque if they do not know where they are missing it in the first place. Disclosing agents are used to identify plaque for the patient, and they serve as an excellent motivational and educational tool. Additionally, they provide the clinician the opportunity to record a plaque index that serves as a historic record of the patient's performance with time. Disclosing agents may be incorporated into oral hygiene instruction for all patients, especially children and for adults with inadequate oral hygiene.

Historically, iodine, food coloring, Bismarck brown, mercurochrome, and basic fuschin have been used as disclosing agents.[1,2] Today, erythrosin is the most widely used agent. The agents are available as liquid or chewable tablets. The liquid is most convenient for dental office use and can be swabbed onto the teeth with a cotton-tipped applicator. The patient rinses with a small amount of water and expectorates. The tablets work best for home use. The chewed-up tablet is swished and expectorated. Both liquid and tablets are available over-the-counter for patient use. Fluorescein disclosing agents are also available. These agents are barely visible under regular light, but fluoresce under blue light. They are ideal for adult patients who find the erythrosin staining objectionable.

# BRUSHING

For a thorough discussion of the many different methods of brushing, the reader is referred to current periodontics and dental hygiene textbooks. The sulcular (Bass) method will be considered in this chapter as the preferred method because it is specifically designed to remove plaque adjacent to and within the sulcus.

The sulcular cleansing technique is usually recommended because of its effectiveness in controlling plaque at the gingival margin.[3] It should be emphasized, however, that brushing instruction should be based on each patient's individual needs. More than one technique may be necessary for a patient to achieve acceptable plaque removal.

To cleanse the teeth using the sulcular technique, the toothbrush bristles should be placed at a 45-degree angle to the long axis of the tooth. When properly positioned, some of the brush's bristles will enter the sulcus. The brush is then gently moved in short, back and forth, almost vibratory strokes to disrupt the organized plaque. Each area is overlapped as the brush is moved.

The modified Bass technique is accomplished by including the rolling stroke after the vibratory stroke. The rolling stroke is designed to cleanse the facial and lingual–palatal surfaces. The rolling stroke is accomplished by resting the toothbrush against the gingiva with the bristles directed apically.[4] The brush is rotated coronally with a sweeping motion until the entire tooth surface is cleansed.

## Manual Toothbrushes

A wide variety of toothbrushes is available to suit any patient's needs. Manufacturers are continually striving to improve brushes by altering size, shape, handle, shape of bristles, and arrangement of bristles. Lack of conformity makes determining the most effective toothbrush difficult. Patient satisfaction should help dictate the type of brush used. The ideal toothbrush should be small enough to reach all areas of the mouth, have soft or extra soft bristles, and effectively remove plaque without causing trauma to the hard and soft tissues.

## Powered (Mechanical) Toothbrushes

Powered or mechanical toothbrushes have undergone considerable evolution since their inception. They can be especially useful for patients with limited dexterity, those who are physically handicapped or mentally retarded, those patients with poor motivation toward plaque control, those with orthodontic appliances, patients with implants, or for any patient who is interested in the plaque control capabilities they provide.

Several varieties of powered brushes are available: rotary and contrarotary, oscillating, sonic, and ultrasonic (Fig. 7-1). More recently, less expensive, battery-powered toothbrushes have been introduced. Results of studies are varied regarding the effectiveness of power toothbrushes, but generally they are considered safe and effective.[5–9] One of the most recent innovations involves a sonic toothbrush that simultaneously delivers a dentifrice to the brush head through an attached reservoir (Fig. 7-2).

## Manual Versus Powered Toothbrushes

Numerous studies have been reported concerning the effectiveness of manual versus powered toothbrushes. Although a large number of these studies indicate statistically better plaque reduction with power brushes,[10–13] meta-analysis and systematic review of the literature determined that, overall, powered toothbrushes did not demonstrate an advantage over manual toothbrushes, and the rotation-oscillation powered toothbrushes achieved a significant but modest decrease in plaque and gingivitis compared with a manual toothbrush.[14–16]

When a patient demonstrates the ability to effectively use a manual toothbrush, there appears to be no need to switch to a powered toothbrush. When a patient has attempted a number of manual techniques and has been unsuccessful in controlling plaque, then a powered toothbrush should be considered. It is often more rewarding, dentally and psychologically, to introduce an entirely new concept of tooth cleansing than to attempt to break bad habits that have developed over the years with a manual toothbrush. There is some indication compliance is improved when powered toothbrushes are introduced, especially in periodontal patients.[17]

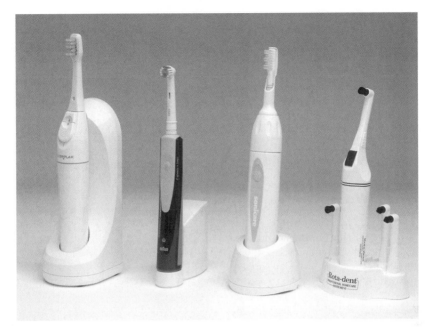

*Figure 7.1* ●

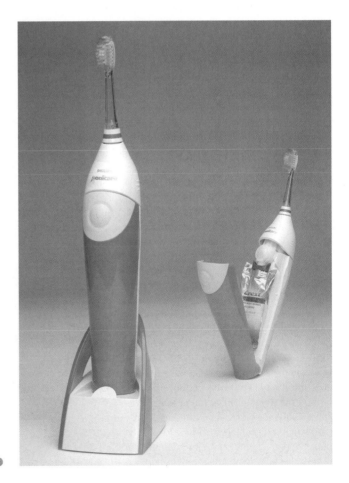

*Figure 7.2* ●

## PROXIMAL CLEANSING

Interproximal plaque removal is crucial to peri-odontal health. The col, the saddlelike depression between the facial and lingual papilla, is nonkera-tinized. Because it is nonkeratinized, the col is more susceptible to bacterial insult and breakdown. The anatomy of the col and the shape of the interdental gingiva allow plaque to harbor and proliferate. No toothbrushing technique, including mechanical toothbrushes, assures interproximal plaque removal.

### Floss and Tape (Waxed and Unwaxed)

Many patients equate flossing with removing food caught between the teeth. Being uninformed, they have no concept of how to clean proximal surfaces and must be instructed in what they are to accom-plish, why, how, and with what devices. Dental floss and tape, either waxed or unwaxed, are equally effective for cleansing proximal sur-faces.[18–20] Individual patient factors, such as con-tacts, restorations, tooth alignment, and manual dexterity, should determine the type of floss used. Unwaxed floss may be recommended for a patient with adequately spaced contact areas, whereas waxed floss may be recommended to a patient with rough interproximal spaces. Floss coated with polytetrafluoroethylene (PTFE—a Teflon-like material) might be suggested for very tight con-tacts. Floss is also available with mint and cinna-mon flavoring, fluoride, and baking soda, and various whitening agents. No additional therapeu-tic benefit has been demonstrated with addition of any of these agents.

Recently an automated interdental device has been introduced that gives the patient the option of using either vibrating floss or a vibrating pick (Fig. 7-3). One study indicates the device is safe and is as effective as flossing in reduction of gin-givitis and bleeding.[21]

Improper flossing can cause tissue trauma and undue discomfort for the patient. "Popping" floss between contact areas of adjacent teeth can lacer-ate papilla. Damage can be avoided by keeping the hands close together, using only a very short zone of floss, exercising control, and sliding the floss back and forth, pressing cervically, until the floss is below the contact area. Once below the contact area, the floss should be wrapped in a 'c' shape around the tooth surface, then moved in an occlu-socervical–incisocervical direction to remove plaque (Fig. 7-4). The floss should be gently maneuvered below the interdental papilla to remove subgingival plaque. Flossing will not

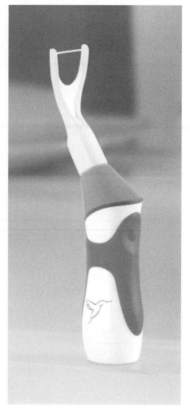

**Figure 7.3** ●

adequately remove plaque from proximal surfaces that are concave and inaccessible to the cleansing fibers (Fig. 7-5). Such surfaces require utilization of other oral hygiene devices discussed below.

The floss-holding devices shown in Figure 7-6 might be helpful for some patients who have diffi-culty in guiding floss with their fingers. Others find it easier to tie the two ends of the floss together to form a circle, then taking up the slack by wrapping the floss around a finger. This technique improves

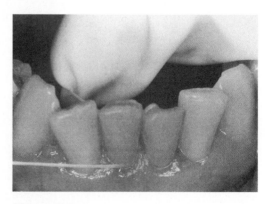

**Figure 7.4** ●

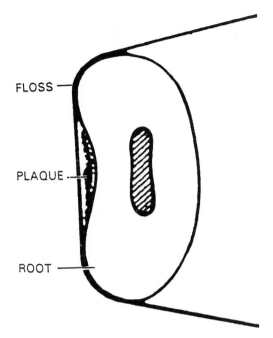

**Figure 7.5** ●

the patient's ability to control the floss. Patients with fixed splinting of the teeth or orthodontic wires are faced with a difficult problem of access to the interproximal region. Floss can be threaded through embrasures by commercially available devices such as those shown in Figure 7-7.

Removing floss in a straight occlusal direction can severely task the retention of restorations when contacts are tight. This problem can be alleviated if the patient either pulls one free end of the floss through the interproximal space or pulls the floss through the contact laterally rather than occlusally.

Superfloss is a variation of dental floss. A strand of Superfloss is stiff on one end for ease of threading under bridge pontics or orthodontic wires. The remainder of the strand is unwaxed dental floss with a portion having a spongelike material.

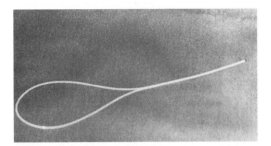

**Figure 7.7** ●

## Gauze

Strips of gauze, in one-inch or one half–inch widths, are particularly effective in removing plaque from proximal surfaces adjacent to an edentulous space or the distal surface of the last molars.

## INTERDENTAL CLEANSERS (RUBBER, PLASTIC, AND WOODEN)

Rubber- or plastic-tipped interproximal devices can be used as aids to clean proximal surfaces. The plastic-tipped devices may be too hard and can cause damage and discomfort. Some clinicians feel that these devices can be used for gingival massage and to maintain healthy interproximal gingival contours,[22] as demonstrated in Figure 7-8. They may also be used for cleansing exposed furcations and cervical areas along the gingival margin. Improperly used, toothpicks can damage the papilla. Some patients have difficulty using them in posterior areas, but these devices are convenient to carry, and their use readily becomes habitual.

Round toothpicks can be used effectively when placed in a special holding device (Fig.7-9). The

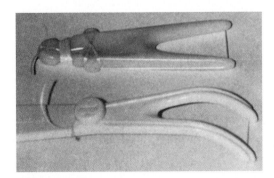

**Figure 7.6** ●

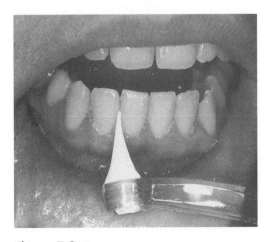

**Figure 7.8** ●

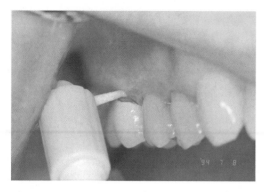

**Figure 7.9** ●

Perio-Aid is one of these devices. The toothpick is moistened with saliva, then used to trace along the gingival margin to remove plaque and debris. These devices are especially effective in cleansing exposed furcations, crown margins, concavities, and areas of gingival recession. The toothpick may also be used to burnish fluoride or other desensitizing agents into the tooth.

## AIDS FOR CLEANSING INACCESSIBLE AREAS

Single-tufted (end-tufted) toothbrushes are highly effective, well accepted by the patient, and safe in cleansing such areas as furcations (Fig. 7-10), concave surfaces, uneven gingival margins, malpositioned teeth, lingual and palatal surfaces, areas of erosion and abrasion, and around fixed prostheses. Patients are instructed to trace the gingival margins with the bristles directed toward the gingiva and to hold the brush in each interproximal area permitting the bristles to work interproximally and subgingivally. Inaccessible areas are dealt with individually. The powered rotary toothbrush has tuft designs that are designed for inaccessible areas and furcations. The powered contrarotary toothbrush will also reach these areas by altering the standard head design by removing the tufts in the second and fourth rows.

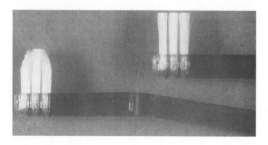

**Figure 7.10** ●

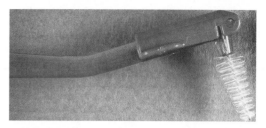

**Figure 7.11** ●

The interproximal toothbrush is a small spiral-type disposable or replaceable toothbrush, resembling a miniature bottle brush, that attaches to a handle (Fig. 7-11). Convenient, completely disposable toothbrush or handle versions are also available. The brushes may be tapered or cylindrical in shape. They are used in wide embrasures or open contacts and conform to concavities on the tooth surface to remove plaque that flossing would not remove. The toothbrush is inserted interproximally and moved in a facial–lingual direction. They are especially useful in periodontal maintenance, implant, and orthodontic patients and demonstrate better removal over dental floss.[23] Only toothbrushes with nylon, plastic, or Teflon-coated wire core should be used with implants.

## ORAL IRRIGATING DEVICES

Oral irrigators, whether of the pulsating or steady stream type, are considered useful *adjuncts* to the toothbrush in patients with poor oral hygiene, for patients with orthodontic bands, or those in fixation after orthognathic surgery.[24–26] They do not remove attached plaque and, consequently, do not replace the toothbrush or interdental cleansing devices. There is some evidence to suggest supragingival oral irrigation may reduce gingivitis in maintenance patients better than regular oral hygiene.[24,27] Patients with healthy gingiva who perform adequate oral hygiene will probably not benefit from supragingival oral irrigation.

There is some evidence that suggests irrigating devices may alter plaque by reducing its toxicity.[27,28] The relationship of this alteration to oral health has not been fully demonstrated except in maintenance patients. Studies have shown that using the pulsating irrigator in the prescribed manner, the solutions penetrated about 3 mm subgingivally, or to about half the pocket depth.[29,30] Specifically designed subgingival tips that can deliver solutions subgingivally are also available. In general, these devices greatly improve penetration depth. Some studies have shown penetration of solutions from 70 to 90% in deep pockets.[29–31]

Some studies suggest that subgingival irrigation with antimicrobials, such as chlorhexidine, phenolic mouth rinses, and others, can result in a greater reduction of gingival inflammation,[32,33] but the results are not conclusive.[25,34,35]

Studies have shown that transient bacteremia may occur with the use of irrigators.[36,37] The effect of such transient bacteremias in a healthy patient is unknown, but caution is urged in patients at risk for bacterial endocarditis. The potential for transient bacteremia is also associated with the use of all plaque control devices.

## MOUTH RINSES

In the past, mouth rinses were considered to be only flavored, breath-freshening solutions with little or no effect on oral health. Today, a number of antimicrobials mouth rinses are available, some of which help control the development of supragingival plaque and gingivitis. These mouth rinses can be valuable *adjuncts* for patients who are poorly motivated or patients whose physical limitations make plaque control difficult or impossible.

Mouth rinses can be divided into two major categories. First-generation mouth rinses are capable of reducing plaque and gingivitis about 20 to 50% when used four to six times a day and have limited or no substantivity. Substantivity is the ability of an antimicrobial to bind to anionic groups on the tooth surface, on the oral mucosa, and on bacterial surfaces and, in effect, produce a sustained release of the active ingredients at therapeutic levels and, therefore, extend the antimicrobial effectiveness of the product. Second-generation mouth rinses are capable of reducing plaque and gingivitis by 70 to 90% when used one to two times a day and have an effective substantivity lasting 12 to 18 hours or longer.

Listerine, Cepacol, and Scope are considered to be first-generation mouth rinses because they lack substantivity. Of these products, Listerine (and its generic equivalents) is the only over-the-counter mouth rinse to receive the ADA seal of approval because of its ability to significantly reduce plaque and gingivitis. Listerine and its equivalents are phenolic compounds, containing four essential oils as their active ingredients: thymol, menthol, eucalyptol, and methyl salicylate. Alcohol content is 27%, with a cool mint version having an alcohol content of 21%.

These essential oil mouth rinses have demonstrated the ability to reduce plaque and gingivitis by approximately 18 to 25%.[38–41] Some patients may experience a burning sensation.

Chlorhexidine preparations containing 0.12% chlorhexidine gluconate are ADA approved, have substantivity lasting between 12 and 18 hours,[41] and are available with a prescription. Alcohol content is 12%. Chlorhexidine has been intensely investigated and is currently the most effective agent available to reduce plaque and gingivitis, between 35 and 45%, rinsing twice daily. Adverse side effects include staining of the teeth and composite restorations, a slight increase in supragingival calculus, and taste alteration.[42] Some patients might experience mucositis.[42,43] Chlorhexidine activity is decreased by blood and purulent material, and toothpaste. Rinsing well with water before rinsing with chlorhexidine is recommended.

More recently, a mouth rinse containing 0.07% cetylpyridinium chloride (CPC) has been introduced, Crest Pro-Health Rinse. CPC has been an ingredient in mouth rinses for many years; however, this product has a higher percentage of CPC. This rinse does not contain alcohol. Independent research is sparse on this product, to date, but preliminary studies by the company indicate this mouth rinse reduces plaque and gingivitis at a level similar to an essential oil mouth rinse.[44,45] Considering the absence of alcohol, this product may show promise if extensive investigation supports these preliminary findings.

## TRICLOSAN

Triclosan is a broad-spectrum agent with mild to moderate antimicrobial properties. It can be found in many mouth rinses and toothpastes available in Europe. Currently, only one oral care product available in the United States contains Triclosan, Colgate Total toothpaste. This toothpaste has demonstrated antiplaque and antigingivitis properties that have earned FDA approval and ADA acceptance for its ability to prevent and reduce gingivitis.[46,47]

## PREBRUSHING MOUTHRINSE

Some products are available as prebrushing mouth rinses and claim to loosen plaque, thereby increasing the effectiveness of toothbrushing. The products contain detergents. Numerous short- and long-term studies have concluded that there is no advantage to using the prebrushing rinse.[48,49] A meta-analysis of the available literature concluded that although Plax may have an effect on plaque and gingivitis reduction, the reductions would not be clinically significant.[50]

Listerine has recently introduced a prebrush rinse, Listerine Whitening. There are no scientific data to support this rinse. It should be emphasized that this product *does not* contain the essential oils like the Listerine antiseptic; therefore, it should not be confused with that product.

# TEACHING PLAQUE CONTROL

There are many approaches to teaching patients effective plaque control. No single technique has been devised that will satisfy the needs of every patient or that can be taught by every clinician. However, there are certain fundamental principles that can be applied to virtually every patient. They are:

1. Keep instructions simple. Remember, practicing plaque control is an exercise in manual dexterity. The more complex the technique the more skill (and time) the patient needs to learn and master it.
2. Do not teach too much at one time. It is far better to introduce the new techniques a few at a time during a longer period, than to expect the patient to remember and practice a long list of procedures that, after a single episode to them, appear very complicated.
3. Encourage the patient. Because of the varied abilities of patients, not every one will perform adequate plaque control at first. With further assistance and continued encouragement almost all patients can be motivated to practice better oral hygiene. Do not, however, excuse lack of effort. One must differentiate between lack of willingness to improve and lack of knowledge and skill.
4. Continue observation and supervision. No matter how well the patient practices plaque control after the initial instructional program, repeated professional evaluation and reinforcement are required to help maintain a high level of performance. The interval between these supervisory evaluations will vary from patient to patient.
5. Be flexible. Although you may teach a specific technique to all patients, remember to individualize based on patient need. Crowded or widely spaced teeth, crown length, presence of fixed prosthetic appliances, and physical disabilities are only some of the variables encountered. Be prepared to alter techniques, and be knowledgeable about products available for use as adjuncts in controlling plaque. Base your recommendations on evidence-based data, not manufacturer claims. Also, do not attempt to change patients to your technique if their present methods are effective.

# REFERENCES

1. Armin SS. Use of disclosing agents for measuring tooth cleanliness. J Periodontol 1963;34:227.
2. Armin SS. Dental caries. Minn Dist Dent J 1953; 37:91.
3. Bass CC. An effective method of personal oral hygiene, part II. J La State Med Soc 1954;106:100–112.
4. Gibson JA, Wade AB. Plaque removal by the Bass and roll brushing techniques. J Periodontol 1977; 48:456–459.
5. Wiliams K, Ferrante A, Dockter K, Haun J, Biesbrock, Bartizek RD. One- and 3-minute plaque removal by a battery-powered versus a manual toothbrush. J Periodontol 2004;75:1107–1113.
6. Soparkar, PM, Rustogi KN, Petrone ME, Volpe AR. Comparison of gingivitis and plaque efficacy of a battery-powered toothbrush and an ADA-provided manual toothbrush. Compend Cont Educ Dent 2000; 21(Suppl):S14–S18.
7. Nathoo S, Rustogi KN, Petrone ME, De Vizio W, Zhang YP, Volpe AR, Proskin HM. Comparative efficacy of the Colgate Actibrush battery-powered toothbrush vs Oral B CrossAction toothbrush on established plaque and gingivitis: a 6-week clinical study. Compend Cont Educ Dent 2000;21(Suppl): S19–S24.
8. Brothwll, DJ, Jutai DKG, Hawkins RJ. An update of mechanical oral hygiene practices: evidence-based recommendations for disease prevention. J Can Dent Assoc 1998;64:295–306.
9. Yukna RA, Shaklee RL. Evaluation of a counter-rotational powered brush in patients in supportive periodontal therapy. J Periodontol 1993;64:859–862.
10. van der Weijden GA, Timmerman MF, Nijboer A, Lie MA, van der Velden U. A comparative study of electric toothbrushes for the effectiveness of plaque removal in relation to toothbrushing duration. J Clin Periodontol 1993;20:476–481.
11. van der Weijden GA, Danser MM, Nijboer A, Timmerman MF, van der Velden U. The plaque-removing efficacy of an oscillating/rotating toothbrush. A short-term study. J Clin Periodontol 1993; 20:273–278.
12. Warren PR. Chater B. The role of the electric toothbrush in the control of plaque and gingivitis: a review of 5 years clinical experience with the Braun Oral-B Plaque Remover. Am J Dent 1996;9(Spec No):S5–S11.
13. Warren, PR, Smith-Ray T, Cugini M, Charter BV. A practice-based study of a power toothbrush: assessment of effectiveness and acceptance. J Am Dent Assoc 2000;131:389–394.
14. Heanue M, Deacon SA, Deery C, Robinson PG, Walmsley AD, Worthington HV, Shaw WC. Manual versus powered toothbrushing for oral health. Cochrane Database Syst Rev 2003(1):CD002281. Available at: www.cochrane-oral.man.ac.uk.
15. Deery C, Heanue M, Deacon S, Robinson PG, Walmsley AD, Worthington H, Shaw W, Glenny A-M. The effectiveness of manual versus powered toothbrushes for dental health: a systematic review. J Dent 2004;32:197–211.
16. Niederman R. Manual versus powered toothbrushes. The Cochrane review. J Am Dent Assoc 2003;134: 1240–1244.
17. Hellstadium K, Asman B, Gustafsson A. Improved maintenance of plaque control by electrical toothbrushing in periodontitis patients with low compliance. J Clin Peridontol 1993;20:235–237.

18. Hill HC, Levi, PA, Glickman I. The effects of waxed and unwaxed dental floss on interdental plaque accumulation and interdental gingival health. J Periodontol 1973;44:411–413.
19. Finkelstein P, Grossman E. The effectiveness of dental floss in reducing gingival inflammation. J Dent Res 1979;58:1034–1039.
20. Ong G. The effectiveness of 3 types of dental floss for interdental plaque removal. J Clin Periodontol 1990;17:463–466.
21. Cronin MJ, Dembling WZ, Cugini MA, Thompson MC, Warren PR. Safety and efficacy of a novel interdental device. J Dent Res 2004;83(Sec Iss A): 0867 (www.dentalresearch.org).
22. Cantor MT, Stahl SS. The effects of various interdental stimulators upon the keratinization of the interdental col. Periodontics 1965;3:243–247.
23. Kiger RD, Nylund D, Feller RP. A comparison of proximal plaque removal using floss and interdental brushes. J Clin Periodontol 1991;18:681–684.
24. Newman MG, Cattabriga M, Etienne D, Flemming T, Sanz M, Kornman, KS, Doherty F, Moore DJ, Ross C. Effectiveness of adjunctive irrigation in early periodontitis. Multi-center evaluation. J Periodontol 1994;65:224–229.
25. Jolkovsky DL, Waki MY, Newman MG. Clinical and microbiological effects of subgingival and gingival marginal irrigation with chlorhexidine gluconate. J Periodontol 1990;61:663–669.
26. Ciancio SG, Mather ML, Zambon JJ, Reynolds H. Effects of a chemotherapeutic agent delivered by an oral irrigation device on plaque, gingivitis, and subgingival microflora. J Periodontol 1989;60: 310–315.
27. Flemming TF, Newman MG, Doherty FM, Grossman E, Mechel AH, Bakdash MB. Supragingival irrigation with 0.06% chlorhexidine in naturally occurring gingivitis. I. 6 month clinical observations. J Periodontol 1990;61:112–117.
28. Derdivanis JP, Bushmaker S, Dagenais F. Effects of a mouthwash in an irrigating device on accumulation and maturation of dental plaque. J Periodontol 1978;49:81–84.
29. Boyd RL, Hollander BN, Eakle WS. Comparison of subgingivally placed cannula oral irrigator tip with a supragingivally placed standard irrigator tip. J Clin Periodontol 1992;19:340–344.
30. Eakle W, Ford C, Boyd RL. Depth of penetration in periodontal pockets with oral irrigation. J Clin Periodontol 1986;13:39–44.
31. Braun RE, Ciancio SG. Subgingival delivery by an oral irrigation device. J Clin Periodontol 1992;63: 469–472.
32. Vignarajah S, Newman HN, Bulman J. Pulsated jet subgingival irrigation with 0.1% chlorhexidine, simplified oral hygiene and chronic periodontitis. J Clin Periodontol 1989;16:365–370.
33. Soh L, Newman HN, Strahan JD. Effects of subgingival chlorhexidine irrigation on periodontal inflammation. J Clin Periodontol 1982;9:66–74.
34. MacAlpine R, Magnusson I, Kiger R, Crigger M, Garrett S, Egelberg J. Antimicrobial irrigation of deep pockets to supplement oral hygiene instruction and root debridement. I. Bi-weekly irrigation. J Clin Periodontol 1985;12:568–577.
35. Linden GJ, Newman HN. The effects of subgingival irrigation with low dosage metronidazole on periodontal inflammation. J Clin Periodontol 1991;18: 177–181.
36. Romans AR, App GR. Bacteremia, a result from oral irrigation in subjects with gingivitis. J Periodontol 1971;42:757–760.
37. Felix JE, Rosen S, App GR. Detection of bacteremia after the use of an oral irrigation device in subjects with periodontitis. J Periodontol 1971;42: 616–622.
38. Menaker L, Weatheford TW, Pitts G, Ross NM, Lamm R. The effects of Listerine antiseptic on dental plaque. Ala J Med Sci 1979;16:71–77.
39. Ross NM, Munkodi SM, Mostler KL, Charles CH, Bartels LL. Effects of rinsing time on antiplaque-antigingivitis efficacy of Listerine. J Clin Periodontol 1993;20:279–281.
40. Mankodi S, Ross NM, Mostler KL. Clinical efficacy of Listerine in inhibiting and reducing plaque and experimental gingivitis. J Clin Periodontol 1987; 14:285–288.
41. Axelsson P, Lindhe J. Efficacy of mouthrinses in inhibiting dental plaque and gingivitis in man. J Clin Periodontol 1987;14:205–212.
42. Flotra L, Gjermo P, Rolla G, Waerhaug J. Side effects of chlorhexidine mouth washes. Scand J Dent Res 1985;79:119–125.
43. Skoglund LA, Holst E. Desquamative mucosal reactions due to chlorhexidine gluconate. Int J Oral Surg 1982;11:380–382.
44. Witt J, Walters, P, Bsoul S, Gibb R, Dunavent J, Putt M. Comparative clinical trial of two antigingivitis mouthrinses. Am J Dent 2005;18:15A–17A.
45. Witt J, Ramji N, Gibb R, Dunavent J, Flood J, Barnes J. Antibacterial and antiplaque effects of a novel, alcohol-free oral rinse with cetylpyridinium chloride. J Contem Dent Prac 2005;6:1–9.
46. Volpe AR, Petrone ME, DeVizio W, Davis RM, Proskin HM. A review of plaque, gingivitis, calculus and caries clinical efficacy studies with a fluoride dentifrice containing triclosan and PVM/MA copolymer. J Clin Dent 1996;7(Suppl):S1–S14.
47. Barnett ML. The role of therapeutic antimicrobial mouthrinses in clinical practice. J Am Dent Assoc 2003;134:699–704.
48. Kozlovsky A, Zubery Y. The efficacy of Plax pre-brushing rinse: a review of the literature. Quintessence Int 1993;24:141–144.
49. Binney A, Addy M, Newcombe R. The plaque removal effects of single risings and brushings. J Periodontol 1993;64:81–185.
50. Angelillo IF. Nobile CG. Pavia M. Evaluation of the effectiveness of a pre-brushing rinse in plaque removal: a meta-analysis. J Clin Periodontol 2002; 29:301–309.

## CHAPTER 7
## REVIEW QUESTIONS

1. The term substantivity can best be described as the:
   a. Prolonged use of an antimicrobial agent
   b. Potential for a substance to cause mucositis
   c. Ability of a substance to adhere to structures in the mouth and be released in therapeutic levels over time
   d. Ability of a substance to be effective without causing side effects

2. Which of the following would be the best choice for cleansing buccal and lingual crown margins?
   a. Proxybrush
   b. Toothpick holder (i.e., Perio-Aid)
   c. Superfloss
   d. Dental floss

3. Once the floss is placed apical to the contact area and wrapped around the tooth, it should be moved in what direction to effectively remove plaque?
   a. Buccolingual
   b. Mesiodistal
   c. Incisocervical (occlusocervical)
   d. The floss is moved in all directions interproximally in an effort to remove the plaque.

4. A proxybrush would be useful for which of the following?
   a. Crowded lower anterior teeth
   b. Deep, narrow pockets
   c. Buccal and lingual crown margins
   d. Large embrasure spaces

5. The best time to perform a plaque index on your patient is:
   a. After data collection, before scaling and polishing
   b. After scaling, before polishing
   c. After scaling and polishing, before fluoride treatment
   d. After the fluoride treatment

6. Specific indications for the Bass technique include plaque:
   a. Adjacent to and directly beneath the gingival margin
   b. On cervical areas beneath the height of contour

   c. Near the coronal third of the tooth
   d. a and b
   e. a, b, and c

7. Research has demonstrated that unwaxed dental floss removes significantly more plaque than waxed dental floss; waxed dental floss is indicated if interproximal restorations are rough.
   a. Both statements true
   b. First statement true; second statement false
   c. First statement false, second statement true
   d. Both statements false

8. Which of the following are purposes of taking a plaque index on your patient?
   (1) Enables the patient to recognize the need to improve oral hygiene
   (2) Reveals degree of effectiveness of patient's present oral hygiene
   (3) Provides a means of motivation for the patient
   (4) Evaluates oral hygiene during a period of time by comparing scores
   a. 1 and 2
   b. 2 and 3
   c. 1, 2, and 3
   d. 2, 3, and 4
   e. All of the above

9. After brushing, a patient should rinse well with water before rinsing with chlorhexidine because chlorhexidine:
   a. Will stain any remaining dentifrice
   b. Is inactivated by dentifrice ingredients
   c. Will cause a burning sensation when mixed with dentifrice
   d. None of the above. It is acceptable to rinse with chlorhexidine immediately after brushing.

10. Which one of the following antimicrobial agents has demonstrated the most significant decrease in plaque and gingivitis?
    a. Chlorhexidine
    b. Triclosan
    c. Essential oils
    d. Prebrushing rinses

# Scaling and Root Preparation

Jane Amme

Scaling and root preparation are essential procedures in all phases of periodontal therapy. Mechanical tooth preparation usually includes scaling and root planing.[1] It is often difficult to determine where scaling stops and root planing begins, and frequently, the two procedures cannot be dissociated.

## SCALING

This is the initial procedure in which the crown and root surfaces of the teeth are instrumented to remove calculus, plaque, accumulated material, and stain.

## ROOT PREPARATION

Root planing with curets and sonic or ultrasonic instruments is a technique designed to remove residual calculus, subgingival microbial biofilm (dental plaque), and endotoxins from the root surface.[2] It appears, however, that periodontal improvement can be achieved without intentional cementum removal. It has been suggested that the term "root detoxification," which is more descriptive of the treatment attempted, supersede the often misunderstood and misinterpreted term of "root planing." Root detoxification can be accomplished by mechanical or chemical techniques, or a combination of these procedures.[3,4] The use of chemical agents to treat the diseased root surface is under investigation. Some examples of these chemical compounds include chlorhexidine gluconate 0.12%, tetracycline hydrochloride, doxycycline hyclate, and minocycline hydrochloride. Future research may provide new and more effective products for root detoxification (see Chapter 10).

## RATIONALE FOR TOOTH PREPARATION

### Supragingival Area

The goal is to obtain a tooth surface that does not encourage the accumulation of deposits and can be maintained by the patient.[5] Scaling and polishing are the indicated procedures to achieve a clean, smooth supragingival tooth surface.

### Subgingival Area

The objective of root preparation is to clean and detoxify the root surface to:

1. Minimize the toxic root contribution as an ongoing insult to the adjacent periodontal tissues.
2. Obtain a biologically acceptable root surface for tissue adaptation and potential new attachment.

## HAND INSTRUMENTATION AND ARMAMENTARIUM

Prerequisites for scaling and root planing are a thorough knowledge of root morphology and effective basic instrumentation skills. The successful practice of periodontics is centered around the skillful use of instruments during scaling and root planing (root detoxification).[6] These instruments generally include scalers, curets, files, and sonic and ultrasonic scaling devices. Calculus deposits can be removed by any of these instruments. Curets, however, are the hand instruments of choice for root detoxification procedures because they are the most effective, with the least amount of trauma to the hard and soft tissues. The shortcomings of using curets are that the process requires physical demands on the clinician and significant time expenditure regardless of the clinician's proficiency. Curets must be sharpened to be effective, and there is limited access in furcation areas and deeper probing sites.[6] Ultrasonic and sonic instruments also are effective root detoxification instruments, especially with new improvements in their longer and narrower tip design.[7,8] Powered instruments and techniques will be addressed later in this chapter.

## PERIODONTAL EXAMINATION INSTRUMENTS

### Periodontal Probe and Nabors Probe

Radiographs alone cannot be relied on to determine the attachment levels in a patient with gingivitis or periodontitis. The periodontal probe is a reliable means of assessing periodontal pocket depths and attachment levels. It also is used for determining bleeding sites. The periodontal probe is manufactured with various designs, single-ended with multiple numerical markings and color-coded variations, working end sizes, and shapes. The Nabors probe is designed to assess the furcation areas. It is a double-ended instrument and is available in one color or color-coded in different numerical variations.

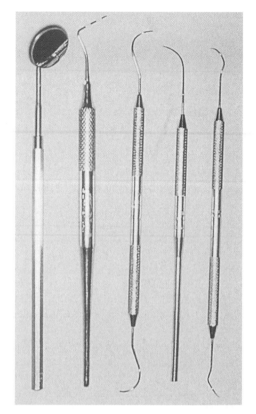

**Figure 8.1** ●

### Explorers

The successful clinician must have the ability to detect calculus and variations in root surfaces with an explorer during scaling and root planing procedures. This important skill is as important as proficiency of root planing instrumentation technique. The development of tactile sensitivity is a key factor to becoming a competent clinician. The explorer is an extremely sensitive instrument because it is wirelike, which permits vibration for detection of tooth surface characteristics and the presence of calculus, caries, furcations, overhanging restorations, and root surface variations. Explorers are available in single-ended, double-ended mirror image, and double-ended designs. The EXD 11/12 explorer (Fig. 8-1) is designed like the Gracey 11/12 curet and is effective for detection in deep periodontal pockets. Newer additions for detecting calculus include the use of endoscopes. This fiberoptic instrument provides visualization and magnification of root deposits. Examples are the Detectar by Ultradentent Products, Inc. and Perioscopy System, produced by DentalView, Inc.

## SUPRAGINGIVAL DEPOSITS REMOVAL INSTRUMENTS

### Scalers, Hoes, Chisels, and Files

Scalers are designed for supragingival deposit removal and are available in straight and curved sickle designs. The straight sickle scaler (the Jacquette scaler is one example) has two cutting edges on a straight blade that ends in a sharp point and is triangular in cross section. The curved sickle has two cutting edges on a curved blade. Scalers feature a rigid shank and a thin face that tapers to a point, which aids in "chipping" off calculus, especially in interproximal areas. The triangular shape and sharp back does not allow for deep submarginal instrumentation without trauma to the soft tissue. Scalers with straight shanks are designed for anterior teeth, whereas angled shanks are for use on posterior teeth (Fig. 8-2).

Other instruments for supragingival deposit removal include (1) hoes for dislodging heavy calculus, (2) chisels for removal of calculus "bridges" from mandibular anterior teeth, and (3) files to

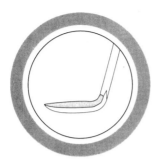

**The Straight Sickle Scaler**
Two cutting edges on a straight blade
that end in a sharp point.
Also known as a Jacquette Scaler

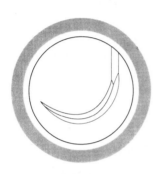

**The Curved Sickle Scaler**
Two cutting edges on a curved blade
that end in a sharp point

*Figure 8.2* ●

**HOES**
*Used to dislodge heavy
supramarginal calculus
deposits.*

**FILES**
*Used to crush and
remove heavy calculus
deposits.*

**CHISELS**
*Used to dislodge bridges
of calculus on Anterior
Mandibular teeth.*

*Figure 8.3* ●

crush and remove calculus deposits supramarginally and also in deep narrow periodontal pockets (Fig. 8-3).

## SUBGINGIVAL DEPOSIT REMOVAL INSTRUMENTS

### Universal and Area-Specific Curets

Curets are the hand instrument of choice for hand root preparation. Curets have flexing shanks for tactile sensitivity and a face that ends in a rounded toe. They are moon-shaped in cross section. The rounded back and toe allow for submarginal instrumentation without trauma to the surrounding soft tissues. There are many types of universal and area-specific (Gracey) curets available with variations to meet almost any clinician's needs.

There are two basic curet designs. The universal curet has a blade with two cutting edges and is designed for general use. This curet can be used on the mesial and distal surfaces of the tooth without changing instrument-working ends. The blade is not offset, and the face of the blade is beveled at 90 degrees to the shank. Both cutting edges are used.

The area-specific (Gracey) curet is designed for specific areas in the mouth. The Gracey curet is honed to offset the blade, and the face of the blade is beveled at 60 to 70 degrees to the shank. The longer angled shank allows for adaptation in deep pockets. One cutting edge of this curet is used.

Several manufacturers make a rigid curet. The rigid curet features a larger, heavier, and less flexible shank than the standard curet. The rigid curet is designed to remove moderate to heavy calculus, but the heavier instrument design decreases the tactile sensitivity (Fig. 8-4).

## AREA-SPECIFIC CURET MODIFICATIONS

### After-Five Curets and Mini-Five Curets

The Hu-Friedy after-five curets are modified area-specific instruments. The terminal shank is elongated by 3 mm to access deep periodontal pockets and root surfaces. The blade is thinned to ease gingival insertion and reduce tissue distention. These curets are available in the rigid and finishing designs.

The mini-five curets are a modification of the after-five design. The blade is reduced by half in length for ease of instrumentation and better adaptation in areas that are difficult to instrument. They are available in finishing and rigid designs (Fig. 8-5).

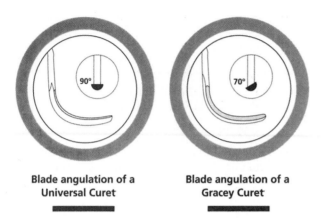

Blade angulation of a
Universal Curet

Blade angulation of a
Gracey Curet

Figure 8.4 ●

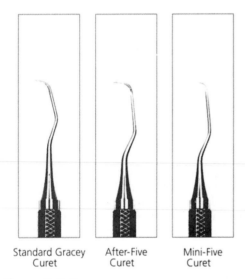

Standard Gracey
Curet

After-Five
Curet

Mini-Five
Curet

Figure 8.5 ●

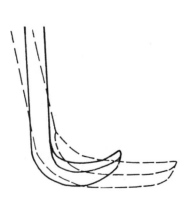

Figure 8.6 ●

## Gracey Curvettes

The American Dental Instrument Gracey curvettes consist of a set of four instruments. The blade length has been reduced to half of the Gracey curet with the blade modified to curve slightly upward. The shorter blade, upward curvature, and blunted tip allow for adaptation in the deep anterior and premolar and line angle of posterior teeth (Fig. 8-6).

## Langer Curets

The three Langer curets combine the advantages of the area-specific shank design with the versatility of the universal blade honed at 90 degrees. This allows for adaptation to both mesial and distal surfaces without changing instruments. The combination of shank design of the Gracey 5-6, 11-12, and 13-14 and the universal curet blade make up the basic Langer set of curets (Fig. 8-7). The Langer curets are also available with the after-five and mini-five modifications, as well as a rigid shank design and Pattison design.

Plastic instruments designed for use on the dental implant surfaces are covered under Dental Implant: Maintenance, in Chapter 22.

## TECHNIQUE FOR HAND INSTRUMENTATION

### Basic Principles

Proficiency in instrumentation is obtained by adhering to general guidelines:

1. Work comfortably. Make the patient comfortable, but mainly, make yourself comfortable.
2. Follow an orderly sequence of instrumentation. This avoids omitting a particular tooth surface.
3. Operate with maximal visibility. When possible, it is best to have direct vision of the

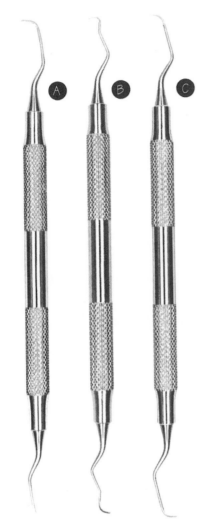

**Figure 8.7** ●

7. Be certain all instruments are sharp. A dull instrument will merely slide over the thinner pieces of calculus, giving the impression that all calculus has been removed. Instruments must be sharp to be effective. Sharpen them after each use. Frequently, instruments require sharpening during the root preparation procedure.
8. Be gentle and careful. Do not confuse roughness with thoroughness.
9. Know the function of each instrument. Using the instrument correctly makes the job quicker and easier.
10. Use as few instruments as possible. You become more efficient and proficient when using fewer instruments.
11. Know the relation of the instrument to the tooth and periodontal structures before activating it. Put the instrument into place slowly and deliberately. This prevents undue injury to the tissues.
12. Check for completeness. Use explorers or endoscopes for this purpose.

## Basic Strokes

There are two basic strokes for scaling and root detoxification (Fig. 8-8):

1. Exploratory stroke. This is used to determine the topography of subgingival deposits. The blade of the instrument is passed along the root surface or calculus deposit, apically, to the depth of the pocket. If any apparent obstruction is encountered during exploration, the blade should be moved laterally from the root surface and, if possible, gently moved further apically. This movement aids in distinguishing between a ledge of calculus and the base of the pocket.
2. Working stroke. Once calculus or roughness is located, it is removed by engaging the root surface and calculus at an 80-degree angle and then deliberately moving the instrument along the root surface. This stroke is followed by a smoothing action performed with absolute control.

operated areas. Also, have a good light source. Fiberoptics are helpful in obtaining direct visibility. They can also be used for transillumination and may show small deposits that might otherwise be overlooked.
4. Obtain maximal accessibility. Use mirror and fingers.
5. Maintain complete control of instruments. Stability is essential for effective controlled action of the instrument.
6. Maintain a clear field. Gauze and cotton rolls, frequent flushing with water, and compressed air may be used. A surgical suction tip is helpful when scaling and root planing or when the tissue is bleeding excessively. Flushing is helpful in ensuring that no calculus or tooth shavings remain in the gingival sulcus or pocket.

Use sharp curets with short strokes in a smooth, rhythmic, and continuous manner to accomplish root detoxification. The instrument should be placed at the edge of the deposit and then there should be "stepping" or overlapping of areas around the tooth to cover the entire surface. Care must be taken to avoid scratching or gouging the root. The shaving action is continued until the root surface is completely smooth (Fig. 8-9).

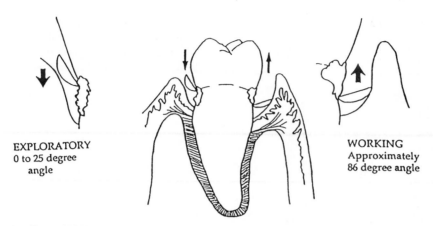

EXPLORATORY
0 to 25 degree
angle

WORKING
Approximately
86 degree angle

*Figure 8.8* ●

## Anesthesia

For most patients, supragingival scaling can be accomplished without anesthesia. Local anesthesia is indicated for proper scaling and root detoxification procedures performed on subgingival root surfaces.

It is recommended that practitioners use block or infiltration anesthesia and limit the appointment to a segment, quadrant, or one-half mouth. The practitioner can then accomplish adequate root preparation with minimal discomfort to the patient.

## ROOT PLANING STROKES

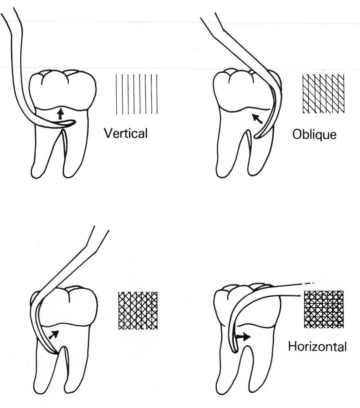

Vertical

Oblique

Horizontal

*Figure 8.9* ●

## Ultrasonic and Sonic Scalers

The sonic and ultrasonic scalers provide a fast and easy means of debridement with a high degree of patient comfort. The combined effects of cavitation by the water and vibration by the instrument against the tooth surface provide the force necessary to dislodge debris and accretions. No damage to soft or hard tissue will occur if light pressure, constant motion of the tip, and adequate water spray are used to prevent heating of the tooth and soft tissue. Several types of devices are available. Many research studies show that ultrasonic scalers are equal in effectiveness when compared with hand instrumentation in removing calculus and biofilm.[9–11] The power instruments' lavage, however, may have additional effects in removing biofilm. Powered scalers may also be more effective when instrumenting class II and class III furcations. However, a significant disadvantage with the use of power instruments is the production of contaminated aerosols.

## Magnetostrictive (Ultrasonic)

The Cavitron operates on the principle of magnetostriction. That is, if a bar of metal (or stack) is placed in a field of alternating current, the stack of metal will vibrate at the speed generated by the field of alternating current. The Cavitron tips vibrate, in an elliptical pattern, at speeds between 18,000 to 45,000 cycles per second (cps) in the newer models. The tips are round shaped in cross section. High to medium power is needed to remove calculus and medium to low power to remove biofilm. The inserts commonly used for effective heavy deposit removal is the #10 universal tip, used on the high or medium power setting (Fig. 8-10). The #10 tip can be used anywhere in the mouth and is effective on subgingival calculus, but the bulky profile may limit access in deeper probing areas. The newest addition of tip design is called Slim Line and consists of a set of slim tips that are designed for root preparation in deep pockets in all areas of the mouth. The longer, thinner tips can be used for more accessible instrumentation in furcations and for calculus and biofilm debridement in deeper probing areas (Fig. 8-10). The tip and corners of all Cavitron inserts are potentially dangerous. Even a dull insert will gouge teeth and restorations if used improperly.

The Cavimed is an instrument that can deliver the operator's choice of antimicrobial through a hollow tip while the instrument tip removes light deposits of calculus and plaque biofilm. The Odontoson is the only magnetostrictive scaler to operate at 42,000 cps. All Odontoson scaler tips are mounted on a ferrite ceramic transducer, similar to the properties of piezo ceramic, ferrite, which allows the Odontoson to generate the higher frequency (Fig. 8-11). This instrument is designed to deliver antimicrobials while scaling subgingivally. The scaling tips are designed similar to hand scaler tips. Other magnetostrictive scalers are produced by Parkell, Coltene, Satelec, and EMS.

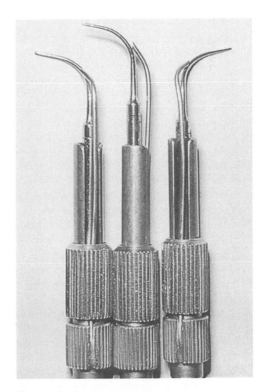

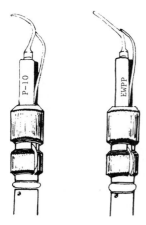

**Figure 8.10** ●

**Figure 8.11** ●

## PIEZOELECTRIC (ULTRASONIC)

The piezoelectric scaler's vibrations are produced by oscillation of a quartz crystal in the handpiece and move at a rate of 25,000 to 50,000 cps in a linear back and forth cycle. The tip is trapezoidal in cross section with angular edges. The quartz crystal generates less heat than the magnetostrictive scaler and, therefore, a lesser volume of water is required to cool the tip. Magnetostrictive tips are usually interchangeable with other brands, but most piezoelectric tips usually are not interchangeable. Studies show nearly equal clinical results when using the piezoelectric and magnetostrictive scalers. Manufacturers include Parkell, Amadent, Prodentec, and Satelec.[12,13]

## TECHNIQUE FOR ULTRASONIC INSTRUMENTATION

### Basic Principles

1. Flush water lines for a minimum of 2 minutes before use to reduce microorganisms.
2. Patients with heart murmurs, hip replacements, past Phen-fen, Redux or Pondimin users, or other patients with bacteremia precautions should be premedicated.
3. Have the patient rinse with chlorhexidine gluconate for 30 seconds before instrumentation. The aerosol that is produced should be taken into consideration if the patient has AIDS, hepatitis, and respiratory or other infectious disease. The patient could aspirate microorganisms, and risks to the operator should be weighed. With such patients, the ultrasonic instrument would be contraindicated or extreme precaution should be taken. High-speed evacuation devices will help reduce the amount of aerosol. Use of the ultrasonic on patients with an infectious disease is contraindicated.
4. The operator and assistant need to wear an overgown, gloves, mask, and safety glasses.
5. Check with a patient's cardiologist before using the magnetostrictive ultrasonic on patients with pacemakers. No such problems have been reported with piezoelectric scalers, but some cardiologists may discourage use of any powered instrument.
6. Always fill the entire handpiece with water before inserting the tip. If the tip becomes hot, stop instrumentation immediately and readjust the water and power settings. Excessive heat can cause damage to the teeth and soft tissue, so you need to use a generous water supply to prevent excessive heating and patient discomfort.

7. Keep the side of the tip in constant motion, using light pressure, during instrumentation.
8. Care should be taken during instrumentation around porcelain, composite, and amalgam restoration margins. Power scalers may cause loss of restoration material or chipping and scratching of the restoration.
9. Ultrasonic instrumentation with metal inserts will damage implant surfaces, and the instrument's vibration can cause damage to implants if used on the teeth adjacent to implants.
10. Always check for completeness of instrumentation with an explorer or endoscope. The EXD 11/12 explorer has a long-angled shank and is very effective for detection in periodontitis patients with deep probing depths.

The ultrasonic and sonic instruments also are highly recommended for use in gross debridement, particularly in cases of necrotizing ulcerative gingivitis or periodontitis, periocornitis, or acute gingivitis, and are effective in removing orthodontic cement and overhanging amalgam restorations. Ultrasonic instrumentation will remove the pocket lining, if subgingival curettage is the objective, and healing of the wound is as rapid as after hand instrumentation.

These instruments dislodge debris rapidly, and the water spray clears the operative site. Some clinicians advocate the use of the ultrasonic or sonic instruments for debridement during periodontal surgery. A washed field with improved visualization is helpful during the surgery; however, the water source from the unit often contains microorganisms that could be introduced into the surgical site. If these instruments are to be used during any surgical procedure, they should be used as a self-contained, sterilized unit with its own source of sterile, distilled water maintained in a sterile pressure tank. Even then, it is necessary to routinely check the tank and hoses leading to the instrument for possible contamination.

Heavy extrinsic surface stain can be removed with these instruments. A great deal of time should not be expended in removing stain that could be removed quickly and more effectively with a rubber cup and polishing agent, or a Prophy-Jet or Prophy-Mate type polishing instrument.

## SONIC SCALER

The Titan-S (Fig. 8-12) scaler tip vibrates at a range from 3,000 to 8,000 cps. The sonic scaler is easily connected to the high-speed handpiece hose and vibrates by air passing over the metal rod, which is contained in the Titan-S handpiece.

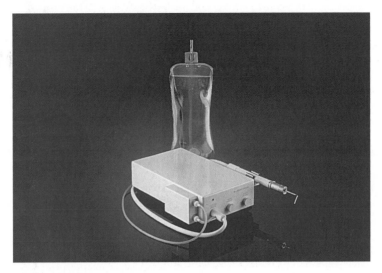

*Figure 8.12* ●

The scaling tip does not produce heat, but water is required to cool the friction between the tip and the tooth. The sonic scalers also produce aerosol contamination. There are three tips available with the unit. The tip action is elliptical. The sonic scaler has less power for rapid calculus removal but is convenient because of its small size and ease of attachment. It also is less expensive than the ultrasonic and easy to sterilize. Other sonic scalers include Quixonic by Midwest/Dentsply, MTI, and KaVo America.

## POLISHING

Several low-abrasive, fluoride-containing agents are commercially available for polishing the supragingival tooth surface with a rubber cup after instrumentation. Care must be taken to select products that are minimally abrasive to avoid excessive loss of tooth surface.

Other instruments that have been introduced for tooth polishing are the Prophy-Jet and the Prophy-Mate (Fig. 8-13). These instruments deliver a sodium bicarbonate–water mixture with a high volume of air and are fast and effective in removing stain and biofilm. They will *not* remove calculus. These instruments are safe to use on sound enamel surfaces but care must be taken when applied to dentin and cementum surfaces and sealants. These polishing instruments also can roughen dental restorations, especially composite and nonmetallic restorations. Care should be taken to prevent the spray from being directed at the soft tissue. The same ultrasonic and sonic precautions are necessary when using these instruments

because of the aerosol contamination inherent with any instrument driven by high volumes of air. Overgowns, gloves, masks, and protective eye gear are mandatory to protect both the operator and the assistant. Care should be exercised when treating patients with sodium-restricted diets or respiratory

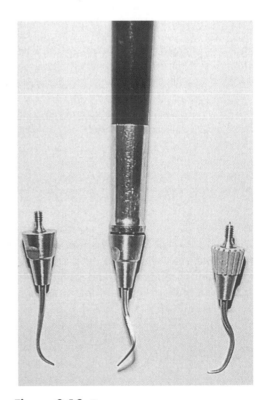

*Figure 8.13* ●

problems, and those patients who wear contact lenses. Premedication is necessary before rubber cup polishing in patients requiring prophylactic antibiotic coverage.

Polishing with the rubber cup, Prophy-Jet, and Prophy-Mate may be contraindicated in the presence of severe inflammation, caries, and decalcification and exposed root surfaces.

## TOPICAL FLUORIDE APPLICATION

Professional topical fluoride treatment is recommended after the polishing procedure. Sodium fluoride 2% applications are highly recommended as they will not harm sealants or ceramic or composite restorations. Sodium fluoride also is called neutral fluoride because it has a neutral pH of 7.0. Acidulated phosphate fluoride (APF) 1.23% acid should be used with care, as APF may cause surface roughening, pitting, or etching of nonmetallic restorations, including sealants. If you use APF, protect these restorations with petroleum jelly. Stannous fluoride preparations may cause staining of decalcified areas. Stannous fluoride is seldom used in clinical practice because of the unpleasant taste and tooth staining. Home fluoride preparations, which contain sodium fluoride, are recommended for patients with rampant caries, root sensitivity, or xerostomia or those patients undergoing radiation therapy.

## REFERENCES

1. Pattison GL, Pattison AM. Periodontal Instrumentation, 2nd ed. Norwalk, CT: Appleton and Lange, 1992.
2. Harper DS, Robinson PJ. Correlation of histometric, microbial, and clinical indicators of periodontal disease status before and after root planing. J Clin Periodontol 1987;14:190–196.
3. Cobb CM. Non-surgical pocket therapy: mechanical. Ann Periodontol 1996;1:443–490.
4. Drisco CL, Cochran DL, Blieden T et al. Position paper: sonic and ultrasonic scalers in periodontics. Research, Science and Therapy Committee of the American Academy of Periodontology. J Periodontol 2000;71:1792–1801.
5. Cercek JF, Kiger RD, Garrett S, Egelberg J. Relative effects of plaque control and instrumentation on the clinical parameters of human periodontal disease. J Clin Periodontol 1983;10:46–56.
6. Wilkins EM. Clinical Practice of the Dental Hygienist, 9th ed. Lippincott Williams & Wilkins, 2005.
7. Smart GJ, Wilson M, Davies EH, Kieser JB. The assessment of ultrasonic root surface debridement by determination of residual endotoxin levels. J Clin Periodontol 1990;17:174–178.
8. Chiew SY, Wilson M, Davies EH, Kieser JB. Assessment of ultrasonic debridement calculus-associated periodontally-involved root surfaces by limulus amoebocyte lysate assay. J Clin Periodontol 1991;18:240–244.
9. Baehni P, Thilo B, Chapuis B, Pernet D Effects of ultrasonic and sonic scalers on dental plaque microflora in vitro and vivo J Clin Periodontol 1992; 19:455–459.
10. Thilo BE, Baehni PC. Effect of ultrasonic instrumentation on dental plaque microflora in vitro. J Periodont Res 1987;22:518–521.
11. Checchi L, Pelliccioni GA. Hand versus ultrasonic instrumentation in the removal of endotoxins from root surfaces in vitro. J Periodont 1988;59:398–402.
12. Loos B, Kiger R, Egelberg J. An evaluation of basic periodontal therapy using sonic and ultrasonic scalers. J Clin Periodontol 1987;14:29–33.
13. Laurell L, Pettersson B. Periodontal healing after treatment with either the Titan-S sonic scaler or hand instruments. Swed Dent J1988;12:187–192.

# CHAPTER 8
## REVIEW QUESTIONS

1. The hand instrument that is designed for crushing calculus deposits is the:
   a. Scaler
   b. File
   c. Hoe
   d. Chisel

2. The magnetostrictive scaler tip shape is:
   a. Trapezoidal
   b. Triangular
   c. Round
   d. Moon

3. Tip motion is a linear back and forth cycle when using the:
   a. Piezoelectric scaler
   b. Magnetostrictive scaler
   c. Sonic scaler
   d. All the above

4. The long-angled shank of the Gracey curet aids in:
   a. Tactile sense
   b. Activation
   c. Adaptation
   d. All the above

5. The abrasive used in the Prophy-Jet is:
   a. Sodium bicarbonate
   b. Coarse pumice
   c. Fine pumice
   d. Flour of pumice

6. The universal curet has an angle between the face of the blade and the shank of the instrument of:
   a. 45 degrees
   b. 80 degrees
   c. 60–70 degrees
   d. 90 degrees

7. Acidulated phosphate fluoride may cause roughening, pitting, or etching of:
   a. Sealants
   b. Composite restorations
   c. Ceramic restorations
   d. All the above

8. The Hu-Friedy after-five curet shanks are elongated by:
   a. 1 mm
   b. 2 mm
   c. 3 mm
   d. 4 mm

9. Sonic and ultrasonic instrumentation may be contraindicated if the patient has:
   a. AIDS
   b. Hepatitis
   c. Respiratory disease
   d. All the above

10. The angle between the instrument and the tooth during the working stroke is approximately:
    a. 0–45 degrees
    b. 60–70 degrees
    c. 80 degrees
    d. 90 degrees

# Instrument Preparation

Elizabeth Hughes

The goal of instrument processing is to provide sterile instruments chair side for use on the next patient (Fig. 9-1). Instrument sterilization is an essential part of a dental practice's infection control program and must be performed properly to better ensure patient and practitioner safety.

Improper technique can lead to a variety of difficulties. For example, instruments may be damaged, discolored, or dulled, or even experience rusting during sterilization, especially if processed through a steam autoclave.[1]

## CATEGORIES OF PATIENT CARE ITEMS

The Centers for Disease Control and Prevention (CDC) has categorized patient care items as critical, semicritical, or noncritical based on the potential risk of infection to patients during their use. The CDC uses a classification system based on one first proposed by Spaulding in 1968 (Table 9-1). The CDC recommends that all critical and semicritical items first undergo a thorough cleaning followed by sterilization. Heat sterilization methods are preferred.[2]

Semicritical items that are heat sensitive must undergo adequate cleaning and treatment with a high-level disinfectant. Cleaning followed by treatment with a low-level disinfectant when no blood is visible is appropriate for noncritical items. Intermediate-level disinfectants must be used when blood can be seen.[2]

## STERILIZATION OF DENTAL INSTRUMENTS

Instrument sterilization involves seven sequential tasks, i.e., chair side and transport; holding (presoaking); cleaning; corrosion control, drying, and

lubrication; packaging; processing; and storage.[3] One must perform each step correctly to keep instrument damage to an absolute minimum, as shown in Table 9-2.

Corrosion associated with moisture and heat affects stainless steel instruments less than some carbon steel instruments. Some instruments are made of stainless steel but have carbon steel cutting edges because they keep their sharpness longer. Unfortunately, carbon steel has a tendency to corrode and lose sharpness during stream sterilization. Dips and sprays can reduce corrosion.[4] Processing in unsaturated chemical vapor or dry heat generally produces less rusting and dulling of carbon steel items.[1] Generous rinsing during holding and cleaning will help remove biologic debris and chemicals that could reduce sterilization efficiency and instrument integrity.

## SHARPENING INSTRUMENTS CHAIR SIDE

How can the clinician effectively maintain aseptic technique and sharpen instruments chair side? We all know that sharp instruments increase our efficiency with scaling, root planing, and debridement. Additionally, sharp instruments are critical for enhancing the level of patient comfort, reducing fatigue, enhancing tactile sense, and increasing refined manipulation. Sharp instruments also can decrease the likelihood of the dreaded burnished calculus.

The ideal safety routine would be to clean, sterilize, sharpen, and resterilize the instruments before the patient arrives (Table 9-3). It would be prudent to have a variety of individually wrapped, sterilized, sharp instruments to replace the unusable instruments during patient treatment.[5] This is

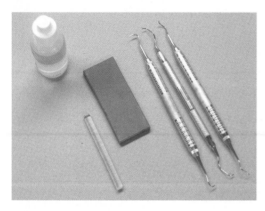

**Figure 9.1** ●

a safer option compared with sharpening orally contaminated instruments chair side. Sharpening of contaminated instruments presents an increased risk for disease transmission through an occupational exposure—cut, abrasion, or puncture.[6]

If you must sharpen chair side with a seated patient, there are techniques to diminish risk. These include the following:

1. Perform sharpening procedures away from patient's view
2. Use armamentarium that can be completely (and easily) sterilized
3. Use safe, stable, sharpening techniques

First, start with a sterile stone. Clean sharpening stones before sterilization (steam, chemical vapor, or dry heat). Again, any sharpening aid, template, or device you may consider using at chair side must also withstand sterilization. Sharpening devices must be disassembled and sterilized after each use.

Sharpening techniques are as varied as the instruments themselves. Sharpening can be achieved by moving the stone across the cutting edge or by moving the cutting edge across the stone (Fig. 9-2). A ceramic stone is best for chair side sharpening because the lubricant used is water. Natural stones require oil lubricants, which cannot undergo sterilization. Thus, natural stones are less desirable for chair side sharpening during patient treatment.[7] Power sharpening devices and sharpening templates should be used according to manufacturer's guidelines. Both methods require a stable, well-lighted, protected working surface to ensure control of sharpening strokes, to aid in maintaining integrity of instrument design, and to guard against injury. To aid in infection control, secure a protective barrier to a flat surface (countertop) with tape.

The clinician must be familiar with the specific features of each instrument's design. The designs of universal and area-specific curets feature a rounded toe and back. These features must be maintained during sharpening. In contrast, scalers have pointed tips, which also must be maintained during sharpening.

## SHARPENING TECHNIQUES

### Sharpening by Moving the Stone

Grasp the instrument in your nondominant hand, place your arm flat on a stable surface parallel to the surface edge, and secure the instrument with your thumb. The surface requiring sharpening will be lower than the countertop edge and will face your dominant hand. Adjust the angle of the cutting edge, not the handle, perpendicular to the flat table surface. It is critical that you recognize the

## TABLE 9.1

### Categories of Patient Care Items

| Category | Definition | Examples |
|----------|------------|----------|
| Critical | Penetrates soft tissue, contacts bone, enters into or contacts the bloodstream or other normally sterile tissue | Surgical instruments, periodontal scalers, scalpel blades, surgical dental burs |
| Semicritical | Contacts mucous membrane or nonintact skin; will not penetrate soft tissue, contact bone, enter into or contact other normally sterile tissue | Dental mouth mirror, amalgam condenser, reusable dental impression trays, dental hand pieces[a] |
| Noncritical | Contacts intact skin | Radiograph heads or cones, blood pressure cuffs, facebows, pulse oximeters |

[a]Although dental handpieces are considered a semicritical item, they should always be heat sterilized between uses and not high-level disinfected.

**TABLE 9.2**

## Suggestions for Protecting Instruments During Processing

| Sterilization Step(s) | Specific Tip |
|---|---|
| Chairside and transport; holding and cleaning | **Keep instruments from knocking into each other as much as possible.** Instruments can be held in cassettes or ultrasonically cleaned in small batches. |
| Chairside and transport; holding and cleaning | **Clean instruments as soon as possible after use.** Materials can affect instrument integrity (e.g., corrosives, blood, and salts). Instrument cleaning should occur as quickly as possible after dismissal of the patient. |
| Holding and cleaning | **Do not let instruments sit in water or chloride solutions for extended periods.** Water can cause corrosion, and chlorine can damage some metals. |
| Holding and cleaning | **Use only cleaning solutions recommended for use on dental and medical instruments.** Such cleaning solutions not only are effective, but also they are gentler to metals because of their neutral pH and because they are easily rinsed away. Some cleaning solutions are also anticorrosive. |
| Holding and cleaning | **Rinse well after cleaning.** Instruments rinsed well are less likely to develop stains or corrosion after processing. |
| Corrosion control, drying, and lubrication | **Spray with or immerse instruments in corrosion inhibitors before sterilization in steam autoclaves.** |
| Corrosion control, drying, and lubrication | **Instruments need to be dried as well as possible before wrapping.** |
| Wrapping and packaging | **Properly wrapped (including cassettes) instruments are less likely to contact other instrument sets.** Instrument damage generally is less when instruments are processed in cassettes. |
| Sterilization | **Use distilled or deionized water in steam autoclaves.** Mineral-rich water can create water spots on instruments and hard water deposits within autoclaves, affecting performance. |
| Sterilization | **Generally, corrosion is less when unsaturated chemical vapor sterilizer or dry heat ovens are used.** Corrosion can affect the performance (dulling) of some instruments. Always dry instruments as well as possible before sterilization. Excessive moisture interferes with the anticorrosion characteristics of unsaturated chemical vapor sterilizers and dry heat ovens. |

instrument design to keep the intended cutting edge intact. Hold the stone in your dominant hand and begin to move the stone in an up and down motion following the lines of the cutting edge. To avoid injury, hold the stone on the edges so that your fingertips do not risk coming into contact with the instrument blade.

## Sharpening by Moving the Instrument

Hold the instrument over the stone, place the stone on a protected flat surface, and move the instrument over the stone toward you. Most instruments can be sharpened by placing the stone either

## TABLE 9.3

### Hand Instrument Sharpening Processes

| Stone | Type(s) | Texture | Lubrication | Sterilization Method(s) |
|---|---|---|---|---|
| Arkansas stone | Natural stone | Fine | Oil | Steam, unsaturated chemical vapor, and dry heat |
| India stone | Natural stone | Medium | Oil | Steam, unsaturated chemical vapor, and dry heat |
| Ceramic stone | Synthetic stone | Medium | Water | Steam, unsaturated chemical vapor, and dry heat |
| Power devices and honing machines | India stone, synthetic stone, Arkansas stone | Coarse, medium, or fine | Water, oil, or none (as directed by manufacturer) | Steam, unsaturated chemical vapor, and dry heat (to use chair side, all removable instrument contact parts must be sterilized) |
| Test stick | Plastic | Smooth | None | Steam, unsaturated chemical vapor, and dry heat |

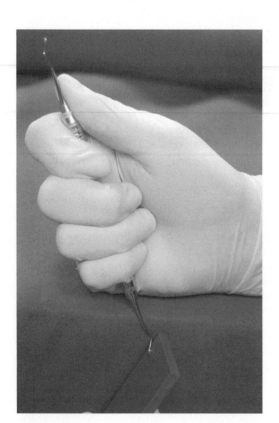

**Figure 9.2** ●

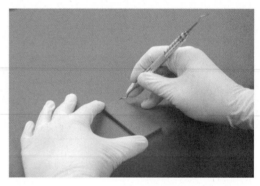

**Figure 9.3a** ●

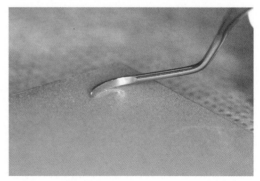

**Figure 9.3b** ●

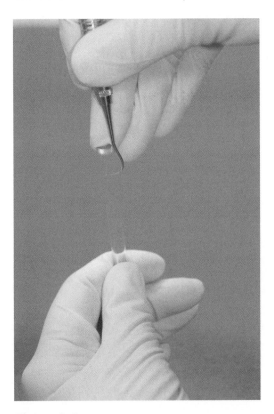

**Figure 9.4** •

perpendicular to the countertop edge or parallel to the edge. With this technique, you will have to change your body position to allow for the best view of the cutting edge. Use a finger or hand fulcrum to prevent instrument slippage and to guide the instrument in a continuous, controlled sweep over the stone. Unless the instrument is in need of recontouring, use only light to moderate pressure. Stabilize the stone with your nondominant hand, making sure to keep fingertips clear of the direction of the sharpening stroke (Fig. 9-3A). The cutting edge of the instrument should be placed at a 75-degree angle to the sharpening stone (Fig. 9-3B).

No matter what your preferred method of sharpening, all chair side methods carry the risk of operator injury. By following simple guidelines for caution, you can protect yourself from disease-promoting injury or merely the inconvenience of a sore finger.

## Testing Sharpness With Acrylic Testing Stick

Carefully wipe residual materials from the instrument using double or triple gauzes. Test the sharpness by adapting the cutting edge to the test stick (Fig. 9-4). Stroke away from yourself and with fingers clear from direction of the sharpened edge. If the instrument is sharp, the cutting edge will catch on the plastic stick. At the end of the appointment, clean and package all instruments for sterilization.

## REFERENCES

1. Stach DJ, Cross-Poline GN, Newman SM, Tilliss TS. Effect of repeated sterilization and ultrasonic cleaning on curet blades. J Dent Hyg 1995;69: 31–39.
2. Center for Disease Control and Prevention. Guidelines for infection control in dental health-care settings—2003. Morbid Mortal Wkly Rep MMWR 2003;52(RR-17):1–68, Also available at: http://wonder.cdc.gov/wonder/prevguid/p0000191/p0000191.asp#head008000000000000
3. Organization for Safety and Aseptic Procedures. From Policy to Practice: OSAP's Guide to the Guidelines. Annapolis, MD: Organization for Safety and Aseptic Procedures, 2004:193–207.
4. Hutcheson CL. Taking care of your instruments, what you need to know to protect your instruments and your patients. Dent Equip Mater 2004;9:22.
5. Marquam B. Keep eye on sharpening techniques to prevent disease transmission. RDH 1992;12:20–23.
6. Miller CH, Palenik CJ. Infection Control and Management of Hazardous Materials for the Dental Team, 3rd ed. St. Louis: Elsevier Mosby, 2005.
7. Rossi R, Smukler H. A scanning electron microscope study comparing the effectiveness of different types of sharpening stones and curets. J Periodontol 1995;66:956–961.

## SUGGESTED READINGS

Darby M, Walsh M. Dental Hygiene Theory and Practice, 2nd ed. St. Louis: Saunders, 2003.
Nield-Gehrig JS. Fundamentals of Periodontal Instrumentation and Advanced Root Instrumentation, 5th ed. Baltimore: Lippincott Williams & Wilkins, 2004.

# CHAPTER 9
## REVIEW QUESTIONS

1. CDC guidelines describe periodontal and surgical instruments used intraorally to be in what category for infection control?
   a. Critical
   b. Semicritical
   c. Noncritical
   d. Intermediate

2. All of the following techniques are important for protecting instruments during holding and cleaning except:
   a. Rinse well after cleaning
   b. Clean instruments as soon as possible after use
   c. Soak contaminated instruments in bleach solutions before cleaning
   d. Keep instruments from knocking into each other during transport

3. It is not necessary to dry instruments thoroughly before sterilization.
   a. True
   b. False

4. Carbon steel instruments should be sterilized by:
   a. Dry heat
   b. Autoclave
   c. Chemical disinfection

5. Ceramic stones are best suited for chair side sharpening because:
   a. They do not require sterilization
   b. They produce a sharper cutting edge
   c. They can be lubricated with water

6. The ideal time to sharpen instruments is:
   a. During patient use
   b. After patient use but before cleaning
   c. After sterilization and before treatment

7. Which sharpening approach best maintains the original instrument design of a curet?
   a. Square toe
   b. Rounded toe
   c. Pointed toe

8. Sharpening stones should be prepared for use by which of the following methods?
   a. Scrubbed with disinfecting soap
   b. Wiped with a high-level disinfectant
   c. Wiped with alcohol
   d. Heat or chemical sterilization

9. To maintain cutting edges that do not require significant recontouring, how much pressure should be applied during sharpening?
   a. Heavy pressure
   b. Moderate pressure
   c. Light to moderate pressure

10. During the sharpening process, it is important to round the toe of:
    a. Curets
    b. Scalers
    c. All periodontal instruments

# Local and Systemic Periodontal Chemotherapy

Steven Blanchard

Periodontal destruction is a result of host inflammatory responses to bacterial plaque biofilms. Although traditional periodontal therapy is largely effective in controlling this disease process, the use of adjunctive antimicrobial therapy can be beneficial in cases that fail to respond or only partially respond to periodontal debridement and periodontal surgery. This chapter will examine the uses of adjunctive antimicrobial therapy and host modulation therapy in periodontal treatment regimens.

## RATIONALE FOR ADJUNCTIVE ANTIMICROBIAL THERAPY

Scaling and root planing have been effective in dramatically reducing the bacterial counts in the subgingival environment. A large body of evidence exists documenting the effectiveness of nonsurgical periodontal therapy,[1] and it remains as the cornerstone of periodontal therapy. However, an equally large number of studies have consistently shown that complete removal of all hard and soft bacterial deposits from root surfaces is virtually impossible.[2–4] Studies have shown up to 99% reduction of the total viable counts of bacteria after thorough subgingival debridement,[5,6] but subgingival recolonization and rebound have been found to occur within 6 weeks.[7,8] Regrowth of bacteria may occur from bacteria residing on the soft tissue pocket wall,[6] from root surface irregularities,[9] or from microbial niches outside of the periodontal pocket such as the dorsum of the tongue, tonsillar pillars, and saliva.[10] Even with improved access to the root surfaces through surgical periodontal therapy, complete removal of all plaque and calculus has been shown to be difficult if not impossible.[11,12] It is not surprising, therefore, that a significant number of patients fail to effectively respond to traditional therapy.

The use of chemotherapeutic agents may be of some benefit in attempting to control and eliminate subgingival periodontopathic flora in patients with destructive periodontal diseases. It is important to keep in mind, however, that antimicrobial agents can only be expected to be effective when used in conjunction with some type of mechanical subgingival debridement. Plaque biofilms are complex bacterial structures surrounded by an extracellular polysaccharide matrix with interspersed channels and pores for nutrient diffusion that allow for growth and interactions between and among the various microorganisms within the biofilm.[13] The nature of these biofilms provides protection against systemic and locally delivered antimicrobials unless the biofilm is first disrupted and reduced in mass by mechanical debridement. Concentrations of antimicrobials against undisturbed biofilms must be up to 500 times greater than that needed to be effective against planktonic levels of the same bacteria.[14]

Chemotherapeutic agents used in periodontal therapy may be divided into antiseptics and antibiotics. Antiseptics are agents that kill or inhibit the growth of microorganisms on surfaces. Antiseptics are powerful antimicrobial agents but are potentially toxic if absorbed systemically and should be restricted to topical use on skin or mucosa. Commonly used antiseptics for oral chemotherapy include chlorhexidine, essential oils, povidone iodine, sodium hypochlorite, fluorides, quaternary ammonium compounds, triclosan, and oxygenating agents. Antibiotics are naturally occurring or synthetic organic compounds that kill or inhibit the growth of microorganisms at low concentrations and may be used either topically or systemically. Antibiotics used for periodontal application include the penicillins, tetracyclines, metronidazole, azithromycin, fluoroquinolones, and clindamycin.

There are a number of delivery systems that can be used for agent application including oral rinses, gels, dentifrices, oral irrigation, controlled-release devices, and systemic delivery. Agent delivery by oral rinsing and through dentifrices is largely directed against supragingival microorganisms but has limited ability to reach the subgingival environment, and their use should be limited to gingivitis. Oral irrigation, controlled-release devices, and systemic use of agents allow for subgingival delivery of antimicrobial agents and, therefore, have applications for the treatment of periodontitis.

Dentifrices are commonly used for the delivery of sodium fluoride (0.24%) for anticariogenic activity. Mouth rinses can be used as an adjunct to mechanical plaque control when oral hygiene is inadequate or difficult to accomplish, after surgical procedures when normal oral hygiene procedures may not be practical, and as a preprocedural rinse to decrease bacterial aerosols and reduce bacteremias.

## TOPICAL APPLICATION OF ANTISEPTICS IN PERIODONTAL THERAPY

Antiseptics for periodontal chemotherapeutic agents are applied in mouth rinses, in dentifrices, and as oral irrigants. Mouth rinses and dentifrices are the most widely used methods for the delivery of oral antimicrobial agents, but have a limited effect on periodontitis because agents in rinses and dentifrices are not able to reach the subgingival environment.

Oral irrigators were introduced in the late 1960s. Initial studies showed limited effectiveness on supragingival plaque removal, but improvements on gingival inflammation and bleeding were evident.[15] Numerous studies have further documented the effect of oral irrigation on reductions in gingivitis, gingival bleeding, and reductions in periodontal pathogens.[16–18] Oral irrigation systems are generally powered water-pulsing devices using water or medicaments. Home irrigation devices using a standard tip have been shown to deliver medicaments 30 to 44% into the depth of 3- to 8-mm pockets.[19] Introducing a needle cannula for in-office irrigation improves penetration of agents up to 75 to 100% of pocket depth in pockets ranging from 3 to 10 mm.[20,21] Irrigation is largely directed against the unattached subgingival plaque flora and also aids in dilution of bacterial byproducts and inflammatory products. This flushing and dilution effect should not be minimized, as many of the irrigation studies have shown that irrigation with water alone was often as effective as was irrigation with various medicaments.[16,22–24]

## Chlorhexidine

Chlorhexidine gluconate is a cationic bisbiguanide that binds to bacterial cell walls and leads to rupture of the cell membrane with leakage of cellular contents, leading to cell death. Chlorhexidine is often considered as the "gold standard" for antiplaque and antigingivitis agents. Chlorhexidine also exhibits substantivity by its ability to bind to teeth and mucous membranes and be released over an 8- to 12-hour period with sustained antimicrobial activity. Chlorhexidine exhibits a wide antimicrobial spectrum and is active against Gram-positive and Gram-negative bacteria, yeasts, and some viruses.[25]

Chlorhexidine is available in the United States by prescription as a 0.12% rinse (Peridex, Zila Pharmaceuticals, Cincinnati, OH; PerioGard, Colgate Oral Pharmaceuticals, Canton, MA; Oris, Dentsply International, York, PA), and studies have demonstrated gingivitis reductions of 35 to 45% and plaque reductions of 50 to 55%.[26] Chlorhexidine is used as a 30-second rinse twice daily or as a preprocedural rinse. Because of its cationic nature, chlorhexidine is inactivated with anionic compounds found in most dentifrices and, therefore, should not be used in conjunction with toothbrushing using a dentifrice or used only after thorough rinsing after dentifrice use. Rinses containing chlorhexidine have been awarded the ADA Seal of Acceptance for its ability to reduce plaque and gingivitis.

Despite the positive benefits of oral rinsing with chlorhexidine, irrigation studies using chlorhexidine have been quite disappointing.[22–24] Repeated professional irrigation with chlorhexidine showed only minor clinical improvements and a transient antibacterial effect whether used in addition to root planing[27,28] or with an ultrasonic scaler.[29,30] The disappointing results of subgingival irrigation with chlorhexidine can possibly be explained by its affinity to bind to salivary or serum proteins,[31] lowering the subgingival concentrations to subtherapeutic levels. Southard and coworkers[28] were able to demonstrate comparable effects of 2% chlorhexidine rinsing to scaling and root planing, but this was at a concentration of 20 times that found in commercially available chlorhexidine rinses.

Chlorhexidine has a wide margin of safety because of its poor absorption through mucous membranes or if swallowed. The most common side effect of chlorhexidine is extrinsic staining of teeth, restorations, and tongue after a few days of use. Staining is exacerbated in smokers. Other side effects are altered taste sensation and increased calculus formation.

## Essential Oils

Essential oils have long been used as antimicrobial agents. Listerine (Pfizer, New York, NY) uses a combination of thymol, menthol, eucalyptol, and methyl salicylate in an alcohol base and has demonstrated plaque and gingivitis reductions of up to 34%.[32] Essential oils have a mechanism of action of cell wall disruption leading to cell lysis and inhibition of bacterial enzymes. Rinses with essential oils demonstrate no substantivity and are to be used as a 30-second rinse twice daily or as a preprocedural rinse. Mouth rinses containing essential oils are the only over-the-counter rinse with the ADA Seal of Acceptance for demonstrated antiplaque and antigingivitis properties. Alcohol concentration varies from 21.6 to 26.9%. Additional effects of subgingival irrigation with essential oils versus rinsing alone have not been reported. Possible side effects from products containing essential oils are a burning sensation, depending on formulation.

## Quaternary Ammonium Compounds

Quaternary ammonium compounds are cationic surface-active agents similar to chlorhexidine that demonstrate slight substantivity for up to 3 hours[33] and demonstrate variable and inconclusive antiplaque and antigingivitis properties.[34] Formulations of quaternary ammonium compounds include cetylpyridinium chloride alone (Cepacol, Combe, White Plains, NY; Viadent, Colgate Oral Pharmaceuticals, Canton, MA) or cetylpyridinium chloride combined with domiphen bromide (Scope, Proctor and Gamble, Cincinnati, OH). Alcohol concentrations vary from 6% (Viadent), to 14% (Cepacol), to 18.9% (Scope). Mechanisms of action of quaternary ammonium compounds are cell lysis from increased cellular permeability and leakage of cellular contents. Adverse side effects have been found to be similar to chlorhexidine and include some staining, mucosal ulceration, and increased calculus formation.

## Povidone Iodine

Iodine is a potent broad-spectrum antimicrobial that has been used by health professionals for more than 150 years. Povidone iodine 10% (Betadine,

Purdue Frederich Co, Norwalk, CT) is an iodophor consisting of elemental iodine and polyvinyl-pyrrolidone that serves to increase the solubility of the iodine while maintaining a sustained iodine release. Iodophors are generally nontoxic and exert a strong antimicrobial effect against Gram-positive and Gram-negative bacteria, fungi, viruses, and protozoans,[35] with virtually no evidence of development of resistant microorganisms.[36] The antimicrobial action of povidone iodine is caused by the leakage of cellular contents through transient and permanent pore formation in bacterial cell walls with resulting rapid cell death.

Povidone iodine can be used as an oral rinse but is more commonly used as a subgingival medicament. Oral rinsing with povidone iodine was able to reduce bacterial levels along the gingival margin by 33% compared with 8% by the control rinse,[37] and adjunctive rinsing with a povidone iodine–hydrogen peroxide solution was able to reduce papillary bleeding by 38% compared with 31% for povidone iodine–water and 18% for water alone.[38] Some studies have indicated that subgingival irrigation with povidone iodine before extractions was able to reduce bacteremias by 30 to 50%,[39,40] but this has not been borne out in all studies.[41] Christersson and colleagues[42] used a 0.5% povidone iodine solution with ultrasonic debridement and, although clinical improvements were comparable to ultrasonic debridement with saline in pockets of 5 mm or less, they found gains in probing attachment of 2 mm or more in 80% of sites irrigated with povidone iodine but only 55% in saline-irrigated sites. Rosling et al.[43] compared the use of ultrasonic debridement with 0.1% povidone iodine with ultrasonic debridement with water and found that the use of 0.1% povidone iodine led to significantly reduced pocket depths and gains in clinical attachment during the first 12 months of the study. Continued use of 0.1% povidone iodine with ultrasonic debridement during maintenance visits led to significantly less attachment loss during the entire 13-year study period compared with ultrasonic debridement with water irrigation.[43] Despite these encouraging results, more studies are needed, including multicenter trials, to further validate the effectiveness of this inexpensive antimicrobial agent (approximately $0.20 per whole-mouth periodontal treatment).[44]

Ten percent povidone iodine (Betadine) can be used undiluted, applied repeatedly with a blunt irrigation needle after scaling and root planing to maintain a contact time of 5 minutes, or may be diluted with nine parts or less of water for use in ultrasonic scalers. Povidone iodine is soluble in water, is nonirritating to healthy or inflamed oral mucosa, and does not exhibit the adverse side effects of tooth staining, tongue discoloration, or taste alteration seen with other antimicrobials. Povidone iodine can stain clothing, but the stains are removed either with soap and water or a sodium thiosulfate solution.[44] Prolonged iodine use has the potential to induce hypothyroidism as a result of excessive thyroid iodine uptake, but short-term use has not been associated with thyroid dysfunction.[45] Iodine hypersensitivity is rare, but iodine is contraindicated in pregnant and nursing women to protect the infant.[46]

## Stannous Fluoride

Stannous fluoride was the first anticaries agent to receive the ADA Seal of Acceptance but has received renewed interest for its effect on gingivitis.[47,48] Two 6-month studies of a 0.454% stannous fluoride dentifrice (Crest Gum Care, Proctor and Gamble, Cincinnati, OH) showed reductions of 20 to 33% in gingivitis and a 20% reduction in gingival bleeding with no resultant improvement in plaque scores,[47,48] but a study by Ciancio and colleagues[49] showed a 29% plaque reduction with a stannous fluoride dentifrice. Antimicrobial properties of stannous fluorides are believed to be related to the tin ion, leading to a reduction of bacterial adhesion to tooth surfaces. Stannous fluorides have been evaluated as a professionally applied subgingival irrigation medicament with only slight improvements in clinical parameters.[50] Commonly reported adverse effects of stannous fluorides include tooth staining and a metallic taste, which has been effectively masked by recent dentifrice formulations.

## Triclosan

Triclosan is a bisphenol compound possessing antimicrobial activity against Gram-positive and Gram-negative bacteria and is a common agent found in soaps and deodorants. An antiplaque and antigingivitis dentifrice (Total, Colgate Oral Pharmaceuticals, Canton, MA) incorporates 0.3% triclosan and 2% polyvinylmethylether–maleic acid, which has demonstrated substantivity up to 12 hours after use.[51] Triclosan reduces plaque biofilm formation and affects the quality of existing plaque. The use of this triclosan dentifrice has shown a 20% reduction in gingivitis and a 25% plaque reduction compared with a placebo dentifrice[52] and has been awarded the ADA Seal of Acceptance. No adverse side effects from triclosan have been reported.

## Sodium Hypochlorite

Chlorine compounds, specifically hypochlorites, have a long history of use as disinfectants and antiseptics. The active component of hypochlorites is undisassociated hypochlorous acid (HOCl), which is a strong oxidizing agent that is lethal to most bacteria, fungi, and viruses.[44] Advantages of hypochlorite are broad antimicrobial spectrum, rapid bacteriocidal activity, low toxicity at low concentrations, and very low cost.[53] Sodium hypochlorite is readily available, and solutions for home use can be prepared by diluting household bleach (5.25 to 6.5%) 1:50 with water, with a resultant solution around 0.1% or 1,000 ppm of available chlorine for use in commercial oral irrigator or oral rinse. This can be done by adding 1 teaspoon (5 mL) of household bleach to 1 cup (250 mL) of water. Disadvantages of sodium hypochlorite include a bleach odor and taste, the need to mix fresh solutions daily, bleaching of fabrics, corroding effects on some metals, and irritation of oral mucous membranes if used at high concentrations. Bacteria have been shown to be inactivated in vitro by chlorine solutions as low as 0.01%,[54] and dilute solutions of sodium hypochlorite applied to extracted tooth roots were able to significantly reduce endotoxin levels by more than 80-fold.[55] Sodium hypochlorite solutions were found to be effective antibacterial agents when used for debridement of wounds and skin ulcers without inhibition of fibroblast activity.[56] Despite potential advantages as a potent antimicrobial, the use of sodium hypochlorite has not been investigated in large-scale periodontal trials.

## Hydrogen Peroxide

Hydrogen peroxide releases oxygen when hydrolyzed and would appear, in theory, to offer some benefit against anaerobic periodontal pathogens. However, when used as an adjunct to scaling and root planing, neither professionally delivered nor patient-delivered hydrogen peroxide irrigation was able to show any significant difference in subgingival microbial shifts compared with saline irrigation.[57] Hydrogen peroxide is an effective debriding agent for wounds and ulcers, including the oral cavity; however, claims of plaque and gingivitis reduction are not well supported. Safety concerns about hydrogen peroxide have been raised. It has been suspected of being a cocarcinogen in animal experiments[58] and has been associated with occasional gingival irritation and delayed wound healing.[59] However, most studies have indicated that 3% hydrogen peroxide was safe with few side effects, but long-term studies have shown no advantages in the use of hydrogen peroxide compared with conventional oral hygiene practices.[59]

## SYSTEMIC ANTIBIOTIC USE IN PERIODONTAL THERAPY

Periodontal diseases are chronic infections, and so it would seem logical that use of systemic antibiotics may be of use in therapy. Systemic antibiotics have been successfully used in the treatment of chronic and aggressive periodontitis in numerous studies.[60–64] An excellent review of studies using systemic antibiotics for periodontal diseases has been conducted by Slots and Ting.[65] There is also a growing body of evidence to suggest that periodontitis is not an innocuous infection and may be associated in the etiology or exacerbation of systemic diseases and conditions.[66–69] Systemic antibiotics may be a useful adjunct to nonsurgical and surgical therapy for patients with aggressive forms of periodontitis, patients with moderate to advanced chronic periodontitis that is not responsive to conventional therapy, and immunocompromised patients. However, the growing problem of bacterial antibiotic resistance has challenged the use of antibiotics for the treatment of periodontal infections. Indiscriminate use of antibiotics contributes to the risk of increasing antibiotic resistance and limits their effectiveness and use for potentially life-threatening infections or leads to overgrowth of resistant bacterial and fungal microorganisms and should be avoided.

Antibiotic selection should ideally be based on culture and sensitivity testing. The expense of testing, however, precludes its widespread use. Because periodontal diseases are predominantly Gram-negative anaerobic infections, the selection of antibiotics that are effective against Gram-negative anaerobes should be of benefit if systemic antibiotics are to be used in therapy. Drug cost may also play a factor in antibiotic selection. Penicillins, tetracyclines, and metronidazole are low-cost antibiotics whereas azithromycin, amoxicillin/clavulanic acid, fluoroquinolones, and clindamycin are considerably more expensive. Antibiotics, notably penicillins and tetracyclines, may interfere with the metabolism of oral contraceptives from alterations of the gastrointestinal flora necessary for metabolism of estrogen to its active form in the stomach. These patients should be cautioned to use alternative forms of contraception while taking antibiotics.

### Penicillins

Penicillins are bacteriocidal (β-lactam antibiotics that act by inhibition of bacterial wall synthesis. Penicillins are among the least toxic antibiotics as mammalian cells do not possess a cell wall. The most commonly used antibiotic for periodontal disease is amoxicillin because of its broad-spectrum antimicrobial activity; most other penicillins have limited effectiveness against Gram-negative bacteria. Widespread use (and abuse) of penicillins has led to development of hypersensitivity reactions in approximately 15% of the population, and bacterial resistance through the production of β-lactamases has restricted their effectiveness. To overcome the susceptibility to β-lactamases, amoxicillin is often used in combination with a β-lactamase inhibitor, clavulanic acid (Augmentin, GlaxoSmithKline, Philadelphia, PA). Generic forms of Augmentin are now available, reducing its cost.

Amoxicillin/clavulanic acid has been shown to be effective in significantly reducing gingival bleeding and pocket depths,[70,71] improving clinical attachment,[71] and reducing levels of most suspected periodontal pathogens.[70,71] Antibiotic levels well above the minimum inhibitory concentration to some periodontal pathogens could be detected in the gingival crevicular fluid after multiple doses of amoxicillin/clavulanic acid.[72] Normal dosing is amoxicillin 250 to 500 mg with clavulanic acid 125 mg taken three times daily for 10 to 14 days. Adverse side effects include hypersensitivity reactions and gastrointestinal upset (nausea and diarrhea).

### Tetracyclines

Tetracyclines are a group of naturally occurring or semisynthetic broad-spectrum bacteriostatic antibiotics that hinder bacterial multiplication through inhibition of protein synthesis by blocking the translation of mRNA. Tetracyclines, especially doxycycline and minocycline, have been frequently used in the treatment of periodontal diseases. Doxycycline and minocycline are completely absorbed by the gastrointestinal tract and are not affected by ingestion of dairy products. Tetracyclines have been reported to be concentrated in gingival crevicular fluid at 2 to 4 times serum levels[73]; however, a more recent report found that crevicular fluid levels of tetracyclines were often lower than serum levels and varied widely among individuals, with 50% of sites sampled exhibiting levels less than 1 μg/mL.[74] These findings might explain the variability seen in clinical responses to individuals taking systemic tetracyclines. Tetracyclines also possess anticollagenase properties from inhibition of destructive host-derived matrix metalloproteinases (MMPs).

Inhibition of MMPs has been found to be independent of the antibiotic's antibacterial activity and has led to the development of subantimicrobial dosing of tetracycline (Periostat, CollaGenex Pharmaceuticals, Newtown, PA) used to modify the host inflammatory responses to periodontal bacterial challenge (see Host Modulation Therapy).

The review article on systemic antibiotics in periodontal therapy by Slots and Ting[65] reports data on more than 20 studies incorporating the use of tetracyclines. Tetracyclines have been found to significantly reduce gingival bleeding and probing depths,[75–77] improve clinical attachment levels,[76–78] and reduce levels of periodontal pathogens.[76,79] Other studies showed improvement of clinical[80–82] and microbial[81,82] parameters after tetracycline use, although the changes did not reach statistical significance. One study found administration of systemic tetracycline for juvenile periodontitis[83] resulted in almost complete regeneration of bony defects, and clinical results remained stable for up to 4 years after therapy. Typical dosing for tetracycline is 250 mg, three to four times daily for 14 to 30 days; 100 mg of doxycycline is taken once daily for 14 to 21 days (often taking 100 mg twice daily for the first day); and minocycline dosing is 100 to 200 mg daily for 14 to 21 days. Adverse side effects from tetracyclines include nausea, vomiting, diarrhea (less frequently seen with doxycycline and minocycline as they are more completely absorbed from the gastrointestinal tract), and photosensitivity. Tetracyclines can stain dentin and enamel during tooth development and should be avoided during pregnancy and for children younger than the age of 10. Ingestion of calcium products (dairy products and antacids) delay the absorption of tetracycline (except doxycycline and minocycline) and should be avoided.

## Metronidazole

Metronidazole is a bacteriocidal nitroimidazole effective against obligate anaerobes, including spirochetes, by inhibition of bacterial DNA synthesis. Metronidazole has been widely used, sometimes in combination with amoxicillin, for periodontal infections. The addition of amoxicillin is used to increase the antimicrobial spectrum to include facultative microorganisms such as *Actinobacillus actinomycetemcomitans* or *Pseudomonas* species.[65] Metronidazole is particularly effective in the treatment of necrotizing periodontal diseases that are caused by anaerobic fusospirochetal infections. Metronidazole is concentrated in the gingival tissues and crevicular fluid[84] and may be effective where bacterial tissue penetration

occurs. Resistance to metronidazole by anaerobic microorganisms is uncommon.

Metronidazole has been shown to be a useful adjunct in the treatment of both aggressive and chronic forms of periodontitis. Metronidazole, used alone or in combination with amoxicillin, significantly reduces gingival bleeding[85,86] and pocket depths,[62,85] improves clinical attachment,[87,88] and reduces anaerobic periodontal pathogens.[88,89] Loesche and colleagues[62,63] have reported that metronidazole use can reduce periodontal surgical needs in cases with advanced periodontitis. However, like other antibiotics, some studies have shown no benefits of metronidazole compared with control subjects.[90,91] Metronidazole 250 mg is taken three times a day for 7 days or may be combined with amoxicillin 375 to 500 mg taken three times daily for 7 to 14 days. Gastrointestinal upset (especially nausea) is frequently reported with metronidazole, along with a metallic taste. Patients should be cautioned about alcohol consumption while taking metronidazole as disulfiram-like reactions of headache, nausea, and vomiting may occur. Metronidazole should be avoided with patients taking oral anticoagulants (warfarin) as it increases the anticoagulant effect.

## Azithromycin

Azithromycin is a second-generation macrolide that has a broad spectrum of action against both Gram-positive and Gram-negative bacteria but fewer side effects than most macrolides. It is bacteriostatic and inhibits bacterial protein synthesis by binding to the 50S ribosome. Azithromycin shows promise in periodontal treatment as it readily penetrates into periodontally inflamed tissue and is concentrated in polymorphonuclear leukocytes (PMNs) and macrophages.[92] Azithromycin is able to maintain tissue levels exceeding minimum inhibitory concentrations for most periodontal pathogens up to 4.5 days after discontinuation of the drug.[92] Although studies have been limited, double-blind, placebo-controlled trials have found that azithromycin can decrease gingival bleeding and probing depths[93] and reduce levels of periodontal pathogens.[94] Azithromycin 500 mg is taken once daily for 3 days. Although an expensive drug, the patient compliance with azithromycin may be improved compared with other antibiotics as it is only taken once daily for 3 days. Adverse side effects from azithromycin are usually limited to gastrointestinal upset, although the severity and frequency of side effects are much lower than those seen with most erythromycins.

## Clindamycin and Fluoroquinolones

Clindamycin is a broad-spectrum bacteriostatic antibiotic that acts by inhibiting bacterial protein synthesis by blocking translation of RNA. It is effective against most periodontal pathogens except *A. actinomycetemcomitans*. Studies evaluating the use of clindamycin for refractory periodontitis have found a decrease in the percentage of active sites (sites losing ≥ 3 mm attachment) from 10 to 0.5%,[95] improved probing depths, decreased gingival bleeding, and decreased levels of spirochetes and Gram-negative anaerobic rods.[95,96] Clindamycin 150 mg is taken four times a day for 7 days. Common adverse side effects from clindamycin include diarrhea, although pseudomembranous colitis has been associated with clindamycin from an overgrowth of *Clostridium difficile.*

Fluoroquinolones, notably ciprofloxacin, are broad-spectrum bacteriocidal antibiotics that have good activity against Gram-negative facultative anaerobes (i.e., *A. actinomycetemcomitans*). They are effective against most bacterial associated with various forms of periodontitis, but clinical studies evaluating their use are lacking. In vitro antimicrobial sensitivity testing on periodontal pathogens suggests a combination of ciprofloxacin 500 mg and metronidazole 500 mg taken twice daily for 8 days should effectively eradicate Gram-negative anaerobic rods and *A. actinomycetemcomitans* and allow growth of nonpathogenic streptococci capable of inhibiting Gram-negative pathogens.[97] Adverse side effects reported from ciprofloxacin include nausea and vomiting, headache, convulsions, dizziness, and photosensitivity. Antacids and dairy products will impair absorption of ciprofloxacin.

## Conclusions Regarding Adjunctive Systemic Antibiotic Use in Periodontal Therapy

Systemic antibiotic use may play a valuable role in the treatment of more advanced or aggressive forms of periodontal diseases. Initial subgingival microbial reduction and disruption of the root-associated biofilms through mechanical instrumentation is imperative before, or in conjunction with, antibiotic administration. Without prior microbiologic testing, a combination of metronidazole and amoxicillin would be a reasonable choice and should prove effective in the majority of advanced periodontitis patients.[65] It appears unlikely that one antibiotic or antibiotic combination will be effective for all patients. A recently published study[98] examined which antibiotics or

antibiotic combinations would be best used against target complexes of bacterial pathogens present in 774 patients with periodontitis. Reported achievable antibiotic gingival crevicular fluid concentrations had to be at least 10 times the minimum inhibitory concentration for pathogen complexes to be judged effective. Antibiotic combinations of metronidazole and amoxicillin, metronidazole and amoxicillin/clavulanic acid, or metronidazole and ciprofloxacin would be effective against 24 pathogen complexes found in 74% of all patients. However, at least 10 different antibiotic regimens would be required to specifically target the more than 45 pathogenic complexes identified.[98] Systemic antibiotic use may be best restricted to patients with aggressive forms of periodontal disease and those with moderate to advanced attachment loss who do not respond to mechanical therapy.

## USE OF PROPHYLACTIC SYSTEMIC ANTIBIOTICS FOR PERIODONTAL AND IMPLANT SURGERY

There is little scientific evidence that warrants the use of prophylactic antibiotics for periodontal surgical procedures in the overwhelming majority of patients. Postsurgical infection rates are low and have been reported to be between 2 and 4% after periodontal surgery.[99,100] The use of prophylactic antibiotics had no effect on the prevalence of infections in these studies. Many clinicians will empirically prescribe antibiotics before regenerative periodontal surgery to avoid infection of implanted materials and enhance clinical outcomes. Again, however, the available evidence does not support this clinical rationale as antibiotic use for regenerative periodontal procedures did not influence probing depth reduction,[101,102] gain of clinical attachment,[101,102] or bone regeneration.[101,103] Data are conflicting (and lacking) concerning the justification for prophylactic antibiotic use when dental implants are placed. Some studies reported a decrease in implant failures when preoperative antibiotics were used,[104,105] but another found no influence of antibiotics on implant survival.[106] An evidence-based review on the use of perioperative antibiotics for dental implants concluded that there is insufficient scientific evidence to recommend or discourage the practice of antibiotic use to prevent complications or failures of dental implants.[107]

There are instances, however, when prophylactic systemic use before surgical procedures is recommended. There are definitive guidelines for the use of antibiotics before invasive procedures for patients at moderate and high risk for infective endocarditis and those at risk of infection because of prosthetic joints.[108,109] There is more confusion about the use of antibiotics to prevent infection or reduce complications in medically compromised patients. This group includes those who have poorly controlled diabetes, organ transplant patients, patients undergoing chemotherapy, patients on long-term, high-dose corticosteroids, patients with other significant immunodeficiencies, and those with other significant metabolic diseases. Prior consultation with the patient's physician is warranted in these instances.

## CONTROLLED DRUG DELIVERY IN PERIODONTAL THERAPY

Previously discussed antimicrobial drug delivery methods, with the possible exception of professional irrigation, are directed against all oral sites uniformly and do not discriminate between healthy and diseased sites. Periodontal disease is a site-specific infection and at any one time in the same mouth there may be sites that are periodontally healthy, sites that are inflamed but stable, and a few sites that are undergoing active periodontal destruction. The ultimate goal of therapy would be to direct periodontal therapy only against those sites that are currently breaking down or will break down in the near future. Although there are no currently available simple methods or tests that will accurately identify active periodontal destructive sites, clinicians concentrate their efforts on sites that have deeper probing depths and demonstrate gingival bleeding on probing. Controlled drug delivery fits well into this treatment philosophy. Controlled drug delivery seeks to deliver sustained high concentrations of antimicrobial agents into the periodontal pocket for prolonged periods at a fraction of the dose required for systemic drug administration. In theory, delivery of high drug concentrations to a specific contained area (i.e., periodontal pocket) would permit eradication of the offending bacteria with minimal systemic absorption and undesirable side effects. Effective killing of bacteria within the pocket would also minimize the development of resistant microorganisms. Controlled drug delivery is best indicated for isolated recurrent or nonresponsive bleeding sites 5 mm or greater in depth. Controlled drug delivery may also be indicated for patients who, for a variety of reasons, may not be good candidates for more aggressive forms of periodontal therapy such as periodontal surgery.

Controlled drug delivery agents that have been available for commercial use in the United States include tetracycline fibers (Actisite, Alza Corp,

Palo Alta, CA), doxycycline polymer gel (Atridox, Atrix Laboratories, Fort Collins, CO), chlorhexidine chip (PerioChip, Dexel Pharma, Edison, NJ), and minocycline microspheres (Arestin, Orapharma, Warminster, PA). Agents available for use outside of the United States include metronidazole gel (Elyzol, Dumex, Copenhagen, Denmark) and minocycline gel (Dentomycin, Cyanamid, Lederlee Dental Division, Wayne, NJ, and Periocline, Sunstar Corp, Osaka, Japan).

### Tetracycline Fibers (Actisite)

Tetracycline fibers were the first controlled delivery product available for commercial use. Flexible ethylene vinyl acetate fibers are impregnated with 25% tetracycline containing 12.7 mg of tetracycline HCl in the 9-inch fiber (Actisite). The fibers are placed subgingivally in an overlapping manner until the pocket is filled to within 1 mm of the gingival margin and sealed in place with cyanoacrylate. Fiber placement may take up to 15 minutes per site. Tetracycline is slowly released during the course of 10 days, after which the nonresorbable fiber is removed. High concentrations of tetracycline ($>1{,}500$ μg/mL) are released during the course of the 10 days the fibers are in place.[110] These levels are in excess of 1,000 times the minimum inhibitory concentrations of most periodontal pathogens, yet serum levels remained less than 0.1 μg/mL during the 10-day period.[111] Several studies evaluated the effect of tetracycline fiber plus scaling and root planing compared with scaling and root planing alone.[112–116] The combined mean results from these studies show a mean probing reduction of 1.8 mm for scaling and root planing plus fiber application compared with a mean probing reduction of 1.5 mm for scaling and root planing alone. Attachment level changes from these same studies show a gain of 1.3 mm for the combined therapy compared with a gain of 0.9 mm for root planing alone. Reductions in gingival bleeding were more pronounced when scaling and root planing was combined with fiber placement.[114,115] Tetracycline fibers are no longer available for use in the United States. The time necessary to place the fibers, the premature loss of fibers from the pocket, and the need to remove the fibers after 10 days, plus the introduction of simplified delivery systems, all led to the removal of Actisite from the U.S. market.

### Doxycycline Polymer Gel (Atridox)

Atridox is a formulation of 10% by weight doxycycline hyclate in a biodegradable polymer.

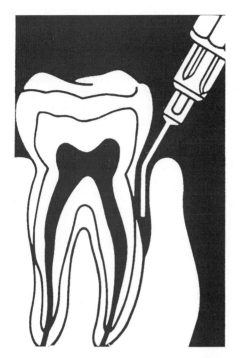

**Figure 10.1** ●

Atridox comes packaged in two syringes, one containing 42.5 mg of doxycycline, the other containing the Atrigel Delivery System consisting of poly (DL) lactide dissolved in *N*-methyl-2-pyrrolidone, and must be stored refrigerated until used.

Activation of the polymer gel is done by coupling the two syringes together and mixing the contents of the syringes back and forth for 100 cycles. A blunt cannula is attached to the syringe, and the gel is extruded into the periodontal pocket. The gel polymerizes on contact with oral fluids. Doxycycline is released from the polymer for the next 7 days. After Atridox placement, doxycycline gingival crevicular fluid (GCF) levels of 1,500 μg/mL have been detected at 2 hours and remained above 1,000 μg/mL for the next 18 hours.[117] At 1 week, doxycycline GCF levels of 250 μg/mL have been found, and serum levels never exceeded 0.1 μg/mL (Figs. 10-1 and 10-2).[118]

Atridox is unique among controlled drug delivery systems in that it can be used to treat multiple sites using the same syringe. Use of the product is moderately technique sensitive, and some users have complained that the polymerized gel will stick to the cannula as the cannula is withdrawn. This can be avoided by turning the tip of the cannula against the root surface as the cannula is withdrawn to pinch off the polymerizing gel. If some material is expressed outside of the pocket, it can be gently packed back into the sulcus with the back of a curet or other instrument. Another technique that has been suggested is to express the material along the gingival margin of each site where product delivery is desired. The material will polymerize and can be packed subgingivally as previously described. Patients should be cautioned against brushing or flossing for the first

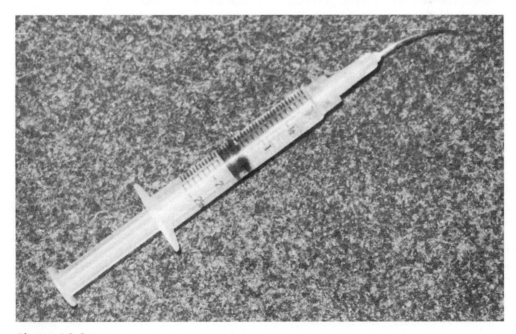

**Figure 10.2** ●

week after placement to minimize dislodgement of the polymerized gel. Atridox is the only controlled-release product that has been tested as a monotherapy, that is, without the use of scaling and root planing. In two multicenter trials, Atridox was compared with a placebo and scaling and root planing alone and found to demonstrate equivalent results with scaling and root planing.[119] At 9 months, mean clinical attachment gain was 0.8 mm for the doxycycline gel alone compared with 0.7 mm for the scaling and root planing alone group in one study, and 0.8 mm and 0.9 mm, respectively, in the second study. Similarly, probing depth reductions were 1.1 mm for Atridox versus 0.9 mm for scaling and root planing in the first trial and reductions of 1.3 mm in both groups for the second study. A similar study investigated the use of Atridox for periodontal maintenance patients.[120] Patients received either doxycycline gel or scaling and root planing on one half of their dentition for all sites 5 mm or greater at baseline and at 4 months. At 9 months, probing depths were 1.3 mm for Atridox and 1.1 mm for scaling and root planing; attachment level gains were 0.7 mm for doxycycline gel and 0.8 mm for scaling and root planing. Although clinical trials tested Atridox as a monotherapy, the product is normally used in conjunction with subgingival root debridement.

## Chlorhexidine Chip (PerioChip)

PerioChip is a biodegradable hydrolyzed gelatin chip impregnated with chlorhexidine gluconate. It measures 5 mm by 4 mm by 0.35 mm thick and contains 2.5 mg of chlorhexidine. It is stored at room temperature and can be inserted into pockets larger than 5 mm with a pair of cotton forceps with the curved end of the chip directed apically. Handling characteristics have been improved from earlier formulations, and no adhesives are required as the chip adheres to the pocket wall after contact with crevicular fluid. Patients should be cautioned against brushing or flossing in the area for 1 week. Chlorhexidine is released in a biphasic manner, with 40% of the chlorhexidine being released in the first 24 hours, then with a more linear release for the next 7 to 10 days.[121] Gingival crevicular levels of chlorhexidine were as high as 2,000 µg/mL 2 hours after placement and falling to less than 60 µg/mL after 1 week.[122] Two double-blind, randomized, controlled trials evaluated the use of the PerioChip in conjunction with scaling and root planing compared with scaling and root planing alone in 5- to 8-mm periodontal pockets.[123] Patients were examined at 3, 6, and 9 months. Any PerioChip site still probing more than 5 mm had additional chips placed; however, no additional root planing was done for either group. At 9 months, sites receiving scaling and root planing alone improved by 0.65 mm and sites that received scaling and root planing plus PerioChip improved by 0.95 mm. Attachment level changes were 0.58 mm for scaling and root planing alone versus 0.75 mm for scaling and root planing plus chlorhexidine chip. The percentage of pockets with 2 mm or more of pocket reduction was 8% for scaling and root planing and 19% for scaling and root planing plus PerioChip. All findings were statistically significant.[123] A more recent study examined the use of the chlorhexidine chip in conjunction with regenerative periodontal surgery.[124] PerioChip placement was performed 1 week before GTR surgery and at 3 and 6 months after surgery at any site of 5 mm or greater. After 1 year, pocket depth reductions and clinical attachment gains were demonstrated with the use of the PerioChip, but results were not statistically significant. However, digital subtraction radiography showed that sites receiving the chlorhexidine chip gained more than 2 mm more bone than the surgery alone sites (3.54 mm versus 1.49 mm).[124] PerioChip may also be effective in reducing MMP levels implicated in periodontal destruction. A study by Azmak and coworkers[125] reported that insertion of a chlorhexidine chip was able to reduce MMP-8 levels in GCF for up to 6 months compared with scaling and root planing alone, although the differences were only statistically significant for the first month after placement.

## Minocycline Microspheres (Arestin)

Minocycline microspheres (Arestin) have been the most recently introduced controlled drug delivery product to the U.S. market. Arestin is minocycline HCl microencapsulated in a bioresorbable polyglycolide-co-DL-lactide polymer. It is stored at room temperature and packaged in a disposable plastic cartridge containing 1 mg of minocycline to be used with a stainless steel syringe. It is perhaps the easiest controlled delivery product to use. The tip of the plastic cartridge is inserted subgingivally to the base of the pocket (≥5 mm). Pressure on the plunger of the syringe expresses the material into the pocket as the tip is withdrawn. The material adheres to the walls of the pocket after contact with moisture. The minocycline microspheres are hydrolyzed by fluids, causing channels to form inside the microspheres, slowly releasing the minocycline for 14 days. At 2 weeks, GCF levels of minocycline of 340 µg/mL were detected.[126] Occasionally, the tip of the plastic cartridge is too big to insert into the pocket orifice. An instrument, such as a periodontal probe, can be used to place gentle lateral forces along the pocket wall, or the plastic tip of the cartridge can be slightly flattened with the handle of a mirror to facilitate tip insertion.

The use of Arestin in addition to scaling and root planing compared with scaling and root planing alone was evaluated in 748 patients from 18 different treatment centers in a random controlled trial.[126] Sites probing 5 mm or more received scaling and root planing plus Arestin or scaling and root planing and placebo control at baseline; additional Arestin or vehicle control was placed in pockets of 5 mm or greater at 3 and 6 months. Approximately 30 sites per patient were treated, more than 23,000 sites in all. Results at 9 months showed statistically significant greater pocket reduction at sites receiving scaling and root planing plus Arestin (1.20 mm) compared with scaling and root planing plus vehicle control (0.90 mm) or scaling and root planing only (1.04 mm). When the data were analyzed based on initial pocket depths, the differences when Arestin was used became more pronounced as pocket depth increased. Differences between Arestin and scaling and root planing compared with scaling and root planing alone were 0.24 mm for pockets of 5 mm or greater, 0.41 mm for pockets of 6 mm or greater, and 1.01 mm for pockets of 7 mm or greater. As the pocket depths increased, the benefits achieved in using minocycline microspheres as an adjunct to scaling and root planing also increased.[126]

## Minocycline Gel (Dentomycin and Periocline)

Two formulations of 2% minocycline gel (Dentomycin and Periocline) are available for use outside of the United States. These products should be considered as sustained-release as opposed to controlled-release, as the drug concentrations are depleted within 24 hours. Multiple applications may be required for optimal effectiveness. These products are applied with a blunt cannula attached to a syringe until the pocket is filled to the gingival margin. GCF concentrations of doxycycline of 1,000 μg/mL were detected 1 hour after administration, and levels in excess of 100 μg/mL were detected for the first 6 hours, whereas systemic minocycline levels remained less than 0.1 μg/mL.[127] Several studies evaluated the effectiveness of repeated subgingival application of 2% minocycline gel as an adjunct to scaling and root planing compared with root planing alone,[128,129] and these studies showed statistically improved

clinical and microbiologic parameters compared with control groups. A 15-month double-blind, random-controlled multicenter study repeatedly applied 2% minocycline gel at baseline, weeks 2 and 4, and at months 3, 6, 9, and 12. At 15 months, 2% minocycline sites showed pocket reductions of 1.9 mm versus 1.2 mm for the control group. Clinical attachment level changes were 0.9 mm for the test sites and 0.5 mm for control sites. Probing depth and attachment level changes were even more significant in pockets of 7 mm or greater. Levels of *P. gingivalis* and *Treponema denticola* were significantly reduced at all times versus controls. Pocket depth reductions of 2 mm or more were noted in significantly more sites when the minocycline gel was used for both moderate (≥5 mm) and deep sites (≥7 mm) compared with control sites (63% versus 43%, 73% versus 53%, respectively).[129] Another study[130] evaluated 2% minocycline gel (reapplied at weeks 2 and 4) along with tetracycline fiber and 25% metronidazole gel as adjuncts to root planing compared with root planing alone. Although all three antimicrobial treatments showed greater pocket reduction than root planing alone, only the root planing plus tetracycline fiber showed a statistical improvement at 6 months.

## Metronidazole Gel (Elyzol)

Another sustained-release product currently not available in the United States is a 25% metronidazole gel in a glyceryl mono-oleate and sesame oil base. Like the 2% minocycline gel, Elyzol is applied using a syringe with a blunt cannula, and repeated applications may be necessary for optimal results. GCF levels of metronidazole were found to exceed the minimum inhibitory concentration for most periodontal pathogens up to 24 hours after application.[131] Two 6-month studies found that application of a 25% metronidazole gel as a monotherapy (repeated at 1 week) was found to have comparable results with scaling and root planing for pocket reduction.[132,133] Another study evaluated 25% metronidazole gel (reapplied at 1 week) along with tetracycline fiber and 2% minocycline gel as adjuncts to root planing compared with root planing alone, but found no differences when the metronidazole gel was used compared with controls.[130]

## Conclusions Regarding the Use of Controlled Drug Delivery

Considerable confusion exists today regarding the use of controlled drug delivery products. There is no doubt that these agents provide some additional benefit to nonsurgical periodontal therapy. The magnitude of additional changes is small, usually less than 0.5 mm, and many have questioned whether this difference is clinically significant. Evidence suggests that the magnitude of change is increased as pocket depths increase, and a greater proportion of sites demonstrate pocket depth reductions of 2 mm or greater when adjunctive controlled-release agents are used. Manufacturers often claim that the evidence supports use of these products at the time of initial therapy in all sites probing 5 mm or greater. Although this may be true, use of these products in this manner would be cost-prohibitive for many patients. Despite the inherent drawbacks of systemic antibiotic use, even the costliest of systemic antibiotics are less expensive than the costs of professional administration of controlled-release agents in just a few sites. For these reasons, the use of controlled drug delivery should probably be reserved for isolated sites that fail to respond to initial therapy, for periodontal maintenance patients with localized areas demonstrating disease recurrence, and for patients who refuse recommended surgical treatment or are not good surgical candidates because of inadequate plaque control, smoking, or systemic disease.

## HOST MODULATION THERAPY

Studies on experimental gingivitis in the 1960s gave the first concrete evidence of the bacterial etiology of periodontal diseases. From these landmark studies and those that were to follow, the universal theme in periodontics was that periodontal destruction was directly related to the presence of subgingival pathogenic bacteria and accumulated bacterial byproducts. If the bacterial challenge could be controlled, periodontal attachment loss could either be prevented or arrested. Treatment focused on the reduction of the bacterial load by nonsurgical or surgical procedures. However, this disease paradigm failed to explain the variance in disease progression and severity of periodontal destruction seen among the population. And providers were often at a loss trying to explain why some individuals were resistant to periodontal breakdown despite abundant plaque accumulation, whereas others failed to respond to all treatment measures despite demonstrating good plaque control. Contemporary research now suggests that bacteria alone are not sufficient for the initiation of periodontal destruction and that the host response to the bacterial challenge appears to be critical in the initiation and progression of periodontal diseases.[134] Although the host inflammatory response to periodontal pathogens is largely protective in preventing periodontal breakdown, a prolonged and exuberant host response to the bacterial challenge can result in loss of connective tissue attachment and alveolar bone. Bacterial antigens (i.e., lipopolysaccharides) from Gram-negative anaerobes in the subgingival flora initiate an inflammatory cascade, resulting in an accumulation of host inflammatory cells, largely PMNs, in the area of challenge. These inflammatory cells respond by the release of inflammatory mediators including proinflammatory cytokines (interleukin 1$\beta$, interleukin 6, and tumor necrosis factor $\alpha$), prostaglandin E$_2$, and proteolytic enzymes known as MMPs. This results in pathologic alterations of bone and connective tissue metabolism, with the end result being loss of collagen from the periodontal ligament and gingiva and alveolar bone destruction.[135]

MMPs are a family of proteolytic enzymes that mediate the turnover of collagen and bone under normal physiologic conditions, but overproduction of MMPs can lead to excessive destruction of collagen. MMP-8, MMP-9, and MMP-13 are most closely linked with active periodontal breakdown. MMP-8 and MMP-9 (collagenase and gelatinase, respectively) are both produced by PMNs and are the predominant MMPs found in the GCF. Another collagenase, MMP-13, is produced by bone and epithelial cells, mediates pathologic bone loss, and is the predominant MMP found in inflamed gingival connective tissue.

Studies by Golub and coworkers[136,137] demonstrated the ability of tetracylines to inhibit connective tissue loss and bone destruction in several inflammatory diseases, including periodontitis. Interestingly, the inhibition of connective tissue and bone destruction was unrelated to the antimicrobial activity of tetracycline.[138] Pilot studies determined that subantimicrobial doses of tetracyclines could reduce GCF collagenases and enhance mechanical therapy by inhibiting MMP production and release. These studies also showed that doxycycline was the most potent among the tetracyclines in inhibiting MMP activity.[138-140] Subantimicrobial levels of tetracyclines also will inhibit osteoclast activation, thereby reducing bone resorption. Clinical trials were undertaken to determine safety and effectiveness of subantimicrobial dose doxycycline (SDD) in conjunction with mechanical therapy in patients with chronic periodontitis.[141,142] The U.S. Food and Drug Administration gave final approval for adjunctive use of subantimicrobial dose doxycycline (Periostat, CollaGenex Pharmaceuticals, Newtown, PA) for the treatment of chronic periodontitis in 1998.

Periostat is 20 mg of doxycycline hyclate to be taken twice daily. This 20-mg doxycycline twice daily dose will achieve a steady-state plasma concentration of 0.40 μg/mL. Plasma levels peak at 0.65 μg/mL 2 hours after ingestion and fall to 0.40 μg/mL in 4 to 6 hours, well below the minimum antimicrobial level for doxycycline of 1 μg/mL. A randomized double-blind, placebo-controlled multicenter study[141] was conducted to evaluate the efficacy of SDD on 190 patients with evidence of chronic periodontitis (clinical attachment level and probing depths between 5 and 9 mm). After scaling and root planing, patients randomly received SDD 20 mg twice daily or a placebo for 9 months. Clinical measurements and microbial assessments were performed at baseline, and at 3, 6, and 9 months. For pockets initially measuring 4 to 6 mm, probing depths and clinical attachment gains were significantly better for the SDD group compared with the control group (0.95 mm versus 0.69 mm, 1.03 mm versus 0.86 mm, respectively). Results were improved for pockets of 7 mm or greater for both pocket depth reduction (1.68 mm versus 1.20 mm) and attachment gain (1.55 mm versus 1.17 mm). Patients treated with SDD showed a higher percentage of sites with pocket depth reductions of 2 mm or more (30% versus 22%) than did the placebo group. Similar to findings with adjunctive use of systemic antibiotics and controlled drug delivery, the clinical improvements, although statistically significant, were relatively small in magnitude after use of SDD. No shifts in the periodontal flora or development of microbial doxycycline resistance were found, confirming that the improvements were not caused by any antimicrobial effects of SDD.

The dosing recommendation for Periostat is 20 mg, twice daily for 3 to 9 months. The proper length of administration of Periostat has not yet been clearly established, and no tests are readily available to monitor clinical GCF collagenase inhibition. Treatment with SDD for 9 months is clearly more expensive than systemic antibiotic therapy, although short-term use of systemic antibiotics have demonstrated at least comparable (and often better) improvement of clinical parameters than SDD.[143] At this time, the best indications for the use of host modulation with SDD is for patients with systemic disease complications (i.e., poorly controlled diabetics), for patients with moderate to advanced periodontitis who have demonstrated minimal to no response to nonsurgical therapy and are not good candidates for surgical intervention because of poor plaque control or smoking, and for maintenance patients demonstrating continued attachment loss despite good compliance.

Other agents that may be of potential benefit in the modulation of the host inflammatory response are the nonsteroidal anti-inflammatory drugs and the bisphosphonates. Nonsteroidal anti-inflammatory drugs are used in medicine and dentistry as analgesics but may offer some hope for treating chronic inflammatory diseases (including periodontitis) because of their anti-inflammatory properties. These drugs inhibit the production of proinflammatory mediators, such as prostaglandin $E_2$ and prostacyclin, which will activate osteoclasts and trigger bone resorption. However, the benefit of nonsteroidal anti-inflammatory drugs in the treatment of periodontal diseases has yet to be determined, as study results on these agents have been mixed. Most studies have shown no differences from control subjects regarding most clinical measurements with the exception of osseous support.[144] These studies consistently demonstrate less alveolar bone loss when nonsteroidal anti-inflammatory agents have been used.

Bisphosphonates are bone-sparing agents that have been used with increasing frequency to treat a variety of metabolic bone diseases, including osteoporosis, and are also used in the management of metastatic malignancies. Bisphosphonates bind to calcium and are concentrated in bone. Although their complete mechanism of action is not fully understood, bisphosphonates decrease bone resorption by inhibiting osteoclastic activity. Preliminary studies using adjunctive bisphosphonates for chronic periodontitis show promise in limiting alveolar bone loss.[145] Recent reports, however, noted an association between bisphosphonate use and alveolar osteonecrosis.[146,147] The largest case series of bisphosphonate-induced osteonecrosis was that of Ruggiero and coworkers,[146] who reported on 63 cases of osteonecrosis of the jaws. Although 56 of the 63 reported cases had received intravenous bisphosphonates for management of osteolytic malignant metastases, 7 of the patients with oral osteonecrotic lesions had taken oral bisphosphonates with no history of malignancy.

Although both nonsteroidal anti-inflammatory drugs and bisphosphonates offer some promise in periodontal disease management, additional studies are needed to fully evaluate their use and safety as adjunctive agents. It is also possible that in the future, these and other drugs may be used not only to prevent bone loss observed in periodontal diseases and even around implants but also to possibly stimulate new bone formation.

## CONCLUSIONS

Inflammatory periodontal diseases are caused by complex interactions among numerous bacterial species, leading to inflammatory host responses that result in destruction of the attachment apparatus of the periodontium. Treatment by traditional methods of subgingival root debridement, sometimes including surgical interventions, is an effective means of adequately controlling the disease process for many patients. Patients need to be informed of their role and responsibility in the treatment of their periodontal problems to include adequate plaque control measures and smoking cessation. The use of topically applied and systemically delivered antimicrobial agents in addition to modulation of the host inflammatory response should be part of the treatment strategy for patients with aggressive forms of periodontal diseases or for those who otherwise fail to respond to mechanical forms of therapy. Disruption and reduction of the subgingival biofilms by root debridement are crucial for optimal effectiveness of adjunctive antimicrobial or host modulation therapy. Because the magnitude of additional clinical improvements from most forms of adjunctive therapy are typically on the range of 0.3 to 0.7 mm more than scaling and root planing alone, the clinical significance of this benefit has yet to be fully explored, and, therefore, the ethical and judicious use of these agents is imperative. Additional developments from clinical research on antimicrobial and host modulation strategies may prove beneficial in arresting and even reversing the damages from periodontal diseases in the future.

## REFERENCES

1. Cobb CM. Clinical significance of non-surgical periodontal therapy: an evidence-based perspective of scaling and root planing. J Clin Periodontol 2002;29(Suppl 2):6–16.
2. Buchanon SA, Robertson PB. Calculus removal by scaling/root planing with and without surgical access. J Periodontol 1987;58:159–163.
3. Kepic TJ, O'Leary, TJ, Kafwary AH. Total calculus removal: an attainable objective? J Periodontol 1990;40:16–20.
4. Rabanni GM, Ash MM, Caffesse, RG. The effectiveness of subgingival scaling and root planing in calculus removal. J Periodontol 1981;52: 119–123.
5. Haffajee AD, Cugini MA, Dilbart S, Smith C, Kent RI, Socransky SS. The effect of SRP on the clinical and microbiologic parameters of periodontal diseases. J Clin Periodontol 1997;24:324–334.
6. Renvert S, Wikström M, Dahlen G, Slots J, Egelberg J. Effect of root debridement of the elimination of Actinobacillus actinomycetemcomitans and Bacteroides gingivalis from periodontal pockets. J Clin Periodontol 1990;17:345–350.
7. Sbordone L, Ramaglia L, Gulletta E, Iacono V. Recolonization of the subgingival microflora after scaling and root planing in human periodontitis. J Periodontol 1990;61:579–584.
8. van Winkelhoff AJ, van der Velden U, de Graaff J. Microbial succession in recolonizing deep periodontal pockets after a single course of supra- and subgingival debridement. J Clin Periodontol 1988;15: 116–122.
9. Adriens PA, Edwards CA, De Boever, JA, Loesche WJ. Ultrastructural observations on bacterial invasion in cementum and radicular dentin of periodontally diseased human teeth. J Periodontol 1988; 59:493–503.
10. Quirynen M, De Soete M, Dierickx K, van Steenberghe D. The intra-oral translocation of periodontopathogens jeopardizes the outcome of periodontal therapy. A review of the literature. J Clin Periodontol 2001;28:499–507.
11. Wylam JM, Mealey BL, Mills MP, Waldrop TC, Moskowicz DC. The clinical effectiveness of open versus closed scaling and root planing on multirooted teeth. J Periodontol 1993;64:1023–1028.
12. Parashis AO, Anagnou-Vareltzides A, Demetriou N. Calculus removal from multirooted teeth with and without surgical access. II. Comparison between external and furcation surfaces and effect of furcation entrance width. J Clin Periodontol 1993;20: 294–298.
13. Socransky SS, Haffajee AD. Dental Biofilms: difficult therapeutic targets. Periodontol 2000 2002; 28:12–55.
14. Brooun A, Liu S, Lewis K. A dose-response study of antibiotic resistance in Pseudomonas aeruginosa biofilms. Antimicrob Agents Chemother 2000;44: 640–646.
15. Lobene RR. The effect of pulsed water pressure cleansing on oral health. J Periodontol 1969;40: 51–54.
16. Flemmig TF, Newman MG, Doherty FM, Grossman E, Mechkel AH, Bakdash MB. Supragingival irrigation with 0.06% chlorhexidine in naturally occurring gingivitis: I. Six month clinical observations. J Periodontol 1990;61:112–117.
17. Chaves ES, Kornman KS, Manwell MA, Jones, AA, Newbold DA, Wood RC. Mechanism of irrigation effects on gingivitis. J Periodontol 1994;65: 1016–1021.
18. Cobb CM, Rodgers RL, Killoty WJ. Ultrastructural examination of human periodontal pockets following the use of an oral irrigation device in vivo. J Periodontol 1988;59:155–163.
19. Eakle WS, Ford C, Boyd RL. Depth of penetration in periodontal pockets with oral irrigation. J Clin Periodontol 1986;13:39–44.
20. Boyd RL, Hollander BN, Eakle WS. Comparison of subgingivally placed cannula oral irrigator tip with a supragingival placed standard irrigator tip. J Clin Periodontol 1992;19:340–344.

21. Braun RE, Ciancio SG. Subgingival delivery by an oral irrigation device. J Periodontol 1992;63: 469–472.
22. Jolkovsky DL, Waki MY, Newman MG, et al. Clinical and microbiological effects of subgingival and gingival marginal irrigation with chlorhexidine gluconate. J Periodontol 1990;61:663–669.
23. Wennström JL, Dahlen G, Gröndahl K, Heijl L. Periodic subgingival antimicrobial irrigation of pockets. II. Microbiologic and radiographical observations. J Clin Periodontol 1987;14:573–580.
24. MacAlpine R, Magnusson I, Kiger R, Crigger M, Garrett S, Egelberg J. Antimicrobial irrigation of deep pockets to supplement oral hygiene instruction and root debridement. I. Bi-weekly irrigation. J Clin Periodontol 1985;12:568–577.
25. Denton GW. Chlorhexidine. In: Block SS, ed. Disinfection, Sterilization and Preservation, 4th ed. Philadelphia: Lea and Febiger, 1991:274–289.
26. Grossman E, Reiter G, Weijden GA, Sturzenberger OP, Bollmer BW. Six-month study on the effects of a chlorhexidine mouthrinse on gingivitis in adults. J Periodont Res 1986;21:33–41.
27. Schlagenhauf U, Stellwag P, Fiedler A. Subgingival irrigation in the maintenance phase of periodontal therapy. J Clin Periodontol 1990;17:650–653.
28. Southard SR, Drisko CL, Killoy WJ, Cobb CM, Tira DE. The effect of 2% chlorhexidine digluconate irrigation on clinical parameters and the level of Bacteroides gingivalis in periodontal pockets. J Periodontol 1989;60:302–309.
29. Grossi SG, Skrepcinski FB, DeCaro T, Robertson DC, Ho AW, Dunford RG, Genco RJ. Treatment of periodontal disease in diabetics reduces glycated hemoglobin. J Periodontol 1997;68:713–719.
30. Reynolds MA, Lavigne CK, Minah GE, Suzuki JB. Clinical effects of simultaneous ultrasonic scaling and subgingival irrigation with chlorhexidine. Mediating influence of periodontal probing depth. J Clin Periodontol 1992;19:595–600.
31. Rolla G, Loe H, Schiott CR. The affinity of chlorhexidine for hydroxyapatite and salivary mucins. J Periodontal Res 1970;5:90–95.
32. Gordon JM, Lamster IB, Seiger MC. Efficacy of Listerine antiseptic in inhibiting the development of plaque and gingivitis. J Clin Periodontol 1985; 12:697–704.
33. Roberts WR, Addy M. Comparison of the in vivo and in vitro antibacterial properties of antiseptic mouthrinses containing chlorhexidine, alexidine, cetyl pyridinium chloride and hexetidine. Relevance to mode of action. J Clin Periodontol 1981;8: 295–310.
34. Lobene RR, Kashket S, Soparkar PM, Shloss J, Sabine ZM. The effect of cetylpridinium chloride on human plaque bacteria and gingivitis. Pharmacol Ther Dent 1979;4:33–47.
35. Schreier H, Erdos G, Reimer K, Konig B, Konig W, Fleischer W. Molecular effects of povidone-iodine on relevant microorganisms: an electron-microscopic and biochemical study. Dermatology 1997;195 (Suppl 2):111–116.

36. Lanker-Klossner B, Widmer HR, Frey F. Nondevelopment of resistance by bacteria during hospital use of povidone-iodine. Dermatology 1997; 195(Suppl 2):10–13.
37. Randall E, Brenman HS. Local degerming with povidone-iodine, I. Prior to dental prophylaxis. J Periodontol 1974;45:866–869.
38. Clark WB, Magnusson I, Walker CB, Marks RG. Efficacy of Perimed antibacterial system on established gingivitis. (I). Clinical results. J Clin Periodontol 1989;16:630–635.
39. Keosian J, Rafel S, Weinman I. The effect of aqueous diatomic iodine mouth washes on the incidence of postextraction bacteremia. Oral Surg Oral Med Oral Pathol 1956;9:1337–1341.
40. Scopp IW, Orvieto LD. Gingival degerming by povidone-iodine irrigation: bacteremia reduction in extraction procedures. J Am Dent Assoc 1971;83: 1294–1296.
41. Witzenberger T, O'Leary TJ, Gillette WB. Effect of a local germicide on the occurrence of bacteremia during subgingival scaling. J Periodontol 1982;53: 172–179.
42. Christersson LA, Rosling BG, Dunford RG, Wikesjo UM, Zambon JJ, Genco RJ. Monitoring of subgingival Bacteroides gingivalis and Actinobacillus actinomycetemcomitans in the management of advanced periodontitis. Adv Dent Res 1988;2:382–388.
43. Rosling B, Hellstrom MK, Ramberg P, Socransky SS, Lindhe J. The use of PVP-iodine as an adjunct to non-surgical treatment of chronic periodontitis. J Clin Periodontol 2001;28:1023–1031.
44. Slots J. Selection of antimicrobial agents in periodontal therapy. J Periodontal Res 2002;37: 389–398.
45. Nobukuni K, Hayakawa N, Namba R, Ihara Y, Sato K, Takada H, Hayabara T, Kawahara S. The influence of long-term treatment with povidone-iodine on thyroid function. Dermatology 1997;195 (Suppl 2):69–72.
46. Linder N, Davidovitch N, Reichman B, Kuint J, Lubin D, Meyerovitch J, Sela BA, Dolfin Z, Sack J. Topical iodine-containing antiseptics and subclinical hypothyroidism in preterm infants. J Pediatr 1997;131:434–439.
47. Beiswanger BB, Doyle PM, Jackson RD, Mallatt ME, Mau M, Bollmer BW, Crisanti MM, Guay CB, Lanzalaco AC, Lukacovic MF, et al. The clinical effect of dentifrices containing stabilized stannous fluoride on plaque formation and gingivitis—a six-month study with ad libitum brushing. J Clin Dent 1995;6(Spec No):46–53.
48. Perlich MA, Bacca LA, Bollmer BW, Lanzalaco AC, McClanahan SF, Sewak LK, Beiswanger BB, Eichold WA, Hull JR, Jackson RD, et al. The clinical effect of a stabilized stannous fluoride dentifrice on plaque formation, gingivitis and gingival bleeding: a six-month study. J Clin Dent 1995;6(Spec No):54–58.
49. Ciancio SG, Shibly O, Mather ML, Bessinger MA, Severo NC, Slivka J. Clinical effects of a stannous

fluoride mouthrinse on plaque. Clin Prev Dent 1992;14:27–30.

50. Mazza JE, Newman MG, Sims TN. Clinical and antimicrobial effect of stannous fluoride on periodontitis. J Clin Periodontol 1981;8:203–212.

51. Volpe AR, Petrone ME, De Vizio W, Davies RM, Proskin HM. Review of plaque, gingivitis, calculus and caries clinical efficacy studies with a fluoride dentifrice containing triclosan and PVM/MA copolymer. Clin Dent 1996;7(Suppl):S1–S14.

52. Cubells AB, Dalmau LB, Petrone ME, Chaknis P, Volpe AR. The effect of a triclosan/copolymer/fluoride dentifrice on plaque formation and gingivitis: a six-month clinical study. J Clin Dent 1991;2:63–69.

53. Slots J, Jorgensen MG. Effective, safe, practical and affordable periodontal antimicrobial therapy: where are we going, and are we there yet? Periodontol 2000 2002;28:298–312.

54. Rutala WA, Cole EC, Thomann CA, Weber DJ. Stability and bactericidal activity of chlorine solutions. Infect Control Hosp Epidemiol 1998;19: 323–327.

55. Sarbinoff JA, O'Leary TJ, Miller CH. The comparative effectiveness of various agents in detoxifying diseased root surfaces. J Periodontol 1983;54: 77–80.

56. McKenna PJ, Lehr GS, Leist P, Welling RE. Antiseptic effectiveness with fibroblast preservation. Ann Plast Surg 1991;27:265–268.

57. Wennström JL, Dahlen G, Gröndahl K, Heijl L. Periodic subgingival antimicrobial irrigation of periodontal pockets (I). Clinical observations. J Clin Periodontol 1987;14:541–550.

58. Weitzman SA, Weitberg AB, Stossel TP, Schwartz J, Shklar G. Effects of hydrogen peroxide on oral carcinogenesis in hamsters. J Periodontol 1986;57:685–688.

59. Marshall MV, Cancro LP, Fischman SL. Hydrogen peroxide: a review of its use in dentistry. J Periodontol 1995;66:786–796.

60. Feres M, Haffajee AD, Allard K, Som S, Goodson JM, Socransky SS. Change in subgingival microbial profiles in adult periodontitis subjects receiving either systemically-administered amoxicillin or metronidazole. J Clin Periodontol 2001;28: 597–609.

61. Haffajee AD, Dibart S, Kent RL Jr, Socransky SS. Clinical and microbiological changes associated with the use of 4 adjunctive systemically administered agents in the treatment of periodontal infections. J Clin Periodontol 1995;22:618–627.

62. Loesche WJ, Giordano JR, Hujoel P, Schwarcz J, Smith BA. Metronidazole in periodontitis: reduced need for surgery. J Clin Periodontol 1992;19: 103–112.

63. Loesche WJ, Giordano JR, Soehren S, Kaciroti N. The nonsurgical treatment of patients with periodontal disease: results after five years. J Am Dent Assoc 2002;133:311–320.

64. van Winkelhoff AJ, Rams TE, Slots J. Systemic antibiotic therapy in periodontics. Periodontol 2000 1996;10:45–78.

65. Slots J, Ting M. Systemic antibiotics in the treatment of periodontal disease. Periodontol 2000 2002; 28:106–176.

66. Offenbacher S, Katz V, Fertik G, Collins J, Boyd D, Maynor G, McKaig R, Beck J. Periodontal infection as a possible risk factor for preterm low birth weight. J Periodontol 1996;67(10 Suppl):1103–1113.

67. Beck J, Garcia R, Heiss G, Vokonas PS, Offenbacher S. Periodontal disease and cardiovascular disease. J Periodontol 1996;67(10 Suppl): 1123–1137.

68. Taylor GW. Bidirectional interrelationships between diabetes and periodontal diseases: an epidemiologic perspective. Ann Periodontol 2001;6:99–112.

69. Kuramitsu HK, Miyakawa H, Qi M, Kang IC. Cellular responses to oral pathogens. Ann Periodontol 2002;7:90–94.

70. Collins JG, Offenbacher S, Arnold RR. Effects of a combination therapy to eliminate *Porphyromonas gingivalis* in refractory periodontitis. J Periodontol 1993;64:998–1007.

71. Winkel EG, van Winkelhoff AJ, Barendregt DS, van der Weijden GA, Timmerman MF, van der Velden U. Clinical and microbiological effects of initial periodontal therapy in conjunction with amoxicillin and clavulanic acid in patients with adult periodontitis. A randomised double-blind, placebo-controlled study. J Clin Periodontol 1999;2:461–468.

72. Tenenbaum H, Jehl F, Gallion C, Dahan M. Amoxicillin and clavulanic acid concentrations in gingival crevicular fluid. J Clin Periodontol 1997; 24:804–807.

73. Gordon JM, Walker CB, Murphy JC, Goodson JM, Socransky SS. Tetracycline: levels achievable in gingival crevice fluid and in vitro effect on subgingival organisms. Part I. Concentrations in crevicular fluid after repeated doses. J Periodontol 1981; 52:609–612.

74. Sakellari D, Goodson JM, Kolokotronis A, Konstantinidis A. Concentration of 3 tetracyclines in plasma, gingival crevice fluid and saliva. J Clin Periodontol 2000;27:53–60.

75. Hellden LB, Listgarten MA, Lindhe J. The effect of tetracycline and/or scaling on human periodontal disease. J Clin Periodontol 1979;6:222–230.

76. Muller HP, Lange DE, Muller RF. A 2-year study of adjunctive minocycline-HCl in *Actinobacillus actinomycetemcomitans*-associated periodontitis. J Periodontol 1993;64:509–519.

77. Ng VW, Bissada NF. Clinical evaluation of systemic doxycycline and ibuprofen administration as an adjunctive treatment for adult periodontitis. J Periodontol 1998;69:772–776.

78. Ramberg P, Rosling B, Serino G, Hellstrom MK, Socransky SS, Lindhe J. The long-term effect of systemic tetracycline used as an adjunct to non-surgical treatment of advanced periodontitis. J Clin Periodontol 2001;28:446–452.

79. Haffajee AD, Socransky SS, Dibart S, Kent RL Jr. Response to periodontal therapy in patients with high or low levels of *P. gingivalis, P. intermedia,*

*P. nigrescens* and *B. forsythus*. J Clin Periodontol 1996;23:336–345.

80. Feres M, Haffajee AD, Goncalves C, Allard KA, Som S, Smith C, Goodson JM, Socransky SS. Systemic doxycycline administration in the treatment of periodontal infections (I). Effect on the subgingival microbiota. J Clin Periodontol 1999;26:775–783.

81. Lindhe J, Liljenberg B, Adielsson B. Effect of long-term tetracycline therapy on human periodontal disease. J Clin Periodontol 1983;10:590–601.

82. Listgarten MA, Lindhe J, Hellden L. Effect of tetracycline and/or scaling on human periodontal disease. Clinical, microbiological, and histological observations. J Clin Periodontol 1978;5:246–271.

83. Novak MJ, Stamatelakys C, Adair SM. Resolution of early lesions of juvenile periodontitis with tetracycline therapy alone: long-term observations of 4 cases. J Periodontol 1991;62:628–633. Erratum in: J Periodontol 1992;63:148.

84. Van Oosten MA, Notten FJ, Mikx FH. Metronidazole concentrations in human plasma, saliva, and gingival crevice fluid after a single dose. J Dent Res 1986;65:1420–1423.

85. Gusberti FA, Syed SA, Lang NP. Combined antibiotic (metronidazole) and mechanical treatment effects on the subgingival bacterial flora of sites with recurrent periodontal disease. J Clin Periodontol 1988;15:353–359.

86. Lopez NJ, Gamonal JA, Martinez B. Repeated metronidazole and amoxicillin treatment of periodontitis. A follow-up study. J Periodontol 2000;71:79–89.

87. Elter JR, Lawrence HP, Offenbacher S, Beck JD. Meta-analysis of the effect of systemic metronidazole as an adjunct to scaling and root planing for adult periodontitis. J Periodontal Res 1997;32:487–496.

88. Winkel EG, Van Winkelhoff AJ, Timmerman MF, Van der Velden U, Van der Weijden GA. Amoxicillin plus metronidazole in the treatment of adult periodontitis patients. A double-blind placebo-controlled study. J Clin Periodontol 2001;28:296–305.

89. Loesche WJ, Syed SA, Morrison EC, Kerry GA, Higgins T, Stoll J. Metronidazole in periodontitis. I. Clinical and bacteriological results after 15 to 30 weeks. J Periodontol 1984;55:325–335.

90. Soder PO, Frithiof L, Wikner S, Wouters F, Engstrom PE, Rubin B, Nedlich U, Soder B. The effect of systemic metronidazole after non-surgical treatment in moderate and advanced periodontitis in young adults. J Periodontol 1990;61:281–288.

91. van Winkelhoff AJ, Tijhof CJ, de Graaff J. Microbiological and clinical results of metronidazole plus amoxicillin therapy in *Actinobacillus actinomycetemcomitans*-associated periodontitis. J Periodontol 1992;63:52–57.

92. Blandizzi C, Malizia T, Lupetti A, Pesce D, Gabriele M, Giuca MR, Campa M, Del Tacca M, Senesi S Periodontal tissue disposition of azithromycin in patients affected by chronic inflammatory periodontal diseases. J Periodontol 1999;70:960–966.

93. Smith SR, Foyle DM, Daniels J, Joyston-Bechal S, Smales FC, Sefton A, Williams J. A double-blind placebo-controlled trial of azithromycin as an adjunct to non-surgical treatment of periodontitis in adults: clinical results. J Clin Periodontol 2002;29:54–61.

94. Sefton AM, Maskell JP, Beighton D, Whiley A, Shain H, Foyle D, Smith SR, Smales FC, Williams JD. Azithromycin in the treatment of periodontal disease. Effect on microbial flora. J Clin Periodontol 1996;23:998–1003.

95. Gordon J, Walker C, Lamster I, West T, Socransky S, Seiger M, Fasciano R. Efficacy of clindamycin hydrochloride in refractory periodontitis. 12-month results. J Periodontol 1985;56(11 Suppl):75–80.

96. Walker C, Gordon J. The effect of clindamycin on the microbiota associated with refractory periodontitis. J Periodontol 1990;61:692–698.

97. Slots J, Feik D, Rams TE. In vitro antimicrobial sensitivity of enteric rods and pseudomonads from advanced adult periodontitis. Oral Microbiol Immunol 1990;5:298–301.

98. Beikler T, Prior K, Ehmke B, Flemmig TF. Specific antibiotics in the treatment of periodontitis—a proposed strategy. J Periodontol 2004;75:169–175.

99. Checchi L, Trombelli L, Nonato M. Postoperative infections and tetracycline prophylaxis in periodontal surgery: a retrospective study. Quintessence Int 1992;23:191–195.

100. Powell CA, Mealey BL, Deas DE, McDonnell HT, Moritz AJ. Post-surgical infections: prevalence associated with various periodontal surgical procedures. J Periodontol 2005;76:329–333.

101. Demolon IA, Persson GR, Ammons WF, Johnson RH. Effects of antibiotic treatment on clinical conditions with guided tissue regeneration: one-year results. J Periodontol 1994;65:713–717.

102. Sculean A, Blaes A, Arweiler N, Reich E, Donos N, Brecx M. The effect of postsurgical antibiotics on the healing of intrabony defects following treatment with enamel matrix proteins. J Periodontol 2001;72:190–195.

103. Vest TM, Greenwell H, Drisko C, Wittwer JW, Bichara J, Yancey J, Goldsmith J, Rebitski G. The effect of postsurgical antibiotics and a bioabsorbable membrane on regenerative healing in Class II furcation defects. J Periodontol 1999;70:878–887.

104. Dent CD, Olson JW, Farish SE, Bellome J, Casino AJ, Morris HF, Ochi S. The influence of preoperative antibiotics on success of endosseous implants up to and including stage II surgery: a study of 2,641 implants. J Oral Maxillofac Surg 1997;55(Suppl 5):19–24.

105. Laskin DM, Dent CD, Morris HF, Ochi S, Olson JW. The influence of preoperative antibiotics on success of endosseous implants at 36 months. Ann Periodontol 2000;5:166–174.

106. Gynther GW, Kondell PA, Moberg LE, Heimdahl A. Dental implant installation without antibiotic prophylaxis. Oral Surg Oral Med Oral Pathol Oral Radiol Endod 1998;85:509–511.

107. Esposito M, Coulthard P, Oliver R, Thomsen P, Worthington HV. Antibiotics to prevent complications following dental implant treatment. Cochrane Database Syst Rev 2003;3:CD004152.

108. Dajani AS, Taubert KA, Wilson W, Bolger AF, Bayer A, Ferrieri P, Gewitz MH, Shulman ST, Nouri S, Newburger JW, Hutto C, Pallasch TJ, Gage TW, Levison ME, Peter G, Zuccaro G Jr. Prevention of bacterial endocarditis: recommendations by the American Heart Association. J Am Dent Assoc 1997;128:1142–1151.

109. American Dental Association; American Academy of Orthopedic Surgeons. Antibiotic prophylaxis for dental patients with total joint replacements. J Am Dent Assoc 2003;134:895–899.

110. Tonetti M, Cugini MA, Goodson JM. Zero-order delivery with periodontal placement of tetracycline-loaded ethylene vinyl acetate fibers. J Periodontal Res 1990;25:243–249.

111. Rapley JW, Cobb CM, Killoy WJ, Williams DR. Serum levels of tetracycline during treatment with tetracycline-containing fibers. J Periodontol 1992; 63:817–820.

112. Goodson JM, Cugini MA, Kent RL, Armitage GC, Cobb CM, Fine D, Fritz ME, Green E, Imoberdorf MJ, Killoy WJ, et al. Multicenter evaluation of tetracycline fiber therapy: II. Clinical response. J Periodontal Res 1991;26:371–379.

113. Heijl L, Dahlen G, Sundin Y, Wenander A, Goodson JM. A 4-quadrant comparative study of periodontal treatment using tetracycline-containing drug delivery fibers and scaling. J Clin Periodontol 1991;18:111–116.

114. Newman MG, Kornman KS, Doherty FM. A 6-month multi-center evaluation of adjunctive tetracycline fiber therapy used in conjunction with scaling and root planing in maintenance patients: clinical results. J Periodontol 1994;65:685–691.

115. Drisko CL, Cobb CM, Killoy WJ, Michalowicz BS, Pihlstrom BL, Lowenguth RA, Caton JG, Encarnacion M, Knowles M, Goodson JM. Evaluation of periodontal treatments using controlled-release tetracycline fibers: clinical response. J Periodontol 1995;66:692–699.

116. Vandekerckhove BN, Quirynen M, van Steenberghe D. The use of tetracycline-containing controlled-release fibers in the treatment of refractory periodontitis. J Periodontol 1997;68: 353–361.

117. Stoller NH, Johnson LR, Trapnell S, Harrold CQ, Garrett S. The pharmacokinetic profile of a biodegradable controlled-release delivery system containing doxycycline compared to systemically delivered doxycycline in gingival crevicular fluid, saliva, and serum. J Periodontol 1998;69: 1085–1091.

118. Polson AM, Southard GL, Dunn RL, Yewey GL, Godowski KC, Polson AP, Fulfs JC, Laster L. Periodontal pocket treatment in beagle dogs using subgingival doxycycline from a biodegradable system. I. Initial clinical responses. J Periodontol 1996;67:1176–1184.

119. Garrett S, Johnson L, Drisko CH, Adams DF, Bandt C, Beiswanger B, Bogle G, Donly K, Hallmon WW, Hancock EB, Hanes P, Hawley CE, Kiger R, Killoy W, Mellonig JT, Polson A, Raab FJ, Ryder M, Stoller NH, Wang HL, Wolinsky LE, Evans GH, Harrold CQ, Arnold RM, Southard GL, et al. Two multi-center studies evaluating locally delivered doxycycline hyclate, placebo control, oral hygiene, and scaling and root planing in the treatment of periodontitis. J Periodontol 1999;70: 490–503.

120. Garrett S, Adams DF, Bogle G, Donly K, Drisko CH, Hallmon WW, Hancock EB, Hanes P, Hawley CE, Johnson L, Kiger R, Killoy W, Mellonig JT, Raab FJ, Ryder M, Stoller N, Polson A, Wang HL, Wolinsky LE, Yukna RA, Harrold CQ, Hill M, Johnson VB, Southard GL. The effect of locally delivered controlled-release doxycycline or scaling and root planing on periodontal maintenance patients over 9 months. J Periodontol 2000;71:22–30.

121. Ciancio SG. Local delivery of chlorhexidine. Compend Contin Educ Dent 1999;20:427–432.

122. Soskolne WA, Chajek T, Flashner M, Landau I, Stabholtz A, Kolatch B, Lerner EI. An in vivo study of the chlorhexidine release profile of the PerioChip in the gingival crevicular fluid, plasma and urine. J Clin Periodontol 1998;25:1017–1021.

123. Jeffcoat MK, Bray KS, Ciancio SG, Dentino AR, Fine DH, Gordon JM, Gunsolley JC, Killoy WJ, Lowenguth RA, Magnusson NI, Offenbacher S, Palcanis KG, Proskin HM, Finkelman RD, Flashner M. Adjunctive use of a subgingival controlled-release chlorhexidine chip reduces probing depth and improves attachment level compared with scaling and root planing alone. J Periodontol 1998;69:989–997.

124. Reddy MS, Jeffcoat MK, Geurs NC, Palcanis KG, Weatherford TW, Traxler BM, Finkelman RD. Efficacy of controlled-release subgingival chlorhexidine to enhance periodontal regeneration. J Periodontol 2003;74:411–419.

125. Azmak N, Atilla G, Luoto H, Sorsa T. The effect of subgingival controlled-release delivery of chlorhexidine chip on clinical parameters and matrix metalloproteinase-8 levels in gingival crevicular fluid. J Periodontol 2002;73:608–615.

126. Williams RC, Paquette DW, Offenbacher S, Adams DF, Armitage GC, Bray K, Caton J, Cochran DL, Drisko CH, Fiorellini JP, Giannobile WV, Grossi S, Guerrero DM, Johnson GK, Lamster IB, Magnusson I, Oringer RJ, Persson GR, Van Dyke TE, Wolff LF, Santucci EA, Rodda BE, Lessem J. Treatment of periodontitis by local administration of minocycline microspheres: a controlled trial. J Periodontol 2001;72:1535–1544.

127. Satomi A, Uraguchi R, Noguchi T, , Ishikawa I, Tanaru H, Kitamura M. Minocycline HCl concentration in periodontal pockets after administration of LS-007. J Jpn Assoc Periodontol 1987;29: 937–943.

128. Murayama Y, Nomura Y, Yamaoka A, Ueda M, Hori T, Minabe M, Umemoto T, Ishikawa I,

Uraguchi R, Ueno K, et al. Local administration of minocycline for periodontitis. Double blind comparative study of LS-007. J Jpn Assoc Periodontol 1988;30:206–222.

129. van Steenberghe D, Rosling B, Soder PO, Landry RG, van der Velden U, Timmerman MF, McCarthy EF, Vandenhoven G, Wouters C, Wilson M, Matthews J, Newman HN. A 15-month evaluation of the effects of repeated subgingival minocycline in chronic adult periodontitis. J Periodontol 1999;70:657–667.

130. Kinane DF, Radvar M. A six-month comparison of three periodontal local antimicrobial therapies in persistent periodontal pockets. J Periodontol 1999;70:1–7.

131. Stoltze K. Concentration of metronidazole in periodontal pockets after application of a metronidazole 25% dental gel. J Clin Periodontol 1992;19:698–701.

132. Ainamo J, Lie T, Ellingsen BH, Hansen BF, Johansson LA, Karring T, Kisch J, Paunio K, Stoltze K. Clinical responses to subgingival application of a metronidazole 25% gel compared to the effect of subgingival scaling in adult periodontitis. J Clin Periodontol 1992;19:723–729.

133. Pedrazzoli V, Kilian M, Karring T. Comparative clinical and microbiological effects of topical subgingival application of metronidazole 25% dental gel and scaling in the treatment of adult periodontitis. J Clin Periodontol 1992;19:715–722.

134. Socransky SS, Haffajee AD. Microbial mechanisms in the pathogenesis of destructive periodontal diseases: a critical assessment. J Periodontal Res 1991;26:195–212.

135. Page RC, Kornman KS. The pathogenesis of human periodontitis: an introduction. Periodontol 2000 1997;14:9–11.

136. Golub LM, Lee HM, Lehrer G, Nemiroff A, McNamara TF, Kaplan R, Ramamurthy NS. Minocycline reduces gingival collagenolytic activity during diabetes. Preliminary observations and a proposed new mechanism of action. J Periodontal Res 1983;18:516–526.

137. Golub LM, Ramamurthy NS, McNamara TF, Greenwald RA, Rifkin BR. Tetracyclines inhibit connective tissue breakdown: new therapeutic implications for an old family of drugs. Crit Rev Oral Biol Med 1991;2:297–321.

138. Golub LM, Lee HM, Ryan ME, Giannobile WV, Payne J, Sorsa T. Tetracyclines inhibit connective tissue break down by multiple non-antimicrobial mechanisms. Adv Dent Res 1998;12:12–26.

139. Golub LM, Wolff M, Roberts S, Lee HM, Leung M, Payonk GS. Treating periodontal diseases by blocking tissue-destructive enzymes. J Am Dent Assoc 1994;125:163–169.

140. Ryan ME, Ramamurthy S, Golub LM. Matrix metalloproteinases and their inhibition in periodontal treatment. Curr Opin Periodontol 1996;3:85–96.

141. Caton JG, Ciancio SG, Blieden TM, Bradshaw M, Crout RJ, Hefti AF, Massaro JM, Polson AM, Thomas J, Walker C. Treatment with subantimicrobial dose doxycycline improves the efficacy of scaling and root planing in patients with adult periodontitis. J Periodontol 2000;71:521–532.

142. Caton JG, Ciancio SG, Blieden TM, Bradshaw M, Crout RJ, Hefti AF, Massaro JM, Polson AM, Thomas J, Walker C. Subantimicrobial dose doxycycline as an adjunct to scaling and root planing: post-treatment effects. J Clin Periodontol 2001;28:782–789.

143. Greenstein G, Lamster I. Efficacy of subantimicrobial dosing with doxycycline. Point/counterpoint. J Am Dent Assoc 2001;132:457–466.

144. Reddy MS, Geurs NC, Gunsolley JC. Periodontal host modulation with antiproteinase, anti-inflammatory, and bone-sparing agents. A systematic review. Ann Periodontol 2003;8:12–37.

145. Rocha M, Nava LE, Vazquez de la Torre C, Sanchez-Marin F, Garay-Sevilla ME, Malacara JM. Clinical and radiological improvement of periodontal disease in patients with type 2 diabetes mellitus treated with alendronate: a randomized, placebo-controlled trial. J Periodontol 2001;72:204–209.

146. Ruggiero SL, Mehrotra B, Rosenberg TJ, Engroff SL. Osteonecrosis of the jaws associated with the use of bisphosphonates: a review of 63 cases. J Oral Maxillofac Surg 2004;62:527–534.

147. Migliorati CA, Casiglia J, Epstein J, Jacobsen PL, Seigel MA, Woo SB. Managing the care of patients with bisphosphonate-associated osteonecrosis. An American Academy of Oral Medicine position paper. J Am Dent Assoc 2005;136:1658–1667.

## CHAPTER 10
## REVIEW QUESTIONS

1. What is(are) the rationale(s) for the use of periodontal chemotherapeutic agents?
   a. Complete removal of all hard and soft bacterial deposits from root surfaces is virtually impossible.
   b. Subgingival recolonization and rebound has been found to occur within 6 weeks after subgingival debridement.
   c. Regrowth of bacteria may occur from bacteria residing on the soft tissue pocket wall, from root surface irregularities, or from microbial niches outside of the periodontal pocket.
   d. All of the above are valid rationales for periodontal chemotherapy.

2. Which of the following topical antimicrobial agents demonstrates substantivity up to 12 hours after use?
   a. Chlorhexidine
   b. Essential oils
   c. Cetylpyridinium chloride
   d. Povidone iodine

3. Topical application of agents for periodontal chemotherapy includes:
   a. Mouth rinses
   b. Dentifrices
   c. Oral irrigation
   d. Systemic antibiotics
   e. All of the above
   f. a, b, and c only

4. There are a number of antimicrobial delivery systems that can be used for agent application including oral rinses, gels, dentifrices, oral irrigation, controlled-release devices, and systemic delivery. Of these, which are *primarily* directed against the subgingival bacterial flora?
   a. Oral rinses, dentifrices, and controlled-release devices
   b. Dentifrices, oral irrigation, and systemic delivery
   c. Oral irrigation, controlled-release devices, and systemic delivery
   d. Gels, controlled-release devices, and systemic delivery
   e. All of these delivery systems are directed against the subgingival flora

5. Valid indications for the use of systemic antibiotics in periodontal therapy include:
   a. As an adjunct to nonsurgical and surgical therapy for patients with aggressive forms of periodontitis
   b. For patients with moderate to advanced chronic periodontitis that is not responsive to conventional therapy

   c. Before any periodontal surgery to decrease the incidence of postsurgical infections
   d. a and b only
   e. b and c only
   f. a, b, and c

6. Whenever possible, selection of an appropriate antibiotic for treatment of periodontal infections should be *primarily* based on:
   a. Culture and sensitivity testing
   b. Effectiveness against Gram-positive bacteria
   c. Avoiding antibiotics that interfere with effectiveness of oral contraceptives
   d. Prescription coverage by the patient's insurance

7. Which group of antibiotics is presently used in periodontics for host modulation?
   a. Penicillins
   b. Tetracyclines
   c. Metronidazole
   d. Fluoroquinones

8. Controlled drug delivery devices include all of the following *except*:
   a. Periostat
   b. Arestin
   c. PerioChip
   d. Atridox

9. Current concepts on the initiation and progression of destructive periodontal diseases include that:
   a. Periodontal destruction is directly related to the presence of subgingival pathogenic bacteria and accumulated bacterial byproducts
   b. Periodontal attachment loss can always be prevented or arrested by adequate control of the bacterial challenge
   c. A prolonged and exuberant host response to the bacterial challenge can result in loss of periodontal attachment and alveolar bone
   d. The host inflammatory response to periodontal pathogens protects against periodontal attachment loss if plaque control is adequate

10. Which of the following may be the most *cost-effective* adjunctive agent(s) to treat a patient with generalized aggressive periodontitis?
   a. Controlled drug delivery
   b. Systemic amoxicillin and metronidazole combination
   c. Host modulation therapy
   d. a and b
   e. a and c

# The Role of the Dental Hygienist in Nonsurgical Periodontal Therapy

Elizabeth Hughes

Comprehensive oral care of patients is a challenge for the dental health profession team. Although periodontal disease is only one of the dental diseases of our patient population, its prevention, care, and maintenance are particularly challenging and time consuming. It is imperative that the periodontium be in stable, healthy condition before providing comprehensive restorative care. After diagnosis by the dentist or periodontist, nonsurgical periodontal therapy is an appropriate function of the dental hygienist (Fig. 11-1). In addition to the mechanical removal of hard and soft deposits, the hygienist is prepared to educate the patient in the oral and systemic origins of the disease process and provide individualized home care strategies.

The therapy provided by the dental hygienist for the periodontally involved patient is referred to as nonsurgical periodontal therapy (NSPT), phase I periodontal therapy, initial periodontal therapy, and soft tissue management. For the purposes of this chapter, this therapy will be referred to as NSPT. This phase of treatment includes therapies and instructions that can help bring oral tissues to an improved state of health.

## DEFINITIONS OF SKILLS

- **Oral prophylaxis** is a preventive procedure used for periodontally healthy patients or for patients with gingivitis. It includes supragingival and subgingival scaling with polishing to remove plaque, calculus, and stain.[1]
- **Scaling** is defined by the American Academy of Periodontology as instrumentation of the crown and tooth surfaces of the teeth to remove plaque and calculus.[1]
- **Debridement** is the treatment of gingival and periodontal inflammation through mechanical removal of tooth and root surface deposits and irregularities.[2]
- **Root planing** is a definitive procedure designed for the removal of cementum and dentin that is rough or permeated by calculus or contaminated with toxins or microorganisms.[1]

NSPT includes supragingival scaling, subgingival debridement, possible root planing, and effective dental biofilm control (plaque control; see Chapter 7). Successful outcomes of this therapy are influenced by the patient's understanding of the disease process, a commitment to good oral hygiene practices, and compliance with scheduled appointments.[3,4] The intent is to eliminate or reduce pathogenic microorganisms and create a healthy environment that may inhibit further loss of attachment. NSPT is most effective for treating patients with mild and moderate chronic periodontitis. Aggressive periodontitis and severe chronic periodontitis may be more effectively treated in collaboration with a periodontist.

## PRACTICE PHILOSOPHY

Every dental practice must have an NSPT plan (Fig. 11-2), even if the plan is to refer all periodontally involved patients to a periodontist. The commitment to treat patients with periodontitis is solely dependent on the skills of both the hygienist and the general practice dentist. If the hygienist or the general practice dentist does not believe that he or she has the necessary skills to successfully treat the periodontal patient, these patients might be better served by a referral to a periodontist. The general practice must be willing to commit the required time to treat these patients adequately. The dentist and the dental hygienist as cotherapists,

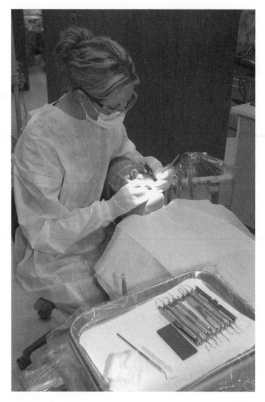

**Figure 11.1** ●

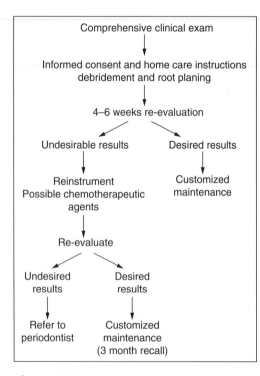

**Figure 11.2** ●

together with all office staff, must develop strategies for patient management (Fig. 11-1). Failure to diagnose and treat periodontal disease puts the practice in legal jeopardy.

The American Academy of Periodontology offers detailed practice parameters to help guide the general practitioner in providing quality, cost-efficient periodontal therapies.[1,5]

Before instituting NSPT, all patients should receive a comprehensive periodontal examination (see Chapter 5). A thorough clinical examination is necessary to determine the severity of disease and to design a therapeutic treatment plan. The examination must include:

- **Chief Complaint:** why is the patient seeking dental care?
- **Medical History**: must be thorough to account for any predisposing conditions that may limit or compromise treatment. Include a consultation with the patient's physician as necessary.
- **Dental History**
- **Clinical Examination**
  - Probing depths
  - Recession
  - Calculation of clinical attachment levels
  - Furcation involvement
  - Mobility
  - Bleeding index
  - Plaque index
  - Hard deposit accumulation
  - Caries
  - Soft tissue lesions
  - Exudates
  - Mucogingival relationships
  - Note any physical disabilities
- **Current Diagnostic Radiographs**

## INFORMED CONSENT

Before initiating the treatment, the patient must be informed of the nature of the disease and the procedures necessary for treatment of their condition. It is imperative that the patient understands the level of commitment required for a successful outcome.[2–4,6] The following items should be included (see Chapter 5):

- Inform the patient of the dentist's diagnosis
- Address all patient concerns; answer patient's questions
- Inform in comprehensible language the recommendations for treatment
- Explain the rationale for treatment recommendations

- Explain the consequences of treatment and of refusal of treatment
- Procure signed and dated written documentation of consent to treat

## PHASES OF PERIODONTAL THERAPY

Traditionally we have separated periodontal therapy into four phases.

- Phase I is nonsurgical periodontal therapy.
- Phase II includes all surgical procedures.
- Phase III addresses all restorative treatment.
- Phase IV is supportive care or maintenance.

The dental hygienist is directly involved in phases I and IV of periodontal therapy.

## GUIDELINES FOR SCHEDULING

Several things should be considered for efficient use of the hygienist's time and to serve the needs of the patient. Sufficient time must be reserved to perform comprehensive NSPT. A variety of treatment experiences within the workday will help diminish operator fatigue. The time reserved for treatment should accommodate the patient's individual requirements, i.e., disease severity, amount of deposits, pain control, and any physical or mental special needs (Table 11-1).

### Phase I

**Patient Education:** Patient education and compliance is important for success in phase I. The dental hygienist is in a unique position on the dental team to help patients understand their responsibility in the healing process. Patients with chronic periodontitis have unique and challenging home care responsibilities. Dental conditions such as furcal involvement, crowding, tooth loss, recession, and deep probing depths require the patient to spend inordinate amounts of time during the at-home cleaning process. Ample time must be allowed in the hygienist's schedule to demonstrate brushing and flossing techniques, the use of any auxiliary aids, and use of any chemotherapeutic agents. It is important to be aware of any physical conditions that could interfere with thorough oral care and to respond to the patient's special needs. During phase I therapy, but not necessarily during the first appointment, the hygienist can offer suggestions for smoking cessation and recommendations for changes in diet, and explain the link between periodontitis and systemic disease (see Chapter 7).

### Instrumentation During Phase I

The dental hygienist should have a variety of hand instruments and powered instruments to address the complex demands of therapy. Meticulous root preparation is very time consuming but essential for soft tissue healing and disease control (see Chapter 8). Typically, the hygienist will schedule a separate appointment for debridement of each quadrant followed by re-evaluation in 4 to 6 weeks.

**Re-evaluation:** The hygienist will compare the attachment levels and number of bleeding sites with the data collected at the initial appointment.

## TABLE 11.1

### Examples of Possible Schedules

| Date | Date | Date |
|---|---|---|
| 8:00 New patient comprehensive examination | 8:00 NSPT Max Rt | 8:00 NSPT re-evaluation |
| 8:30 | | |
| 9:00 Recall patient | | 9:00 NSPT Mand Left |
| 9:30 | 9:30 Recall patient | |
| 9:50 Maintenance patient | | |
| 10:00 | 10:15 Recall patient | 10:00 Recall |
| 10:30 | | |
| 11:00 | | |

Mand Left = left mandible; Max Rt = right maxilla; NSPT = nonsurgical periodontal therapy.

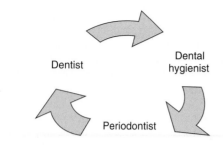

***Figure 11.3*** ●

An evaluation is made of the patient's home care and the thoroughness of the mechanical instrumentation. Additional root planing may be indicated in specific sites that did not respond to the initial instrumentation. The dentist may refer the patient to a specialist for treatment of sites that have not responded, or the patient may be deemed controlled within the general practice.

## Phase IV

This phase of therapy includes those procedures provided after completion of active therapy (see Chapter 23). The customary time between maintenance appointments is generally 3 months, but each patient should be considered according to individual needs.[2-4,6-8] The patient who is unable to achieve adequate oral hygiene may require more frequent visits. If the patient has been treated by a periodontist, it is a common practice to alternate maintenance appointments between the general practice dentist and the periodontist Figure 11.3.

## REFERENCES

1. American Academy of Periodontology 1995; The American Academy of Periodontology. Proceedings of the World Workshop in Clinical Periodontics. Chicago: The American Academy of Periodontology, 1989:1–22; http://www.perio.org/ resources-products/pdf/parameters.pdf; www.perio.org.
2. Stutsman-Young N, O'Hehir TE, Woodall I. Periodontal debridement. In: Woodall I, ed. Comprehensive Dental Hygiene Care, 4th ed. St. Louis: Mosby-Year Book, Inc, 1993.
3. Ramfjord SP. Maintenance care for treated periodontitis patients. J Clin Periodontol 1987;14:433–437.
4. Ramfjord SP, Morrison EC, Burgett FG, Nissle RR, Shick RA, Zann GJ, Knowles JW. Oral hygiene and maintenance of periodontal support. J Periodontol 1982;53:26–30.
5. Parameter on comprehensive periodontal examination. J Periodontol 2000;71(Suppl):847–848; Parameter on periodontal maintenance. J Periodontol 2000;71(Suppl):849–850; Parameter on plaque-induced gingivitis. J Periodontol 2000;71(Suppl):851–852; Parameter on chronic periodontitis with slight to moderate loss of periodontal support. J Periodontol 2000;71(Suppl): 853–855; Parameter on chronic periodontitis with advanced loss of periodontal support. J Periodontol 2000; 71(Suppl):856–858; Parameter on aggressive periodontitis. J Periodontol 2000;71(Suppl):867–869.
6. Wilson TG, Glover ME, Schoen J, Baus C, Jacobs T. Compliance with maintenance therapy in a private periodontal practice. J Periodontol 1984;55:468–473.
7. Wilson TG. Compliance. A review of the literature with possible applications to periodontics. J Periodontol 1987;58;706–714.
8. Wilson T, Hale S, Temple R. The results of efforts to improve compliance with supportive periodontal treatment in a private periodontal practice. J Periodontol 1993;64:311–314.

## SUGGESTED READINGS

1. Darby M, Walsh N. Dental Hygiene Theory and Practice, 2nd ed. Philadelphia: Saunders, 2003: 457–492.
2. Hodges K. Concepts in Nonsurgical Periodontal Therapy. Delmar, 1997:507–527.

## CHAPTER 11
## REVIEW QUESTIONS

1. The general recommendation for maintenance of a periodontally involved patient after initial therapy is:
   a. 1 month
   b. 3 months
   c. 6 months
   d. 12 months

2. Design a comfortable workday schedule of patients for a hygienist in a general dental practice setting. Use an 8-hour workday scheduled in 15-minute intervals. Consider a variety of patient types.

3. The phase(s) of periodontal therapy in which oral hygiene instructions would be given is (are):
   a. Phase I
   b. Phase II
   c. Phase III
   d. Phase IV
   e. Phase I and IV

4. A periodontal treatment plan is not necessary in a general dental practice because the focus of a general practice is restorative dentistry.
   a. True
   b. False

5. The preventive procedure used for periodontally healthy patients or for patients with gingivitis is:
   a. Oral prophylaxis
   b. Debridement
   c. Root planing
   d. Scaling

6. The intentional removal of cementum is part of which procedure?
   a. Scaling
   b. Prophylaxis
   c. Root planing
   d. Debridement

7. The patient returns for an appointment after the initial examination. This is considered consent for treatment.
   a. True
   b. False

8. The dental hygienist may diagnose periodontal disease. The dental hygienist may treat periodontal disease.
   a. Statements 1 and 2 are correct.
   b. Statements 1 and 2 are incorrect.
   c. Statement 1 is correct and statement 2 is incorrect.
   d. Statement 1 is incorrect and statement 2 is correct.

9. Failure to diagnose and treat periodontal disease is a major reason for lawsuits against dentistry.
   a. True
   b. False

10. Severity of periodontitis is measured by:
    a. Recession
    b. Probing depths
    c. Bleeding on probing
    d. Probing depths and recession

# Wound Healing

John Rapley

Surgery causes a disruption of the existing relationship of various cells and tissues of the body. Healing is that phase of the inflammatory response that results in the restoration of the disrupted body elements into a new or restored physiologic and anatomic relationship. It generally includes all of the following:

1. Clot formation
2. Granulation tissue development
3. Epithelialization
4. Collagen formation
5. Regeneration
6. Maturation

Understanding wound repair processes will permit the surgeon to design and perform the proper surgical procedures to support overall therapeutic objectives and to ensure that the patient's healing period will be as brief and comfortable as possible.

Periodontal surgery can be broadly classified into two categories: procedures designed to correct soft tissue defects, and those designed to manage defects of the alveolar bone.

## HEALING OF SOFT TISSUE WOUNDS

### Excision of Gingiva (Gingivectomy)

After the excision of a portion of gingiva (Fig. 12-1A), clot formation occurs with the fibrin clot overlying the exposed connective tissue (Fig. 12-1B). Within hours, the connective tissue begins to produce granulation tissue "buds" (proliferating connective tissue characterized by increased mitotic activity in the fibroblasts, endothelial cells and capillaries, and undifferentiated mesenchymal cells).[1] This is soon covered and infiltrated by neutrophils. The healing wound surface consists of a base of moderately inflamed connective tissue covered with granulation tissue, then a layered zone of neutrophils, and finally a clot.[2] Epithelium begins to proliferate from the wound margins and migrates cell by cell (at about 0.5 mm per day) under the clot, through the neutrophil zone, and over the granulation tissue (Fig. 12-1C). Epithelium continues to proliferate in a thin layer until it reaches the surface of the tooth.[3] While this is occurring, fibroblasts in the granulation tissue begin to produce immature, incompletely polymerized collagen. At this point the clot has been exfoliated, having served its function as a biologic bandage. Proliferation and maturation of both the collagen and epithelium continue until there is a covering of epithelium overlying mature collagen.[4] The gingival crevice is re-formed by coronal growth of connective tissue and apical migration of the junctional epithelium. If healing has progressed relatively free from destructive bacterial products, the lining of the sulcus is composed of a flattened, intact, stratified squamous epithelium.[2] If bacterial products have been present, rete pegs form along the basal layer of the epithelium.

The granulation tissue matures so that the newly formed collagen is indistinguishable from the collagen fibers of original gingiva (Fig. 12-1D). The tissue clinically resembles normal gingiva within a few weeks, although it takes several months for complete healing and organization of the fiber bundles.[4]

Even though the gingival excision surgery has not directly involved bone, there will be some osteoclastic activity on the cortical surface followed by a rebound in osteoblastic activity.[2] This bone remodeling is on a microscopic level and is not usually of clinical significance as long as a sufficient thickness of connective tissue was retained over the bone.

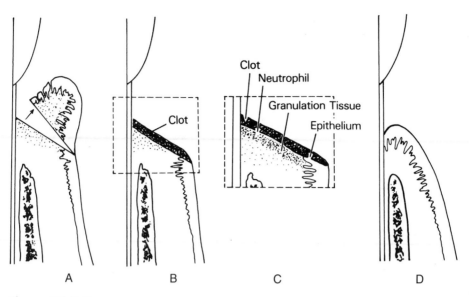

**Figure 12.1** ●

## Simple Incision

When a sharp instrument incises the gingiva, a similar healing process occurs with slight differences based on the architecture of the wound. After an incision, if the incised edges are closely approximated, only a small space exists between the wound surfaces in which a clot can form (Fig. 12-2A). This clot serves only as a "plug" through which granulation tissue grows. It is advantageous to have as small a clot as possible because it must be ultimately resorbed.[5] Healing by the union of approx-

imated wound surfaces is termed healing by primary intention.[5] This is the rationale of primary wound closure in surgical procedures. The better the wound edge approximation and thus the smaller the clot, the more rapid the epithelial bridging between the incised soft tissue surfaces, thereby sealing off the slower maturing connective tissues from the oral environment[6] (Fig. 12-2B).

Clot absorption is concurrently occurring in the depth of the incision, by macrophages removing the fibrin and fibroblasts producing collagen.[5]

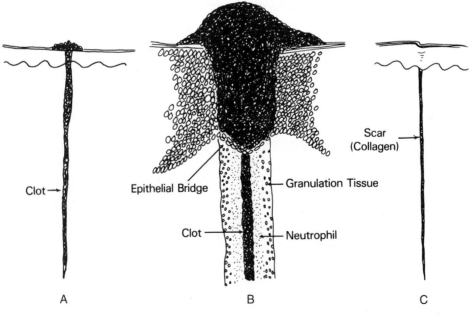

**Figure 12.2** ●

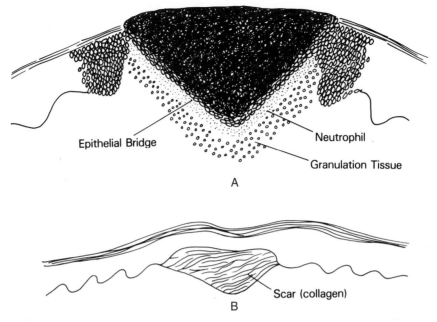

**Figure 12.3** ●

Collagen maturation occurs, which is clinically indistinguishable from the collagen of the normal gingiva after a few months (Fig. 12-2C).

In a poorly approximated wound, the epithelium will migrate into the space created by the gap between the incised surfaces, covering the exposed maturing granulation tissue and lining the wound (Fig. 12-3A). This is often termed healing by second intention, and eventually a relatively large clot is sloughed (Fig. 12-3B).

Epithelial cells require energy for survival, proliferation, and migration. Their nutrients are derived by diffusion from the blood vessels. These cells can travel only a finite distance from the

capillaries, beyond which they lose their source of nutrition. Therefore, the proximity of capillaries (granulation tissue) determines the route of epithelial proliferation.

## Reattachment (Presurgical Level)

Reattachment is defined as the reestablishment of a soft tissue interface on the uninvolved root surface after surgical detachment (connective tissue attachment of the biologic width). When the gingiva is surgically reflected from a tooth surface, some collagen fibers will remain embedded in and extending out of the cementum (Fig. 12-4A), just

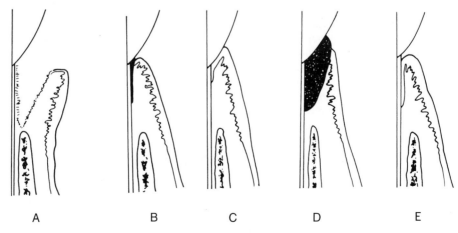

**Figure 12.4** ●

coronal to the alveolar crest.[7] If the tissue is carefully replaced onto the unaltered tooth surface, a small clot will be interposed between the collagen fibers in the cementum and the collagen of the wound surface of the gingiva (Fig. 12-4B).[8] Granulation tissue will form and penetrate the thin clot, and permit the fibers extending from the cementum to unite with new collagen formed by gingival fibroblasts.

The epithelial attachment will usually remain at its original position on the tooth, or it may migrate a few cells apically, and is dependent on the clot size (Fig. 12-4C). If a large clot is formed (Fig. 12-4D), epithelium may migrate apically over the wound surface, resulting in a junctional epithelium that is considerably longer and more apically positioned (Fig. 12-4E).[9] This occurrence is less likely if there is appropriate flap stabilization with sutures, application of gentle pressure for 2 to 3 minutes, and proper placement of a periodontal dressing if needed.

## New Attachment

Soft tissue new attachment implies formation of new cementum, connective tissue fibers, and junctional epithelium at a more coronal level on previously diseased root surfaces. To achieve a more coronal attachment of connective tissue to the tooth, cells capable of producing new cementum and collagen must have access to the tooth surface coronal to the existing level of the junctional epithelium.

The alveolar crest fibers and the transseptal fibers also prevent the fibroblasts and cementoblasts within the periodontal ligament from gaining access to the tooth surface coronal to the original position of the junctional epithelium. When the root has been properly detoxified by mechanical root planing, the instrumentation also has interrupted the integrity of the soft tissue attachment. If the wound surface is then closely readapted to minimize clot size, cellular elements of the periodontal ligament may migrate coronally and may produce new cementum and new Sharpey's fibers, thus establishing a new soft tissue attachment.[9]

However, there is considerable evidence that after attempted new attachment procedures repair instead results via a long thin junctional epithelium adherent to the tooth. Clinical experience and longitudinal studies suggest that this epithelial adherence may be maintainable with time.

Confusion has existed for years as to whether new cementum will form on pulpless teeth or teeth with endodontic fillings. Animal studies indicate that new attachment or regeneration can occur on either pulpless teeth or those with root canal fillings, but with a lower predictability compared with teeth with healthy pulps and with less overall success.

## Open Wounds

At the completion of certain surgical procedures (gingivectomy, gingivoplasty), some areas of the wound will be denuded of epithelium and part of the mucosa. The type of tissue that will be produced during healing depends primarily on the type of tissue underlying the wound. For example, a gingivectomy wound is usually performed on gingival tissue (dense collagenous connective tissue covered by keratinized epithelium), and, predictably, similar tissue will re-form because the remaining underlying connective tissue will be coded for keratinization.

After certain flap procedures, areas of bone may be left with only a very thin covering of connective tissue.[10,11] If gingiva originally covered the bone, then gingiva will re-form. If alveolar mucosa originally covered the bone, then alveolar mucosa will re-form.

## Flaps

A flap is defined as that portion of the gingiva, alveolar mucosa, or periosteum that is reflected or dissected from the tooth and alveolar process and retains a blood supply. Many surgical procedures involve the use of flaps of various designs. There are two methods of reflecting a flap:

1. Blunt elevation (full-thickness or mucoperiosteal flap) exposing the bone surface (Fig 12.5).
2. Sharp dissection (partial thickness or mucosal flap) leaving a varying thickness of connective tissue covering the alveolar process (Fig. 12–6). When flaps are replaced to cover the bone (whether at the original or at a different position), healing is similar to that of a simple incision in that one connective tissue wound surface is placed against another with a small intervening blood clot.[11] The rationale and technique for the full-thickness (mucoperiosteal) and partial-thickness (mucosal) flap are discussed in Chapter 14.

## Free Gingival Grafts (Free Soft Tissue Autograft)

Free grafts, in contrast to flaps, are completely separated from their blood supply and are placed in a different recipient site. The vasculature at the recipient site ultimately provides all the

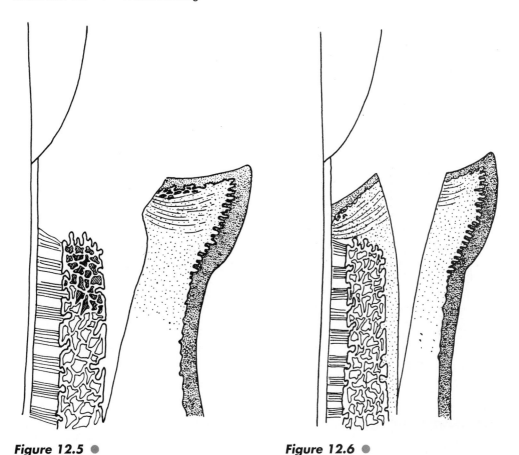

**Figure 12.5** ●                         **Figure 12.6** ●

nourishment for the graft with initial nourishment by diffusion from the underlying tissue.[12] In the case of connective tissue grafts, the diffusion occurs from both the underlying and overlying tissue.

The blood clot at the recipient site should be as thin as possible to permit ready diffusion of nutrients from the recipient site through the clot to the graft.[13] The graft should be in intimate contact with the recipient site and completely immobile to decrease the chance of large clot formation. Because the survival of the graft depends on revascularization, the graft must be immobilized for the first 7 to 10 days at the recipient site.[14]

## Root Detoxification

It has been demonstrated that the removal of plaque, toxins, and calculus from exposed root surfaces results in beneficial changes in the periodontium. This sequence of events is depicted in Figure 12-7. During chronic inflammation, an intact periodontium (Fig. 12-7A) progresses to pocket formation

(Fig. 12-7B) with depolymerization of some gingival fibers, the apical migration of the junctional epithelium, and some loss of crestal bone. The gingiva itself is enlarged as a result of edema. New vascular connective tissue is present within the gingiva, as are many lymphocytes, plasma cells, fibroblasts, and neutrophils (all the elements of defense and repair).[8,9]

This granulomatous tissue has little chance to repair because of continued tissue damage from products produced by the plaque microorganisms. If the local etiologic factors are removed by root detoxification procedures (mechanical root planing) with the establishment of effective plaque control procedures, then the disease process will begin to resolve. The edema will subside, and the granulomatous tissue will be converted to granulation tissue and can proceed to repair with regeneration of gingival collagen.[15] As maturation progresses free from the effects of plaque, further shrinkage will occur until a condition similar to that shown in Figure 12-7C is reached.

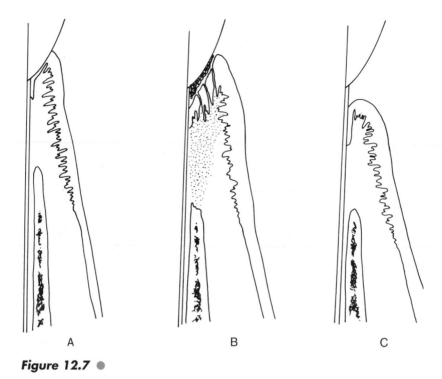

A                                    B                                    C

*Figure 12.7* ●

## HEALING INVOLVING BONE

### General Principles

Bone undergoes remodeling throughout life. In health, osteoblastic activity and osteoclastic activity are in balance. This balance can be disturbed by changes in functional demands on the bone and by disease. Furthermore, any surgical procedure affects bone to some extent. The severity of the change depends on several factors, including the type of bone (cortical or cancellous), the thickness of bone, procedures done to the bone during the surgical procedure, and what type of tissue covering it has after surgery.[16] For example, if thin radicular bone overlying a maxillary canine were exposed during surgery and were left without soft tissue coverage after surgery, one could expect that during the healing process most of the exposed bone would be either resorbed or sequestered, with minimal regeneration. However, if mostly cancellous interproximal bone were treated similarly, some resorption would occur during initial healing, but the vast majority of the bone would regenerate.

When performing periodontal surgery, one should remember that:

1. Bone should be covered by soft tissue after surgery.[16]

2. The thicker the soft tissue covering bone during and after the procedure, the less the bone is affected by surgery.[16]

3. Thin bone will be permanently lost more easily than thick bone.[16]

Thick interproximal bone has sufficient intra-alveolar blood supply (cancellous bone) to withstand the loss of the vascular supply from the supraperiosteal vessels as a result of flap surgery. Conversely, thin radicular bone (minimal or no cancellous bone) is almost totally dependent on the blood supply from the supraperiosteal vessels and can be readily lost if this blood supply is compromised.[10] Canines, first premolars, and the mesial roots of maxillary first molars usually have thin bone. These teeth may even have bony dehiscences or fenestrations, as discussed in Chapter 1. The thickness of the radicular bone over all facial root surfaces should be considered carefully in the design and execution of surgical procedures.

### Infrabony Defects

Many periodontal procedures are performed to stimulate new bone formation for repair of an osseous defect. Figure 12-8 represents a mesiodistal section through the proximal surfaces of two teeth and the interproximal bone and gingiva.

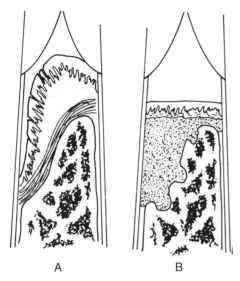

A    B

***Figure 12.8*** ●

An infrabony defect is diagrammed to illustrate three conditions common to most such chronic lesions.

1. Transseptal fibers are present as discrete bundles extending into the defect, and continue to the cementum of the adjacent tooth.
2. A cortical surface may be present on the bony surface that forms the walls of the defect.
3. The junctional epithelium is apical to the crest of the bone and near the base of the defect.

If regeneration is to occur and provide increased support to the tooth, cells must produce new cementum, new collagen fibers, and new bone. Complete debridement of the osseous defect and the root surface creates the conditions suitable for regeneration.[17]

After the soft tissue has been removed, any cortical bone lining the defect should be perforated (intramarrow penetration) to permit egress of pluripotential marrow cells for re-formation of the attachment apparatus (Fig. 12-8).

Ideally, complete restoration of cementum, bone and periodontal ligament occur. However, usually only partial regeneration may result. The predictability of success for such procedures is discussed in Chapter 17.

## Bone Replacement Grafts

There are various types of bone replacement grafts used in surgery, and each type may have different advantages and disadvantages. An autograft is tissue transferred from one site to another in the same individual and has been used successfully for many years in the management of osseous defects of the periodontium. Another popular bone replacement graft is an allograft, which is a tissue graft between individuals of the same species and is harvested from cadavers and prepared by freeze-drying to prevent disease transmission. The alloplast is an inert biocompatible material that acts as a scaffold for bone formation. There are various types of materials used as alloplasts, and all are synthetic. Finally, the last type of graft is a xenograft, which is a tissue graft between members of differing species (such as bovine bone), which is processed by freeze-drying to prevent any disease transmission. The main advantage of allografts, alloplasts, and xenografts is that they are commercially available and can be readily used during surgery.

## Fate of Bone Replacement Grafts

The fate of the calcified portions of bone replacement grafts has been documented as follows:

1. The graft may retain vital osteoblasts and osteocytes as an autograft and thus be **osteogenic.** Such osteocyte viability is maintained only when the cells are close enough (within 1 mm) to a nutrient source, which suggests that osteocytes deep within a comparatively large fragment will not survive.
2. The graft may be completely resorbed, releasing biologic substances (bone morphogenic protein) that induce bone formation, thus be **osteoinductive** as an autograft or allograft.
3. The graft may be completely resorbed during healing but be **osteoconductive** in that it acts as a scaffold for new bone formation as a resorbable alloplast or xenograft.
4. The graft may remain as an inert, nonvital fragment, playing no apparent role in the healing process but acting as a scaffold for bone formation (**osteoconductive**) with the inert particles remaining in the bone as an inert alloplast.
5. The graft may play no apparent role, and be exfoliated during healing. Exfoliation may occur months after the surgical procedure.

## Guided Tissue Regeneration Healing

Animal studies have suggested that wound healing was dependent on the cell types that initially repopulated the surgical area and their ability to progress. Different tissue types migrate into the surgical wound at different rates, and if it were possible to delay some tissue types (as epithelium and connective tissue) and allow other cell types to enter the surgical site (as undifferentiated mesenchymal cells from the periodontal ligament and osteoblasts), then regeneration may occur. This concept was called guided tissue regeneration and used a barrier membrane to exclude the connective tissue and epithelium. Wound healing occurred in the protected area beneath the barrier membrane as previously outlined.

## OTHER CONSIDERATIONS IN WOUND HEALING

### Nutrition and Systemic Disorders

Healing occurs on a cellular or molecular level, requiring the expenditure of energy and the utilization of nutrients as required for anabolic and catabolic activities. Any disorder that interferes with ingestion, digestion, absorption, or effective transport and utilization of nutrients will interfere with healing. Such disorders as diabetes, deficiencies in vitamins, minerals, and foods (especially protein), and severe hormonal imbalances can be expected to retard overall healing.

### Age

Age by itself seems to have no bearing on healing after periodontal surgery. General health without major systemic disease is more important.

### Asepsis

Asepsis is a basic requirement for success in all surgery performed in the oral cavity. Periodontal surgery must be performed in a manner that will prevent introduction of foreign pathogens into the surgical field, which could result in infection and delayed healing. In addition to necessary infection control procedures, sterile gloves, instruments, and drapes should be routine in the performance of all surgical procedures.

### Healing Rate

It seems that there is a maximal speed at which various cells can dispose of cellular debris, produce new materials, move through tissue, or perform reparative tasks. Currently there is no way to accelerate this process, and the best one can do is to avoid slowing the healing rate. Therefore, factors such as nutrition, trauma, smoking, or alcohol consumption should be controlled during the healing period. Smoking has been shown to be the major patient habit that will affect not only the healing rate but also the overall success of a surgical procedure.

## WOUND HEALING APPLIED TO PERIODONTAL SURGERY

A review of this chapter will serve as a reminder that there are many principles of wound healing that apply directly to the success or failure of periodontal surgery. A summary of the more important principles that have been discussed follows:

1. A gingival wound may appear clinically normal within a few weeks; however, it will be a number of months before healing is complete and fiber bundles have formed.
2. The closer the approximation of two soft tissue wound edges and the smaller the clot, the more rapid epithelialization occurs, thereby sealing off the slower maturing connective tissues from the oral environment.
3. In flap procedures, clot thickness should be kept at a minimum between tooth and wound surface to permit reattachment of connective tissue fibers at their original level or new attachment to possibly occur at a more coronal level.
4. Keratinized gingival tissue should be maintained on the margin of the flap for predictable maturation of gingival tissue in apically positioned flaps.
5. Free soft tissue grafts on a recipient site with a thin intervening blood clot afford an excellent opportunity for graft survival.
6. Plaque, calculus, and contaminated cementum must be removed or detoxified for successful wound healing against the tooth surface.
7. Bone should be covered by soft tissue when the surgical procedure is completed.
8. The thicker the soft tissue covering the bone during and after the procedure, the less the bone will be affected.
9. Thin bone is permanently lost more easily than thick bone.
10. In the management of infrabony defects, it is necessary to remove the soft tissue portion of the defect. Also, any cortical bone lining the defect should be perforated to permit egress of pluripotential cells.

## REFERENCES

1. Novaes A, Kon S, Ruben M, Goldman H. Visualization of the microvascularization of the healing periodontal wound. III. Gingivectomy. J Periodontol 1969;40:359–456.

2. Ramfjord SP, Engler WO, Hinkler JJ. A radioautographic study of healing following simple gingivectomy, II: the connective tissue. J Periodontol 1966; 37:179–189.

3. Engler WO, Ramjord SP, Hiniker JJ. Healing following simple gingivectomy. A tritiated thymidine radioautographic study, I. Epithelialization. J Periodontol 1966;37:298–308.

4. Stahl SS, Witkin GJ, Cantor M, Brown R. Gingival healing. II. Clinical and histologic repair sequences following gingivectomy. J Periodontol 1968;39: 109–118.

5. Wilderman M, Wentz F, Orban B. Histogenesis of repair after mucogingival surgery. J Periodontol 1960;31:283–299.

6. Mormann W, Ciancio SG. Blood supply of human gingiva following periodontal surgery. A fluorescein angiographic study. J Periodontol 1977;48:681–692.

7. Frank R, Fiore-Donno G, Cimasoni G, Ogilvie A. Gingival reattachment after surgery in man: an electron microscopic study. J Periodontol 1972;43: 597–605.

8. Cutright DE. The proliferation of blood vessels in gingival wounds J Periodontol 1969;40:137–141.

9. Listgarten M. Electron microscopic study of the junction between surgically denuded root surfaces and regenerated periodontal tissues. J Periodontal Res 1972;7:68–90.

10. Wilderman M. Exposure of bone in periodontal surgery. Dent Clin North Am 1964;2:23–36.

11. Wilderman M, Pennel B, King K, Barron J. Histogenesis of repair following osseous surgery. J Periodontol 1970;41:551–565.

12. Oliver R, Loe H, Karring T. Microscopic evaluation of the healing and revascularization of free gingival grafts. J Periodont Res 1968;3:84–95.

13. Nobuto T, Imai H, Yamaoka A. Microvascularization of the free gingival autograft. J Periodontol 1988;59:639–646.

14. James WC, McFall WT, Burkes EJ. Placement of free gingival grafts on denuded alveolar bone. Part II: microscopic observations. J Periodontol 1978;49: 291–300.

15. Stone S, Ramfjord S, Waldron J. Scaling and gingival currettage: a radioautographic study. J Periodontol 1966;37:415–430.

16. Wood D, Hoag P, Donnenfeld O, Rosenfeld L. Alveolar crest reduction following full and partial thickness flaps. J Periodontol 1972;43: 141–144.

17. Egelberg J. Regeneration and repair of periodontal tissue. J Periodontal Res 1987;22:233–242.

## CHAPTER 12
## REVIEW QUESTIONS

1. The tissue that migrates first into the wound is (are):
   a. Epithelium from the flap margin
   b. Connective tissue from the flap margin
   c. Osteoclasts from the underlying wound
   d. Connective tissue from the underlying wound
2. The newly formed collagen in a wound is indistinguishable from the collagen fibers of the original gingival in:
   a. 1 week
   b. 3 weeks
   c. 6 weeks
   d. 12 weeks
3. Healing by the union of approximated wound surfaces is termed healing by primary intention. The size of the clot between the wound edges does not affect the length of healing time.
   a. Both statements are true.
   b. Both statements are false.
   c. The first statement is true and the second statement is false.
   d. The first statement is false and the second statement is true.
4. The epithelium receives nutrition during wound healing from the proliferation of new epithelial capillaries. Clot resorption occurs by macrophages in the depth of the wound removing the fibrin.
   a. Both statements are true.
   b. Both statements are false.
   c. The first statement is true and the second statement is false.
   d. The first statement is false and the second statement is true.

5. The reestablishment of a soft tissue interface on the uninvolved root surface after surgical detachment is termed:
   a. Repair
   b. Regeneration
   c. Reattachment
   d. New attachment
6. New attachment implies new formation of all of the following tissues except:
   a. Bone
   b. Cementum
   c. Junctional epithelium
   d. Connective tissue fibers
7. A bone replacement graft that is osteoinductive is:
   a. Allograft
   b. Alloplast
   c. Xenoplast
   d. Xenograft
8. Factors that affect the rate of healing include all of the following except:
   a. Age
   b. Smoking
   c. Nutrition
   d. Alcoholism
9. The first stage in the healing of a gingivectomy wound is:
   a. Production of granulation tissue "buds"
   b. Covering of a thick layer of neutrophils
   c. Fibrin clot overlying the exposed connective tissue
   d. Proliferation of epithelium from the wound edges
10. A bone replacement graft that can be considered osteogenic is:
    a. Alloplast
    b. Allograft
    c. Autograft
    d. Xenograft

# Principles of Periodontal Surgery

Jonathan Gray

The principal goal of periodontal surgery is to create an oral environment that is conducive to maintaining the patient's dentition in health, comfort, and function for life.

## RATIONALE FOR SURGERY

### Provide Access

Surgery provides the clinician with increased access to the root surface and alveolar bone. This access permits meticulous root preparation with the elimination of all hard deposits, contaminated cementum, and bacterial and tissue products from the root surfaces. Removal of toxic products from the root surface assists in controlling the inflammatory process. In addition, the reduction in probing depths after surgical therapy allows the patient better access to all surfaces of the teeth for more effective plaque removal.

### Regeneration of the Periodontium

In later chapters, surgical methods designed to restore soft tissue and bone destroyed by disease is described. This surgery consists primarily of hard and soft tissue grafting techniques to restore the periodontium to a state that approaches the predisease level.

### Modification of Bony Architecture

Osseous defects and deformities create aberrations in the physiologic contour of the periodontium that contribute to plaque retention and are not consistent with a state of good health. Contouring the bone to eliminate osseous defects reduces plaque-retentive areas and allows the patient better access to the tooth surfaces for more effective plaque control.

### Periodontal Pocket Reduction

Periodontal pockets may not always be eliminated, but they may be reduced by a variety of resective and regenerative techniques (Chapters 14 through 20). The primary goal is to reduce pocket depths to a manageable level for the dental team and for the patient.

## PRESURGICAL CONSIDERATIONS

### Patient Consent

Informed consent is essential before any treatment is undertaken.[1] The patient should clearly understand the benefits and the possible risks or complications of any proposed procedures. The alternatives to surgery should be carefully explained to enable the patient to give an informed consent to the operative plan. Informed consent must be in language that the patient can understand. A written entry of the discussion and patient agreement should be made in the dental record as well as the actual document. A copy of the signed document must be given to the patient.

### Contraindications for Periodontal Surgery

There are many reasons for not performing periodontal surgery. The existence of certain medical problems could make periodontal surgery inadvisable (such as uncontrolled diabetes or blood pressure). A complete and thorough medical history must be taken before the performance of any periodontal treatment (see Chapter 3). Excellent plaque control is mandatory for success of periodontal surgery (see Chapter 7). The patient must be informed, at an early stage of the treatment, that no surgery will be performed unless the plaque is adequately controlled before surgery and until the patient understands and is committed to long-term maintenance care.

The magnitude of the existing periodontal destruction must be considered. Surgery performed in an attempt to treat severe periodontal destruction could result in further mutilating the tissues, rather than restoring the periodontium to health, comfort, and function. Extraction of teeth is the treatment of choice in managing the severely involved patient in many instances.

Some patients prefer to forego surgery, even after the advantages of surgery have been explained carefully. The best course of action with these patients is to cease further discussion of surgery and to determine an alternative type of treatment to maintain the existing dentition.

Thorough understanding of the anatomy of the surgical procedure is essential.[2] A practitioner who does not feel capable of the surgical management of the patient's condition or will not accept the responsibility of a satisfactory maintenance program for the patient should attempt no periodontal surgery. The dentist loses no status or prestige in the eyes of the patient in referring the advanced case to a trained specialist.

## Smoking Cessation

Although smoking is not an absolute contraindication to periodontal surgery, research has shown that smoking impairs wound healing. Patients should be encouraged to stop smoking for 2 to 4 weeks before surgery. If a patient is unwilling or unable to comply with this request, alternative treatment should be considered.[3,4]

## Infection Control, or Phase I Therapy

Infection control, often referred to as initial preparation or phase I therapy, should be completed before the final decision is made to perform surgery. Infection control therapy is one of the most valuable components of periodontal therapy. During this phase of treatment, it is possible to:

1. Assess the patient's commitment to periodontal therapy
2. Observe the patient's healing potential
3. Reinforce plaque control instruction
4. Reduce the need for surgery
5. Improve tissue tone, which facilitates soft tissue management at the time of surgery

The rationale is that single-appointment treatment is less likely to leave reservoirs of bacteria that might reinfect treated areas between sessions. Although there may be merit to this approach, it does not give the clinician the chance to evaluate the patient's plaque control for a longer period, and provide oral hygiene education and reinforcement.

Four to six weeks after completing the infection control phase of therapy, the patient is re-examined thoroughly to determine what changes have occurred and what further periodontal therapy is required. On the basis of this examination, a decision must be made regarding further treatment. Table 13-1 is a decision matrix that takes into consideration the findings and the possible treatment alternatives one may make at this stage of treatment.

## Antibiotic Prophylaxis

Antibiotic prophylaxis is usually provided for patients at risk for bacterial endocarditis and after joint replacement surgery.[5,6] Premedication with appropriate antibiotics must be provided for the first five systemic conditions listed:

1. Most congenital heart disease
2. Rheumatic heart disease or other acquired valvular heart disease
3. Idiopathic hypertrophic subaortic stenosis
4. Mitral valve prolapse syndrome with mitral insufficiency
5. Prosthetic heart valves
6. Patients with joint prostheses (see below)
7. Patients with compromised immune systems (consult or refer to physician)

The recommendations of the American Dental Association, the American Medical Association, the American Heart Association, and the American Association of Orthopedic Surgeons are discussed in more detail in Chapter 5. There are different opinions regarding antibiotic coverage of patients with joint prostheses. The patient's orthopedist should be consulted to determine the choice of antibiotic for these patients.

There is a minimal amount of evidence to support the concept of prophylactic administration of antibiotics to prevent infection after periodontal surgery.[7] The use of broad-spectrum antibiotics to suppress plaque and to improve healing after bone grafting procedures has merit. Tetracycline is selectively excreted in gingival fluid in a concentration 2 to 10 times the concentration found in plasma. This high concentration in the target gingival sulcular area makes tetracycline particularly appropriate to prescribe after bone grafting procedures. The usual dosage is 250 mg four times per day, starting on the day of surgery and for 7 to 14 days thereafter. Tetracycline should not be taken with food because

## TABLE 13.1

**Decision Matrix**

| Probing Depth Change Compared With Initial Examination | Bleeding | Localized | Generalized |
|---|---|---|---|
| Decreasing | No | Routine maintenance procedures | Routine maintenance procedures |
| | Yes | Consider: 1.Reinforce oral hygiene | Consider: 1. Plaque control may be inadequate—retrain |
| | | 2. Scaling and root planing 3. Site-specific treatment 4. Shorten maintenance intervals | 2. Plaque control adequate: a. Systemic antibiotics b. Referral to a periodontist |
| Unchanged | No | Routine maintenance procedures | Routine maintenance procedures |
| ± 1 mm | Yes | Consider: 1. Reinforce oral hygiene 2. Scaling and root planing 3. Site-specific treatment (may include surgery) 4. Referral to a periodontist | |
| Increasing 2 mm or more | No | Consider: 1. Surgery 2. Referral to a periodontist | Consider: 1. Systemic antibiotics 2. Surgery 3. Referral to a periodontist |
| | Yes | Consider: 1. Surgery 2. Referral to a periodontist | Consider: 1. Systemic antibiotics 2. Surgery 3. Referral to a periodontist |

of the likelihood of impaired absorption. In addition, this antibiotic may cause discoloration of developing teeth; therefore, caution should be observed in prescribing it for pregnant women, or for children with developing dentitions. Tetracycline is also contraindicated in patients with impaired liver and kidney function and those with known allergies to the medication. However, concerns about overuse of antibiotics and the creation of resistant strains of bacteria have merit. In the final analysis, the decision whether or not to use postoperative antibiotics is up to the individual practitioner.

## Asepsis

**Universal precautions:** It is imperative that periodontal surgery be performed under aseptic conditions.[8,9] It is not possible to sterilize the oral cavity, but precautions should be taken to prevent cross-contamination and to preclude the introduction of extraneous bacteria into the patient's mouth. All instruments must be sterilized and placed on a sterile operating tray. The operator should wear a surgical cap. It is mandatory that the operator wear face mask and gloves. A sterile towel can be clipped to the front of the surgeon's clinic clothing. The patient should be draped with sterile towels, and the patient's hair and eyes may be wrapped with sterile towels. Great care should be taken to ensure that nonsterile items are not introduced into the operating field. Whenever aerosols are generated, special precautions must be taken, including face shields, disposable gowns, and high-speed evacuation to minimize splatter.

## Local Anesthesia

Periodontal surgery is usually performed under local anesthesia. The periodontal surgeon should use the minimum of local anesthetic required to keep the patient comfortable during the surgical procedure. The clinician should be aware that the dosage, the method of injection, and the vascularity at the injected site have an effect on the patient.[10]

The action and safe dose range of the anesthetic selected should be well known. The maximal dosage of lidocaine hydrochloride for a healthy person, when used with 1:100,000 epinephrine, is 3.2 mg per pound of body weight. A 1.8-mL dental cartridge with 2% lidocaine hydrochloride contains 36 mg of lidocaine hydrochloride (20 mg/mL). By using this information, it is possible to calculate the maximal dose of lidocaine for a healthy patient. For example, 12 cartridges of 2% lidocaine hydrochloride (36 mg/cartridge) is the maximum that could be used for a 140-pound person (140 × 3.2 mg = 448 mg; therefore, 448 mg = 12.4 cartridges).[11]

It is usually unnecessary for the epinephrine concentration to be greater than 1:100,000 (0.01 mg/mL) in local anesthetic agents used for periodontal surgery. The maximal dosage of epinephrine for a healthy adult patient is 0.2 mg of epinephrine per dental appointment (10 cartridges of lidocaine with an epinephrine concentration of 1:100,000). Patients with severe cardiovascular problems should receive no more than 0.04 mg of epinephrine per dental appointment (two 1.8-mL cartridges of anesthetic with 1:100,000 epinephrine concentration).

**CAUTION: Injection of any local anesthetic in dentistry should be accomplished with aspirating syringes, and at a rate that approximates 1 mL/min.**

## Anxiety Control

Most anxiety can be controlled by managing the patient in a kind and considerate manner. The periodontal surgeon should project a calm confidence in his or her ability to accomplish the surgical procedure. However, there are a few patients whose anxiety cannot be controlled without the utilization of some form of tranquilizing or sedative therapy. A variety of medications and methods are available for this purpose. Incumbent with use of sedation or drug therapy is the responsibility of the clinician to be thoroughly familiar with all aspects of the regimen being considered and the knowledge and the equipment to manage the unexpected adverse reactions.[12]

Inhalation sedation with nitrous oxide and oxygen is straightforward and presents few difficulties with modern equipment. However, it does not provide profound sedation. Oral sedation is the next most effective treatment. Benzodiazepines are generally used. Diazepam (Valium) was commonly used at one time; however, it has a long half-life (30 to 70 hours), which is an undesirable characteristic. Lorazepam (Halcion) provides profound sedation, and the half-life is only 1.5 to 5.5 hours, much more suitable for dental treatment. Unfortunately, not all patients respond predictably to oral sedation. Stomach contents, age, weight, and so forth are all factors that make each sedation experience unique for every patient. Intravenous sedation using a benzodiazepine with or without a narcotic is occasionally required. Some practitioners choose to use intravenous sedation on a routine basis. Intravenous techniques require a much higher level of training, and in most cases, special certification and emergency equipment. Some patients require treatment under general anesthesia, which may be performed in a hospital. An anesthesiologist or nurse anesthetist usually performs the anesthesia. Hospital privileges may be required for operating room procedures.

## Emergencies

The clinician must know and take measures to minimize adverse patient reactions to any administered medication. All office personnel must have ready access to the emergency cart and be competent in the proper use of emergency equipment. Periodic inspection of emergency equipment must be made to ensure that the equipment is in good working condition. Each member of the office staff should be currently certified in basic life support. It is good policy to have periodic drills in emergency procedures so that each staff member will have the confidence to perform effectively in an emergency.[13]

## SURGICAL CONSIDERATIONS
### Surgical Plan

Before surgery, the clinician should carefully review the patient's radiographs and information regarding probing depths, amount of attached and keratinized tissue, and bony contours. These data are used to plan the proper surgical procedure carefully. Although a specific surgical plan is necessary, the clinician should be flexible enough to change the plan if an unsuspected problem is encountered during the surgery. In addition, the clinician must be aware of the anatomic structures that may influence the surgical plan. Dental casts (models) offer a unique view of the surgical site, and can be valuable in planning a procedure.

## Instrumentation and Flap Design

Cutting and root planing instruments must be sharp. Dull instruments traumatize tissue, complicate healing, and frustrate the operator. If dull instruments are found in a surgical set, it should be sharpened or a sterile sharp instrument should be obtained before proceeding. Extra scalpel blades should be readily available. Continuous awareness of the location of the cutting edge of a knife will prevent conversion of a flap into a free graft. Cells die when abused. This basic fact suggests respect for tissue during its manipulation. When a flap is being retracted after elevation, for example, there will be less trauma if the retractor is held gently but firmly against bone instead of against the undersurface of the flap.

Vertical relaxing incisions or access incisions extending toward the palatal vault or along the lingual alveolar plate in the mandible should be avoided.[14,15] These incisions should be made at a 45-degree angle to the surface of the flap. This provides greater surface area for healing. A 90-degree incision should be avoided. Vertical relaxing incisions, particularly on the palate or lingual surface of the mandible, can interfere with the blood supply to tissue medial to the incision. In addition, the greater palatine artery or lingual artery may be severed by injudicious use of these incisions. Hemorrhage from these vessels can be of major proportions. These incisions may also be difficult to suture and often heal slowly with noticeable discomfort to the patient, especially those incisions in the mandible. These problems can usually be avoided by extending the initial flap incision to include a few teeth mesial or distal to the area of instrumentation. If vertical incisions are used on the facial side, they should be designed so as not to compromise the blood supply of the flap (Fig. 13-1). Vertical incisions should be made at line angles of teeth to preserve the interdental papillae for suturing and to prevent necrosis of the wound edge. Under no circumstances should vertical incisions be made over midfacial (radicular) surfaces of roots[16] (Fig. 13-2).

Incisions should be made two or three times with the blade. The first incision rarely severs all connective tissue fibers. If resistance is encountered during elevation, the best course is often to discontinue elevation, and incise the recalcitrant site again until it elevates with little or no effort. Care must be taken to avoid tearing flaps during elevation. If a flap is torn or perforated, it is usually wise to suture the area as soon as possible and not wait until the procedure has been completed. If a periodontally compromised tooth is used as a fulcrum for elevation of a flap (especially a palatal flap), accidental removal of a tooth can result.

It is essential that good visibility of the surgical site be maintained at all times. Blood and saliva may be eliminated from the operative area with good aspiration or by applying intermittent pressure with moist gauze sponges and using periodic irrigation. The gauze sponges should not have a cotton fiber liner.

Bone contouring can be done with sharp chisels or rotating instruments. Caution should be exercised, especially if hand pressure is used, to prevent slipping of the instruments. If a handpiece and burs or stones are used, a sterile saline or water coolant should bathe the area. A fiberoptic handpiece is useful for improved visibility when contouring bone. Ultra-high-speed cutting should be done with the lightest pressure and intermittent contact.

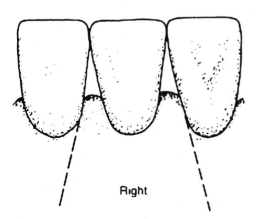 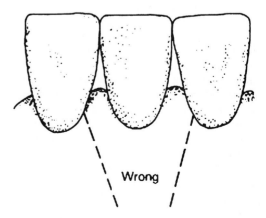

*Figure 13.1* ●

## INCORRECT VERTICAL INCISIONS

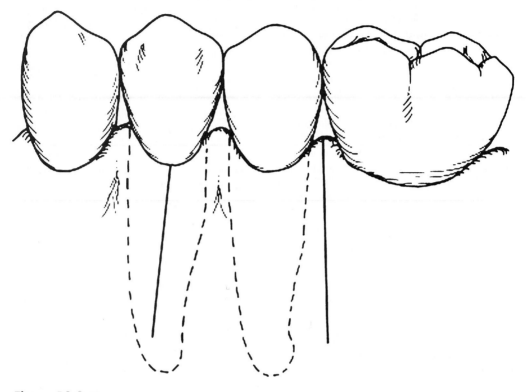

*Figure 13.2* ●

## Control of Bleeding

Frank hemorrhage during or after periodontal surgery is rare. However, excessive bleeding can occur. There can be considerable variation in the amount of blood lost during periodontal surgery. Studies have shown a range in blood loss of 16 to 592 mL per surgical procedure. The mean blood loss per tooth has been reported to be approximately 24 mL. Usually a healthy adult can have a 1-L loss of blood before experiencing hypotension. However, an estimated loss of 500 mL of blood usually requires fluid replacement.

Bleeding may be controlled by putting pressure directly on the bleeding site with a saline-moistened gauze sponge. Bleeding control during flap surgery may be accomplished by replacing the flap and applying pressure to the flap with moistened gauze sponges. The pressure on the flap should be sufficient to overcome capillary or arteriolar pressure, but not be so heavy as to cause tissue damage. Many times, heavy bleeding occurs from the interproximal tissues after flap elevation. This bleeding usually stops as soon as all of the granulomatous tissue has been removed. A suture can also be placed to stop bleeding from vessels in soft tissue. Bleeding from a nutrient canal in the bone can be controlled by crushing the adjacent bone into (swaging) the canal with pressure applied by a metal instrument.

Table 13-2 is a list of some of the commercially available hemostatic agents. For example, thrombin-impregnated oxidized cellulose (Surgicel) strips may be placed over the bleeding site, with gentle pressure applied. These strips may be reapplied as necessary and will resorb in a short time. Microfibrillar collagen hemostat (MCH-Avitene) is another effective hemostatic agent. This material is a dry, sterile, shredded fluff, which is placed with a dry cotton forceps on the bleeding site as required. MCH is resorbable and causes no adverse tissue or systemic reaction.

The use of topically applied epinephrine is not recommended as a hemostatic agent. Epinephrine is readily introduced into the systemic circulation and can cause significant elevation of blood pressure, cardiac arrhythmias, and possibly ventricular fibrillation. Patients with cardiovascular disease could be placed in an acute life-threatening situation from the use of topical epinephrine.

## TABLE 13.2

**Hemostatic Agents**

| Drug | Mechanism of Action | Duration of Action | Laboratory Test |
|---|---|---|---|
| Warfarin (Coumadin) | Warfarin interferes with vitamin K–dependent carboxylation of several coagulation factors including II, VII, IX, and X, as well as anticoagulant proteins C and S. Reversible with administration of vitamin K | 2–5 days | PT, INR |
| Aspirin | Irreversible inhibitor of cyclooxygenase (COX), which prevents formation of the platelet-aggregating substance thromboxane $A_2$ | 7–10 days | Platelet aggregation |
| Clopidogrel (Plavix) | Irreversibly blocks the platelet ADP receptor and prevents activation and aggregation | 7–10 days | Platelet aggregation |
| Ticlopidine (Ticlid) | Irreversibly blocks the platelet ADP receptor and prevents activation and aggregation | 7–10 days | Platelet aggregation |
| Dipyridamole (Persantine®) | Irreversibly blocks the platelet ADP receptor and prevents activation and aggregation | 7–10 days | Platelet aggregation |

ADP = adenosine diphosphate; INR = international normalized ratio; PT = prothrombin time.

Bleeding should be stopped before the dressings are placed. The hemostatic effect of periodontal dressing is not great, nor are they adequate pressure dressings. Remember to strive for minimal blood clots in new attachment procedures. This goal is accomplished by applying gentle pressure to the flap or graft, with gauze soaked in sterile saline solution, for 2 to 3 minutes before the placement of the dressing. When the patient leaves the operative suite, there should be no bleeding from the surgical site.

### Anticoagulant Medications— Hemostasis

Several anticoagulants are commonly used to treat conditions such as heart disease, stroke, and peripheral artery disease. Warfarin (Coumadin), clopidogrel (Plavix), and low-dose aspirin are the drugs that are encountered most often in dental practice (Table 13-2). Medications other than aspirin are generally discontinued before surgery after consulting with the patient's physician. The international normalized ratio (INR) or the

prothrombin time (PT) is used to determine when it is safe to perform surgery for patients taking warfarin. The INR should be 3.0 or less.[17]

Low-dose aspirin is used alone or in conjunction with other anticoagulants. Despite earlier concerns, low doses of aspirin taken daily (81 to 325 mg) do not significantly increase intraoperative bleeding. Furthermore, recent evidence suggests that discontinuing low-dose aspirin places patients at increased risk of a thromboembolic event after 2 weeks without the medication. Patients with coronary artery disease seem to be at particularly high risk. Therefore, aspirin should not be discontinued without consulting the patient's physician.[18,19]

### Wound Closure

Wound closure is important to the success of new attachment procedures and bone grafting. The flap should be designed to permit maximal opportunity for primary closure in the interproximal region. As much interdental papilla as possible must be maintained, which is achieved by using a scalloped

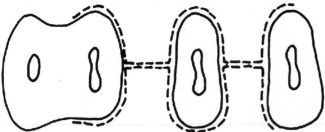

**Figure 13.3** ●

incision (Fig. 13-3). Proximal osteoplasty may be performed to improve approximation of the wound edges when performing new attachment procedures (Fig. 13-4).

## Suturing

Suturing is performed to:

1. Provide proper wound closure
2. Position tissues
3. Control bleeding
4. Help reduce postoperative pain

As stated above, primary wound closure is necessary for successful new attachment and bone grafting techniques. Precise suturing is imperative in mucogingival surgical procedures to maintain the tissues at the desired position.[20]

## Choosing the Right Suture Material

The ideal suture[21] would be:

1. Biologically inert
2. Very strong but able to simply dissolve at a uniform rate
3. Easy to handle and tie
4. Unproblematic, not prone to complications

## Absorbable and Nonabsorbable

Sutures can be divided into two groups: absorbable and nonabsorbable. **The tissues react to all suture materials as foreign bodies.** Gut suture is gradually digested by tissue enzymes. Absorbable synthetic sutures are hydrolyzed. Nonabsorbable sutures are encapsulated by fibroblasts. Nonabsorbable sutures must be removed or they cause chronic sepsis.

## Monofilament and Braided

Sutures may also be classified as monofilament or braided. The former consists of a single strand. It does not "wick" or retain bacteria, and ties easily. However, the knots come untied more frequently than braided suture. A braided suture consists of multiple fibers twisted together. This gives good handling and tying qualities, but does retain bacteria. There is no evidence that wicking impairs healing in periodontal surgery.

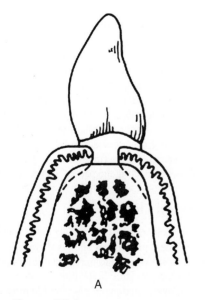

A

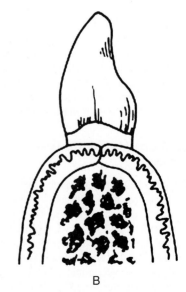

B

**Figure 13.4** ●

## Natural and Synthetic

The most commonly used natural fiber is gut. Gut sutures are particularly advantageous in mucosa because removal of sutures in that tissue can be very painful. There are many synthetic fibers, including nylon and polyglactin (Vicryl and Vicryl Rapide). The latter two are commonly used in periodontics.

## Suture Diameter and Strength

The sizes and tensile strengths are determined by U.S.P. regulations. Size of the suture equates to the diameter: 5-0 is smaller than a size 4-0 which is smaller than 3-0. The smaller the diameter, the smaller the amount of tensile strength. When using a surgical microscope, surgeons may use 9-0 or 10-0 suture, which requires special instruments for handling.

**Certain basic principles must be followed for successful suturing:**

1. Use the least number of sutures necessary to accomplish the desired result.
2. Tension on the suture should be sufficient to hold the tissue in place, but not so great that tissue necrosis may result. In addition, too much tension may cause the suture to tear through the flap.
3. The sutures should be placed in keratinized tissue whenever possible.
4. Take an adequate "bite" of tissue with the suture needle to prevent the suture from tearing through the flap.

Sterile (generally 0-4 or 0-5) prepackaged swaged 1/2- to 3/8-circle reverse cutting or tapered needles are recommended for most periodontal surgical procedures. Numerous suturing techniques are applicable to periodontal surgery. The four most common techniques are the interrupted suture, the sling suture, the continuous suture, and the vertical mattress suture.

1. Interrupted suture. The interrupted suture can be used for virtually all flap and graft surgery. It has its greatest application when both tissue margins require the same amount of tension, as in interproximal tissue approximation (Fig. 13-5).
2. Sling suture. The sling suture encircles the tooth and is used primarily when a flap has been raised on one side of the tooth and it is undesirable to tie it to the opposite side. These sutures are often used as suspensory sutures to hold a flap coronally, such as the laterally positioned flap (Fig. 13-6).
3. Continuous suture. The continuous suture is similar to the sling suture. It is used when

numerous teeth are involved in the surgery, but a flap was elevated on only one side of the teeth. There is a variation, the double continuous suture, that may be used to suture flaps that have been elevated on both the facial and lingual surfaces of the teeth (Fig. 13-7).
4. Mattress suture. The mattress suture (vertical or horizontal) offers the advantage of keeping the suture material out from under the margin of the flap. This suture is often used for interproximal tissue approximation over bone grafts, in excisional new attachment procedures, and for replaced flaps (Fig. 13-8A, horizontal mattress; Fig. 13-8B, vertical mattress).

## Dressing the Wound

The use of periodontal dressings is controversial. Those who advocate using them do so for three reasons:[22]

1. To protect the wound area
2. To enhance patient comfort
3. To help hold flaps in position

The two dressings most commonly used are zinc oxide–eugenol dressings and zinc oxide–non-eugenol dressings. Currently, the non-eugenol dressings are the most popular, and it is becoming more difficult to purchase the eugenol type dressings. Many clinicians believe the use of periodontal dressing after flap surgery is not necessary. A variety of periodontal dressings are available commercially. These dressing materials should be prepared according to the manufacturer's directions. A lubricant should be placed on the gloved fingers before handling the dressing. The dressing should be formed into small rolls approximately the same length as the surgical site. The dressing is adapted over the surgical area so that the apical one-third of the clinical crown is covered, and it should be extended apically to ensure coverage of the surgical area without impinging on the mucobuccal fold or the floor of the mouth. A slightly dampened cotton tip applicator is used to apply gentle pressure to the dressing interproximally. Care should be taken to ensure that the dressing is not forced under the flaps. Use a minimal amount of dressing material to cover the surgical site adequately.

The initial dressing is left in place for about 1 week. When it is removed, the entire area is cleansed with warm water or diluted hydrogen peroxide. Any dressing fragments found embedded in soft tissue or in interproximal areas are removed. The tooth surfaces are carefully examined, and any accumulated plaque, debris, or remaining calculus

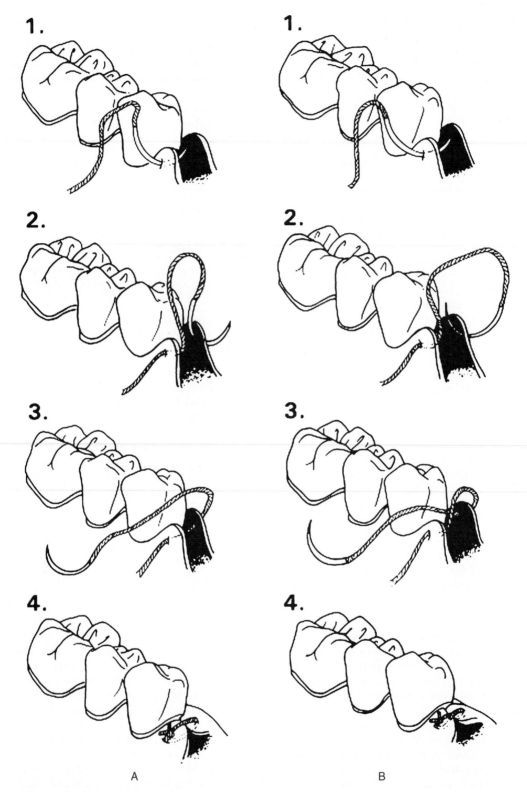

A                                                          B

*Figure 13.5* ●

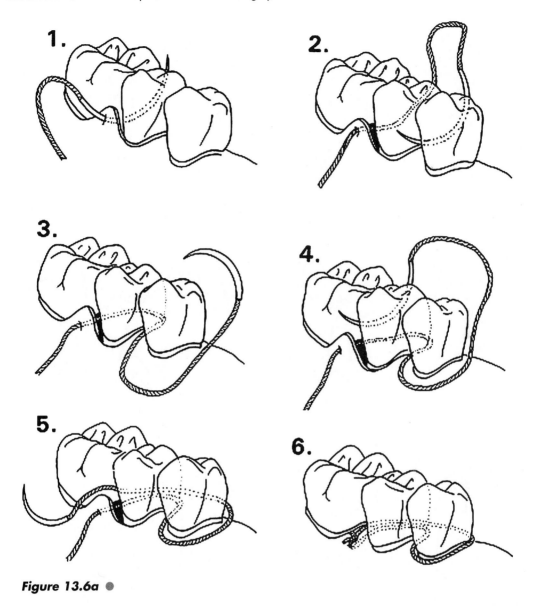

*Figure 13.6a* ●

or dressing material is removed coronal to the gingival margins by using an appropriate low-abrasive prophylactic paste. The patient is instructed in plaque control. The principal criteria for replacement of the dressing are the patient's comfort and the ability of the patient to remove plaque without damaging the healing tissue. Ideally, the patient should receive weekly recalls for polishing and plaque control instruction during the first month(s) after surgery. Additionally, the gelatin-based dressings, such as Stomahesive, are excellent for use after soft tissue augmentation procedures. This

material has good stability properties and dissolves in 24 to 48 hours.

## Analgesics

If the patient and the tissues are treated with care, postoperative pain is generally not a major problem after periodontal surgery. Nonsteroidal analgesics are usually sufficient for postoperative pain management. However, at the time of this printing, there is considerable uncertainty about the safety of some of these drugs, specifically some of the

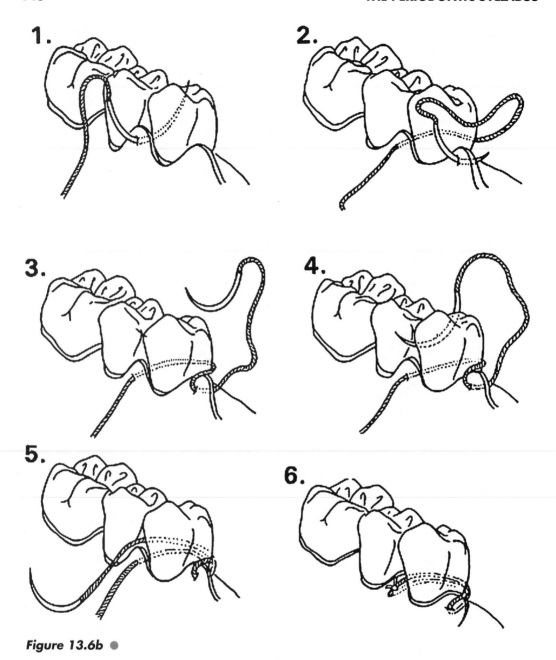

*Figure 13.6b* ●

Cox-2 inhibitors and naproxen sodium. Further research is required. At this time, there are no significant concerns with acetaminophen, aspirin, ibuprofen, or narcotic analgesics, including propoxyphene, for most patients, considering the fact that these prescriptions are for very short periods. As always, a complete medical and drug history is required to determine the safety of any medication for a particular patient. When in doubt, consult with the patient's physician.

## POSTSURGICAL CONSIDERATIONS

### Postoperative Instructions

The patient should be provided with written postoperative instructions. The written instructions must be carefully reviewed with the patient before dismissal from the dental office. Written instructions need not be elaborate and can be tailored to the individual. For example, a patient who has undergone surgery can be given the following instructions:

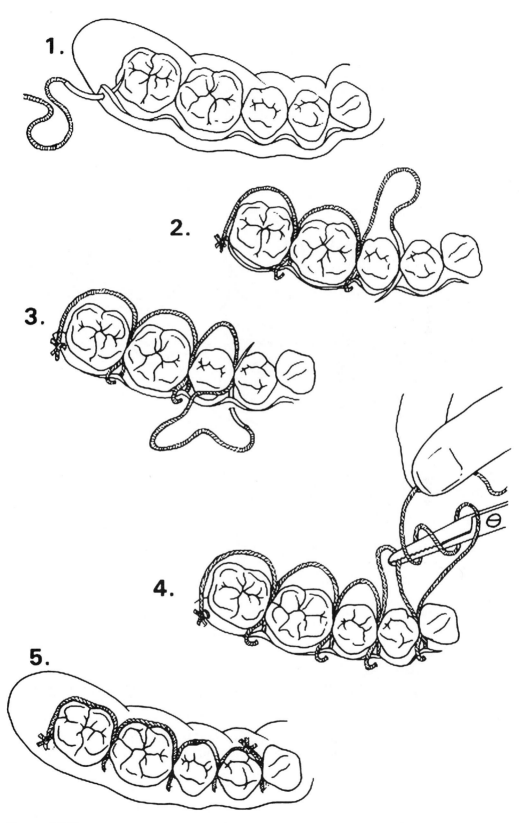

**Figure 13.7a** ●

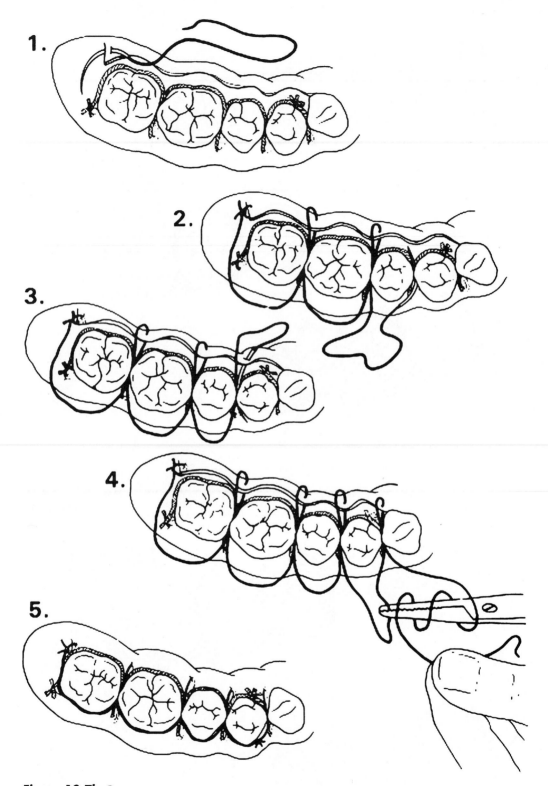

**1.**

**2.**

**3.**

**4.**

**5.**

*Figure 13.7b* ●

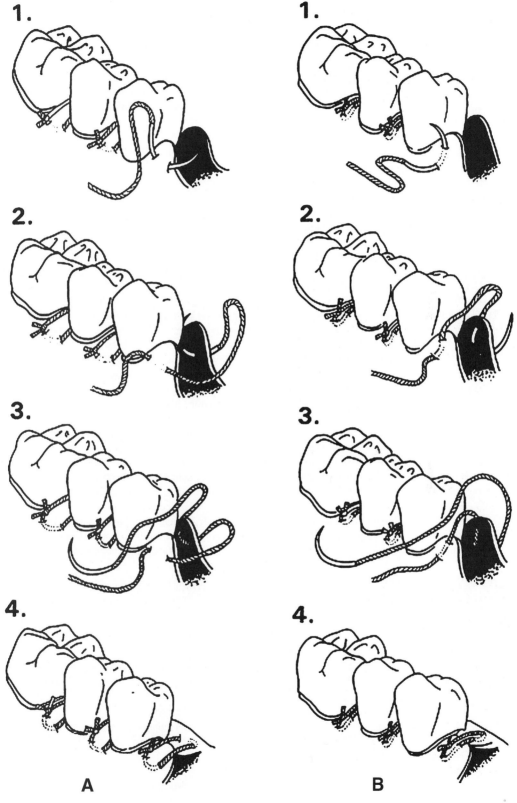

**A**

**B**

**Figure 13.8** ●

## INSTRUCTIONS AFTER PERIODONTAL SURGERY

Read and follow these guidelines for maximum comfort and fewer problems:

1.  BLEEDING: We expect minor oozing for up to 24 hours after surgery, but if heavy bleeding occurs, contact us.
2.  SWELLING: Some swelling is NORMAL after surgery. If swelling is expected, you will be given an ice pack to place adjacent to the surgery site(s) for the next 2 to 3 hours. Use the pack 15 minutes on, 15 minutes off, and so on.
3.  MEDICATIONS: Take your pills as instructed. Do not drink alcoholic drinks or take other medicine without checking. Take pills with a full glass of water or juice to lower the chance of getting nauseated. If you do become sick and it continues, notify us.
4.  FLUIDS: Drink plenty of fluids for the next few days. DO NOT USE A STRAW!
5.  DIET: Eat whatever feels comfortable, such as soups and soft foods, for a few days (e.g., instant breakfast foods).
6.  ACTIVITY: Reduce your activities for the next few days. Avoid running or strenuous activity.
7.  BRUSHING: A clean mouth heals faster! Exercise caution not to injure the surgery site(s).
8.  MOUTH RINSES: Gently rinse your mouth with warm water after each meal to keep the areas clean. You need not add salt to the water. **Use any prescribed mouth rinse as directed.**
9.  AVOID: Smoking, alcoholic drinks, and peroxide rinses for at least 72 hours after surgery—ideally longer!
10. DRESSING: If a dressing was placed, it is intended to remain in place for 1 week. A few pieces may break off and are of NO concern. If the dressing seems loose or is missing, contact our office.
11. SUTURES:
    *   No sutures were placed.
    *   Sutures will dissolve; removal is only required if they become untied and dangle down.
    *   Sutures will not dissolve—your appointment for suture removal is:

    _____.
12. PROBLEMS: If you have any problems about your healing, contact Dr._____ at

    _____.
13. Additional instructions:

    _____

## Postoperative Problems

Bleeding and loose or lost dressings are infrequent problems after surgery, but they are the most common problems. When a patient returns to the dental office because of bleeding, the dressing should usually be removed entirely. The source of bleeding should be located by gently removing any clots that conceal it. Pressure applied to the site with gauze soaked in saline solution about 5 minutes usually stops the bleeding. If it does not stop, another 5-minute application is indicated. If the source of the bleeding is the flap, or other soft tissue location, it may be possible to place a suture that will stop the bleeding. If the source of the bleeding is from the bone, burnishing the site of the bleeding with an instrument may also stop the bleeding. Injection of the bleeding site with an anesthetic containing 1:50,000 epinephrine will stop the bleeding. However, after the epinephrine is metabolized, bleeding may recur. As mentioned previously, topical epinephrine should be avoided. If the above procedures do not control the bleeding, several hemostatic agents can be used (Table 13-3).

## TABLE 13.3

### Hemostatic Agents

| Brand Name | Generic Name |
| --- | --- |
| ARC Dressing | Dry fibrin dressing |
| CollaCote, CollaTape, CollaPlug | Microfibrillar collagen |
| Gelfoam | Absorbable gelatin sponge |
| HemCon | Chitosan (made from shrimp shells and potentially allergenic) |
| Hemarrest | Epsilon aminocaproic acid and thrombin |
| Hemostatin Dressing | Propyl gallate |
| Oxycel, Avitene | Oxidized cellulose |
| Surgicel | Oxidized regenerated cellulose |
| Thrombostat | Thrombin |

Uncontrolled bleeding may be an indication of a deficiency in bleeding or clotting mechanism, and an evaluation of these systems may be required, including questioning the patient about aspirin intake. If the problem is a loose dressing, the dressing should be entirely removed and a new dressing should be placed after cessation of any resultant bleeding.

Infection rarely occurs after careful periodontal surgery. When a patient returns after surgery with a suspected infection, it is essential to take and record the vital signs, especially the temperature. Indurated swelling, severe pain, obvious purulence, lymphadenopathy, fever, or malaise indicate infection, which should be treated promptly and vigorously. Antibiotics such as penicillin, clindamycin, or other appropriate drugs should be used. In some instances, drainage may be necessary. Swelling that compromises the airway is a life-threatening emergency. The patient should be transported to the nearest emergency room in an ambulance.

Postoperative root sensitivity may occur after dressings have been removed, and usually results from ineffective plaque control. Treatment of root sensitivity is discussed in Chapter 25. Because of greater emphasis on plaque control and on new attachment procedures rather than on resection, root sensitivity is not as common a complaint as in years past.

Tooth mobility may occur after periodontal surgery. In most cases, mobility will return to baseline levels within 2 to 4 weeks.[23,24]

## LIMITATIONS OF SURGERY

Periodontal surgery is not curative. It is a means of providing access to the deeper tissues and to the root surface, and of restoring missing parts of the periodontium. When skilled, knowledgeable practitioners perform surgery for motivated, cooperative patients, it is an important part of periodontal treatment.

## REFERENCES

1. Greenwell H, Committee on Research, Science and Therapy. American Academy of Periodontology. Position paper: guidelines for periodontal therapy. J Periodontol 2001;72:1624–1628.
2. Clarke MA, Buetelman KW. Anatomical considerations in periodontal surgery. J Periodontol 1971;42:610–625.
3. Scabbia A, Cho KS, Sigurdsson TJ, Kim CK, Trombelli L. Cigarette smoking negatively affects healing response following flap debridement surgery. J Periodontol 2001;72:43–49.
4. Tobacco use and the periodontal patient. J Periodontol 1999;70:1419–1427; http://www.perio.org/resources-products/pdf/22-Tobacco.pdf.
5. American Dental Association Statement on Antibiotic Prophylaxis; http://www.ada.org/prof/resources/pubs/jada/reports/report_endocarditis01.pdf.
6. Advisory Statement Antibiotic Prophylaxis for Dental Patients with Total Joint Replacements. American Dental Association; American Academy of Orthopaedic Surgeons; http://www.ada.org/prof/resources/pubs/jada/reports/report_prophy_statement.pdf.
7. Systemic antibiotics in periodontics. J Periodontol 2004;75:1553–1565; http://www.perio.org/resources-products/pdf/46-antibiotics.pdf.
8. Centers for Disease Control and Prevention. National Center for Chronic Disease Prevention and Health Promotion. Bloodborne Pathogens and Aerosols; http://www.cdc.gov/OralHealth/infection-control/faq/aerosols.htm.
9. Molinari JA. Centers for Disease Control and Prevention. Updated CDC infection control guidelines for dental health care settings: 1 year later. Compend Contin Educ Dent 2005;26:192, 194, 196.
10. Malmed SF. Handbook of Local Anesthesia. St. Louis: CV Mosby, 2004.
11. Davenport RE, Porcelli RJ, Iacono VJ, Bonura CF, Mallis GI, Baer PN. Effects of anesthetics containing epinephrine on catecholamine levels during periodontal surgery. J Periodontol 1990;61:553–558.
12. Malmed SF. Sedation: A Guide To Patient Management. St. Louis: CV Mosby, 2004.
13. ADA Council on Scientific Affairs. Office emergencies and emergency kits. J Am Dent Assoc 2002;133:364–365.
14. Goldman HM, Cohen DW, eds. Periodontal Therapy. St. Louis: CV Mosby, 1973;840–859.
15. Kon S, Caffesse RG, Castelli WA, Nasjleti CE. Vertical releasing incisions for flap design: clinical and histological study in monkeys. Int J Periodontics Restorative Dent 1984;4:48–57.
16. Messadi DV, Bertolami CN. General principles of healing pertinent to the periodontal problems. Dent Clin North Am 1991;35:443–456.
17. Blinder D, Manor Y, Martinowitz U, Taicher S. Dental extractions in patients maintained on oral anticoagulant therapy: comparison of INR value with occurrence of postoperative bleeding. Int J Oral Maxillofac Surg 2001;30:518–521.
18. Fischer LM, Schlienger RG, Matter CM, Jick H, Meier CR. Discontinuation of nonsteroidal anti-inflammatory drug therapy and risk of acute myocardial infarction. Arch Intern Med 2004;164:2472–2476.
19. Periodontal management of patients with cardiovascular diseases. American Academy of Periodontology Position Paper. J. Periodontol 2002;73:954–968.
20. Nelson EH, Funakoshi E, O'Leary TJ. A comparison of the continuous and interrupted suturing techniques. J Periodontol 1977;48:273–281.

21. Selvig KA, Biagiotti GR, Leknes KN, Wikesjo UM. Oral tissue reactions to suture materials. Int J Periodontics Restorative Dent 1998;18:474–487.

22. Sachs HA, Farnoush A, Checchi L, Joseph CE. Current status of periodontal dressings. J Periodontol 1984;55:689–696.

23. Burch JG, Conroy CW, Ferris RT. Tooth mobility following gingivectomy. A study of gingival support of the teeth. Periodontics 1968;6:90–94.

24. Persson R. Assessment of tooth mobility using small loads. III. Effect of periodontal treatment including a gingivectomy procedure. J Clin Periodontol 1981;8:4–11.

## CHAPTER 13
## REVIEW QUESTIONS

1. A rationale for periodontal surgery is to provide access to the root surface and bone.
   a. True
   b. False
2. _____ is the primary goal of pocket reduction surgery.
   a. Regeneration
   b. Pocket elimination
   c. Pocket reduction
   d. Repair
3. Phase I therapy always eliminates the need for periodontal therapy.
   a. True
   b. False
4. _____ to _____ weeks after phase I therapy, the effect of therapy is re-evaluated.
   a. 1, 3
   b. 2, 4
   c. 3, 5
   d. 4, 6
5. After periodontal therapy, if probing depth is decreasing and there is no bleeding, one may consider which of the following?
   a. Shorter maintenance intervals
   b. Systemic antibiotics
   c. Site-specific therapy
   d. Routine maintenance therapy
6. Antibiotic prophylaxis is required for each of the following except:
   a. Acquired valvular disease
   b. Cardiac stents
   c. Mitral valve prolapse
   d. Prosthetic heart valves
7. The maximum dosage of epinephrine for a healthy adult for one appointment is _____ mg.
   a. 0.1
   b. 0.2
   c. 1.0
   d. 2.0
8. Nitrous oxide and oxygen does not provide profound sedation.
   a. True
   b. False
9. Vertical releasing incisions can be placed over the mid radicular surface of tooth roots.
   a. True
   b. False
10. Frank hemorrhage during or after surgery is rare.
    a. True
    b. False

# Management of Soft Tissue: Gingivoplasty, Gingivectomy, and Gingival Flaps

Donald Newell

## GINGIVOPLASTY AND GINGIVECTOMY

The main purpose of a gingivoplasty is to reduce gingival enlargement and create more normal gingival contours that will make plaque control easier for the patient and help prevent periodontal disease rather than eliminating pockets.[1] In the anterior areas of the mouth, an improved aesthetic appearance also is an important goal.[1,2] If there are moderate, suprabony, soft tissue pockets as a result of attachment loss or pseudopockets caused by gingival enlargement, gingivectomy is required.[1] Gingivectomy is the excision of the gingival walls of suprabony, periodontal pockets and results in the elimination of the pockets with some gingival recession.[1] Both procedures should result in increased access for plaque control by the patient.[3]

## GINGIVOPLASTY

### Indications

Gingivoplasty is primarily indicated to correct abnormal gingival contours such as the recontouring of enlarged, bulbous interdental papillae. These types of enlarged gingival contours frequently result from long-standing, chronic inflammation that has become somewhat fibrotic, especially with occurring hormonal changes during puberty and in mouth breathers.[4] Gingival enlargement also can develop in some patients on medications, such as phenytoin (Dilantin), cyclosporine, and calcium-channel blockers.[3,5]

If the tissues are firm and fibrotic, they are easily excised and contoured. When pseudopockets are present in addition to abnormal buccolingual gingival contours, gingivectomy is indicated in combination with the gingivoplasty.[1] In fact, the two procedures are frequently performed together[1,4,6] (Fig. 14-1).

### Technique

Gingivoplasty entails the beveling of the gingival margin or interdental papillae, creating interdental spillways by blending the contours of the interdental papillae with the interdental grooves (festooning).[4] Gingivoplasty is usually performed with a periodontal knife or coarse diamond stones.[5,7,8]

1. A periodontal knife, such as the Kirkland No. 15/16 or the Goldman-Fox No.7, is used to excise or shave the enlarged gingival tissues to establish the desired basic contours. The Goldman-Fox knife has special blade angulations, which enable it to be more easily positioned to make a beveled cut through the gingiva, especially on the lingual aspects of the mandibular teeth. The knife is then used like a hoe to scrape the tissues to achieve the final knife-edged gingival architecture[6,8] (Fig. 14-1).
2. Coarse diamond stones may also be used[7,8] (Fig. 14-1). The stones may be of various shapes depending on the need and preference of the clinician. A steady stream of sterile saline solution or sterile water must be used, along with adequate aspiration, to prevent burning of the tissue and clogging of the stone. Whether knives or stones are used, the soft tissue will often show minute shreds or tags, which must be removed. Fine scissors or nippers are usually used to perform tissue tag removal.

After the gingiva has been contoured by either of the techniques described, a periodontal dressing, preferably non-eugenol, is placed over the surgical site.[4] The dressing is changed weekly until

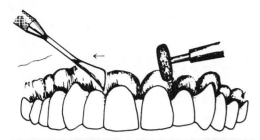

**Figure 14.1** ●

sufficient healing has occurred to permit plaque control by the patient. At each dressing change, the operator should gently remove any accumulated plaque and debris with floss or tape and a curet. The teeth in the operative site should then be polished with a low-abrasive polishing agent, such as toothpaste, both facially and lingually, avoiding damage to the healing tissue. At the time of final dressing removal, all teeth are polished again. Because there is usually a significant postoperative change in the gingival contours, the patient's plaque control often suffers, and he or she must be reinstructed in plaque removal procedures.

## GINGIVECTOMY

### Indications

The gingivectomy was commonly performed for many years in the past, but increased knowledge of wound healing and the development of more sophisticated flap procedures have made its use less frequent today.[3]

Gingivectomy may be indicated for elimination of suprabony periodontal pockets, with or without clinically evident gingival enlargement, when excision of the pocket wall will not result in an inadequate zone of attached gingiva. In cases in which gingival enlargement results in pseudopockets, rather than true pockets from periodontal disease, an adequate zone of keratinized gingiva usually remains after excision of the tissues.

Gingivectomy can be performed on gingiva that is soft and edematous but is better performed after scaling and root planing to reduce inflammation. When any gingival enlargements remain, they are mostly fibrotic, and surgical removal is the treatment of choice.[3]

Some examples of disease entities that usually can be treated by gingivectomy are:

1. Phenytoin (Dilantin)-induced gingival enlargement[7,9,10]
2. Cyclosporine-induced gingival enlargement[11,12]

3. Gingival enlargement associated with calcium-channel blockers[11,13]
4. Chronic, inflammatory gingival enlargement[4]
5. Delayed passive eruption[8,14–16]
6. Hereditary gingivofibromatosis[17]
7. Crown lengthening by removal of soft tissue only[4]
8. Gingival (not periodontal) abscesses[3]
9. Gingival craters with no underlying interproximal bony craters[8]

Gingival enlargement associated with medications, especially phenytoin, is usually followed by progressive regrowth, especially in less compliant patients.[8,10] Good patient plaque control will minimize regrowth, but it still tends to recur.[8] It was hoped that gingivoplasty by an internal beveled gingival flap (described later in this chapter), leaving a mature, epithelialized surface instead of a large exposed connective tissue surface, would retard regrowth.[8] However, there is no evidence to support this idea, but there is usually less postoperative pain and discomfort with this technique, making it a worthwhile surgical approach.[8]

The successful use of a positive-pressure appliance on the gingiva to prevent recurrence of enlargement caused by phenytoin has been reported in the literature.[18,19] An impression is taken immediately after the gingivectomy, and a cast is poured to fabricate the appliance.[18,19] It is worn at night when the concentration of phenytoin in saliva is at its peak.[8]

### Contraindications

Gingivectomy is not recommended in certain instances.[1–4]

1. When the pocket depths are deep enough to be at or apical to the mucogingival junction or when there is an inadequate amount of keratinized gingiva associated with shallower pockets. This will result in a gingival margin composed of alveolar mucosa after completion of the gingivectomy.
2. When the alveolar mucosa forms the soft tissue wall of the pocket.
3. When frenum or muscle attachments are in the area of surgery.
4. When treatment of bony craters by osseous resection or infrabony defects by regenerative procedures are indicated.
5. When an esthetic deformity may result because of the resulting gingival recession.
6. Surgery of any kind is not recommended in a totally noncompliant patient.[20] Initial therapy consisting of scaling and root planing with maintenance visits every 3 months or less will be necessary.

## Technique

The gingivectomy technique as it is used today was described by Goldman.[21]

1. The first step in gingivectomy is to obtain satisfactory anesthesia by either the block or infiltration technique.

2. After the patient is sufficiently anesthetized, the pocket depths in the surgical site are measured at the same six sites probed during an examination, and external puncture marks (bleeding points) are made in the gingiva. This can be accurately accomplished with either Crane-Kaplan (C-K) pocket markers or with a calibrated periodontal probe.[2,7,8] The C-K pocket markers resemble cotton pliers but have one straight prong and one that has a 90-degree bend at the tip with a sharp point that is at the same level as the tip of the straight prong. These pocket markers come in mirror image pairs to measure pocket depths on buccal and lingual surfaces in all quadrants of the dentition. The pocket depth levels are marked with these instruments by placing the straight prong into the gingival crevices to the apex of the pocket with the bent, sharp pointed end external to the gingiva. The prongs are then squeezed together, and the sharp, bent tip punctures the outer wall of the gingival tissue, leaving a bleeding point at the level of the base of the pocket.[2,3] The calibrated periodontal probe can be used as a pocket depth marker by placing it into each of the six pocket sites per tooth and measuring the depths in millimeters. The probe is then withdrawn and positioned over the external surface of the gingiva to the same depth as when in the pocket. Keeping the tip at the same position, the probe is then rotated 90 degrees, and the gingiva is punctured by the probe tip causing an external bleeding point at the level of the base of the pocket.[1] When the entire area has been adequately measured and marked, the bleeding points will outline the required incision[1-3] (Fig. 14-2).

3. Make the initial incision apical to the bleeding points with a broad-bladed knife such as the Kirkland No. 15/16 (Fig. 14-2) or the Goldman-Fox No.7[2,4] (Fig. 14-2). The incision should be beveled externally to about a 45-degree angle to the root of the tooth and should end on the tooth at a depth not farther than the apical end of the epithelial attachment (junctional epithelium).[2] The supracrestal fibers should be left intact so that no bone will be exposed. It is often prudent to repeat the initial incision to ensure that the gingival collar, which will be removed, has been completely cut through to the teeth. When the gingiva is thick, lengthen the bevel to eliminate a plateau or shoulder. Sometimes, access may be so limited or difficult that a proper bevel cannot be obtained with the initial incision. In this case, the bevel can be corrected later by gingivoplasty, either with a broad-bladed knife used as a scraper or with coarse abrasive rotary diamond stones.[7,8]

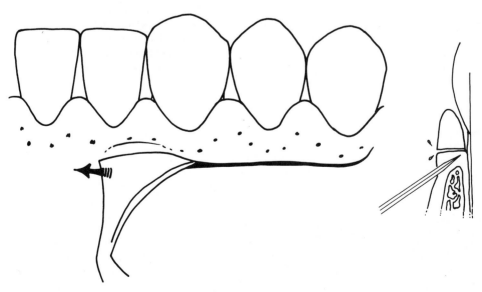

*Figure 14.2* ●

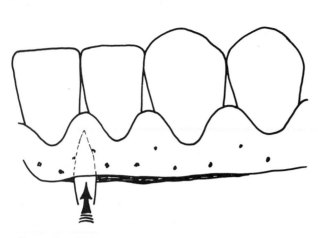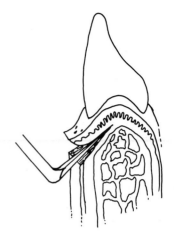

**Figure 14.3 ●**

4. Use narrow-bladed knives, such as the Orban No. 1/2, to excise the tissue interproximally[6,7] (Fig. 14-3). Note that the blade is positioned into the initial incision interproximally so that the angle of the blade is approximately the same as that made with the broad-bladed knife.

5. If the initial marginal and interproximal incisions have been made completely through the gingiva to the base of the pockets and not into the supracrestal fibers, the incised gingival tissue will be easily removed with curets (Fig. 14-4). If any supracrestal fibers remain attached to the gingival collar, it will resist easy removal and the attached fibers will need to be cut cleanly with sulcular incisions.

6. Even though initial scaling and root planing should have been performed before surgery, some subgingival plaque and calculus often remain. Remove these accretions from the root surfaces by scaling and root planing.[2]

Removal of the soft tissue walls of periodontal pockets renders the root surfaces more accessible and visible to the operator now than at any other time. Success or failure of the entire procedure depends on how well the operator performs root preparation to remove residual plaque, calculus, and endotoxin.[6]

7. Complete further contouring as needed by using coarse diamond stones or a broad-bladed knife to scrape the tissue (Fig. 14-5). If diamond stones are used, take care not to damage the tooth surfaces.

8. Remove tissue tags with scissors or nippers.

9. Flush the surgical site with sterile water or sterile saline solution to remove foreign particles.[2]

10. To stop the bleeding, apply constant pressure against the wound for 2 to 3 minutes with cotton-free gauze sponges saturated with sterile water or sterile saline solution.[2]

11. A well-adapted, non-eugenol periodontal dressing should be placed for patient comfort

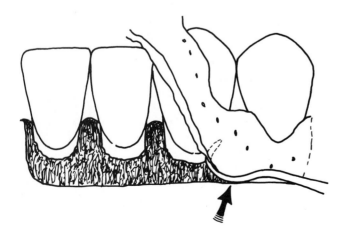

**Figure 14.4 ●**

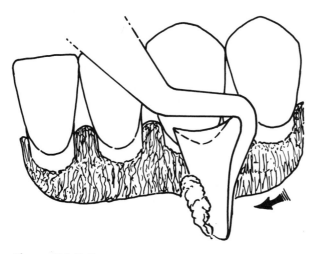
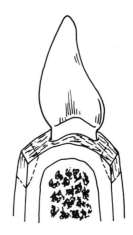

**Figure 14.5** ●

and to prevent formation of exuberant granulation tissue.[2] Apply the dressing by initially placing small, pointed sections of the dressing interproximally with a plastic instrument.[2] Next, place longer strips on the facial, lingual, and palatal aspects and join them to the interproximal sections.[2] The teeth surfaces should be as dry as possible to ensure tacky adhesion of the dressing to the teeth in addition to the interlocking, interproximal retention. Cover the entire wound area with the dressing, taking care not to let the dressing interfere with occlusion or muscle attachments.[2] A common error is making the dressing too large. Manually trimming the dressing while it is still soft and pliable will prevent overextension.[2] If some dressing is to be removed near or over the occlusal surfaces of the teeth, it is carefully removed with a curet directed toward the teeth, not away from them, so that the dressing is not loosened or pulled away from the wound area.

12. Instruct the patient to avoid eating or drinking for 1 hour after surgery to allow the dressing to set. Tart or spicy foods should be avoided.[2] Mouth rinses with 0.12% chlorhexidine gluconate will reduce plaque around the dressing and surgical site and aid healing.[22–24] Medications for discomfort are written, and oral and written postoperative instructions are given to the patient along with the dentist's home phone number. Although the chances of postoperative complications are small, having a contact phone number will make the patient feel more confident.[2]

13. Change the dressing and debride the wound weekly until the tissues have healed suffi-

ciently for the patient to accomplish plaque control. Remember, epithelium will cover a wound at the rate of 0.5 mm/day after an initial 24 hours' postoperative absence of mitotic epithelial activity, so the dressing is often permanently removed in 2 weeks.

14. After the dressing is removed, polish the teeth and instruct the patient in plaque control, making technique adjustments to accommodate the new gingival contours. The patient should be counseled to continue to brush with an extra-soft brush (Butler Gum, Sensodyne Gentle, or Lactona Softex brushes).[2] Good plaque control during the early postoperative period will enhance healing.[2,25]

Other techniques that have been advocated to perform gingivectomy are the use of electrosurgery and lasers.[26,27] Both of these techniques permit adequate contouring of the gingival tissues and control hemorrhage,[28–30] but there are several problems with their use. Electrosurgery should not be used in patients wearing incompatible or poorly shielded cardiac pacemakers.[7] The procedure produces an unpleasant odor, and, when used close to bone, the heat generated can cause tissue damage and loss of periodontal support.[7,31–33] If the electrode touches the tooth root, areas of cementum burn occur.[31] The $CO_2$ laser has been advocated for the excision of gingival growths, but healing is delayed compared with healing after conventional gingivectomy with a scalpel or knife.[34] Presently, the use of lasers for routine periodontal surgery is not supported by research, and caution in its use is recommended pending further well-designed studies.[35]

## GINGIVAL FLAP

The gingival flap is subgingival curettage performed with a knife.[36,37] Subgingival curettage was used extensively in the past and consisted of removal of the inner surface of the soft tissue wall of the pocket containing epithelium, epithelial attachment, and granulomatous tissue by the use of a curet. Even though some inadvertent curettage occurred during routine root planing, subgingival curettage was usually done as a separate procedure to more completely remove the contents of the soft tissue wall of the pocket after scaling and root planing had rendered the gingival tissues more firm and fibrotic.[38] It was thought that removal of these inflamed contents would result in new attachment of connective tissue or a healthy long junctional epithelial adhesion to the tooth root.[38,39] Curettage is no longer frequently used[40] because

the result is the same as with scaling and root planing.[41] This procedure is no longer listed in the ADA Procedural Code as a specific procedure. Some of the reasons for this are that:

1. The complete removal of subgingival deposits by scaling and root planing results in optimal healing without curettage[41]
2. The procedure is technically difficult and time consuming, and the results are similar after flap surgery and curettage[36]
3. More effective methods are available to remove pocket epithelium and adjacent connective tissue by means of internal (reverse) bevel incisions,[42] although crestal and subcrestal incisions have been shown to incompletely remove pocket epithelium[43]

The gingival flap is basically similar to the excisional new attachment procedure (ENAP).[37]

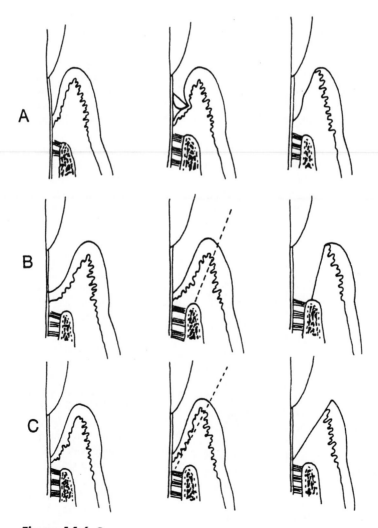

*Figure 14.6* ●

The inner aspect (epithelium, epithelial attachment, and the granulomatous tissue) of the periodontal pocket is excised with a scalpel, and the remaining gingival tissue is closely approximated against and between the detoxified roots of the teeth, thus creating the potential for formation of a new attachment during healing.[37] The gingival flap is not elevated if the remaining gingival tissue approximation is good. If thick, underlying bone prevents close approximation, a flap may be elevated to thin the crestal bone, but the gingival flap is never elevated beyond the mucogingival line.[37] Otherwise, the gingiva remains attached to the alveolar bone.

## Indications

The gingival flap is indicated in[7,37]:

1. Suprabony pockets of shallow to moderate depths (5 mm or less) that have an adequate width and thickness of keratinized tissue
2. The anterior region, where esthetics is a consideration and access to the root for root planing is needed

## Contraindications

The gingival flap is contraindicated when the following conditions are present[7,37]:

1. There is an inadequate zone of keratinized tissue
2. There are osseous defects present that need correcting
3. Pseudopockets are present and need correcting

## Objective

The objective of the gingival flap is pocket reduction by establishing a new attachment (epithelial or connective tissue) to the tooth at a more coronal level. There is little question that some gingival shrinkage occurs with this surgical procedure, but long-term clinical studies also indicate a more coronal attachment of soft tissue.[36,44,45]

## Surgical Procedure

Figure 14-6B illustrates the gingival flap technique. Once the patient has established adequate plaque control and the bacterial control phase is complete, the following should be done[37]:

1. Anesthetize the area.
2. Make an internally beveled incision with a surgical blade from the margin of the gingival tissue apically to the crest of the alveolar bone (Fig. 14-7).

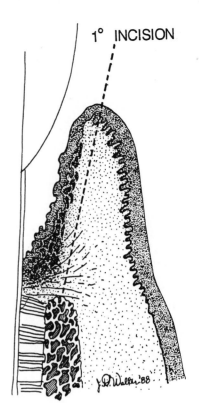

**Figure 14.7** ●

3. Carry the incision interproximally on both the facial and lingual sides, attempting to retain as much of the interdental papilla as possible (Fig. 14-8). The intent is to cut out the inner portion of the soft tissue wall of the pocket all around the tooth. No attempt is made to elevate

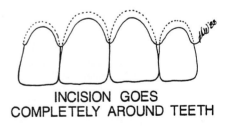

INCISION GOES
COMPLETELY AROUND TEETH

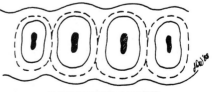

INCISIONS MEET
IN THE INTERPROXIMAL

**Figure 14.8** ●

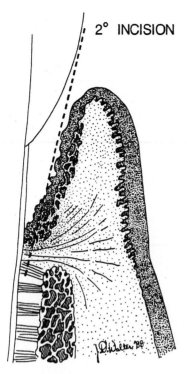

**Figure 14.9** ●

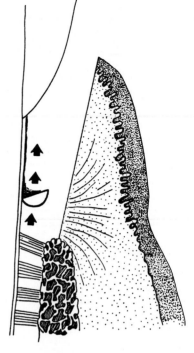

**Figure 14.10** ●

the flap completely away from its attachment to the alveolar bone (a gingival flap rather than a mucoperiosteal or mucosal flap).

4. A secondary sulcular incision is made from the bottom of the pocket through the alveolar crest fibers (and interproximally, through the transseptal fibers) to the crest of the alveolar bone (Fig. 14-9).

5. Remove the excised pocket lining tissue with a curet.

6. Carefully detoxify all cementum that has been exposed to the environment of the pocket. Attempt to create a smooth hard root surface, free of plaque and calculus (Fig. 14-10). Do not attempt to remove the supracrestal connective tissue fibers that constitute the biologic width and are still attached to the tooth about 1 to 2 mm coronal to the crest of the bone. There should be no plaque or calculus in the biologic width zone.

7. Rinse the area with sterile water or sterile normal saline solution, and examine the root surface to ensure that no calculus or plaque remains and that no large blood clots are present.

8. Approximate the wound edges (Fig. 14-11). If the edges do not meet passively, reflect the flap enough to contour the bone until good adaptation of the wound edges is achieved but not past the mucogingival junction.

9. Suture interproximally with interrupted or internal vertical mattress sutures.

10. Apply firm but gentle pressure for 2 to 3 minutes to the operative site from both the facial and lingual aspects with saline-soaked gauze to permit only a small blood clot to form between the tissue and the tooth.

11. Place a periodontal dressing over the site, being careful not to force the dressing between the tooth and the gingival tissue.

12. Remove the dressing and sutures in 7 to 10 days and polish the area.

13. Carefully review plaque control of the surgical site with the patient. Advise the patient to brush and floss the area carefully and meticulously. A roll toothbrushing technique and utilization of interproximal flossing to the gingival margin during the initial period of healing will provide adequate plaque control without disrupting the healing process of the gingival tissue to the tooth surface. Success is dependent on controlling plaque formation during the critical first 4 weeks of healing.

14. Perform postoperative polishing once a week for 4 weeks.

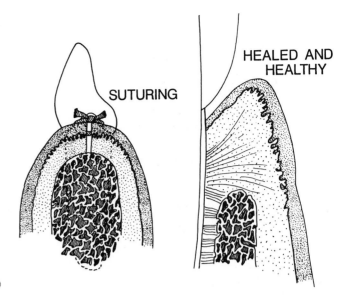

SUTURING

HEALED AND HEALTHY

*Figure 14.11* ●

15. Do not probe for 3 months to permit complete attachment of the epithelium and connective tissue fibers to the tooth.

The gingival flap, or ENAP, is not commonly used today because of its limited access to bone defects.[37,40] However, it can be useful in reducing probing depths and gaining clinical attachment levels for a long period of time when there are moderate suprabony pockets present.[44,45]

## DEEP POCKET RETROMOLAR AREA (DISTAL WEDGE PROCEDURE)

A deep pocket in the retromolar area may be corrected by a distal wedge[46,47] or a distal box procedure[48] in conjunction with facial and lingual flaps.

### Technique

There are various ways of performing the distal wedge procedure. One technique is as follows[6,49]:

1. With a No. 12a or 12b scalpel, outline a narrow triangle approximately 3 mm deep into the gingival tissue distal to the terminal molar, with the base of the triangle at the distal surface of the molar and the apex 10 to 12 mm distal to the tooth (Fig.14-12, A–C). Do not extend the incisions toward the base of the triangular wedge to the buccal and lingual line angles of the terminal molar. Doing so will make it very difficult to approximate the wound edges close to the molar during suturing. The base of the triangular wedge should not measure more than 3 to 4 mm buccolin-

gually. In dissecting the wedge to bone, use undermining incisions with a No. 12a or 12b scalpel blade to prepare partial thickness flaps on the facial and lingual surfaces of the retromolar area as shown in Figure 14-12A. This will result in the wedge being wider at its apical base than it is at the gingival surface (Fig. 14-12a). This triangular distal wedge works better in the mandibular retromolar area, where there is more underlying flexible alveolar mucosa, than it does in the maxillary tuberosity area. The tissue in the maxillary tuberosity is denser, and undermining the buccal and lingual flaps is difficult near the narrow apex of the triangle. In the maxillary tuberosity, if desired, parallel, undermining facial and lingual incisions may be used, followed by a connecting incision at the distal aspect of the two parallel incisions extending slightly to the buccal and lingual as releasing incisions[48]. This results in a rectangular box, rather than a wedge (Fig. 14-12B), and makes undermining more even throughout the wedge.[48]

2. Grasp the wedge of tissue at the distal edge with a curved hemostat and sever its connection from the bone crest (Fig. 14-12C). If the patient is a smoker with clinical evidence of hyperkeratosis in the retromolar or tuberosity areas, it may be desirable to place the excised tissues in formalin for microscopic study. In that case the wedge should be grasped with a tissue pickup forceps. A hemostat will likely crush the specimen and make microscopic cellular examination difficult.

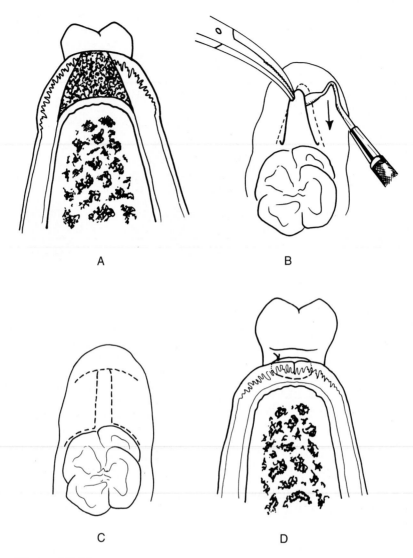

A                                     B

C                                     D

**Figure 14.12** ●

3. Scale and root plane the distal surface of the molar.
4. Perform osseous surgery, if indicated. The distal surface of the second molar is a common area for a deep osseous defect, which may respond to bone grafting procedures.
5. Approximate the wound edges and suture with interrupted sutures (Fig. 14-12D).
6. Protect the area for 7 to 10 days. Then remove the sutures and polish the teeth in the surgical site.

# REFERENCES

1. Grant DA, Stern IB, Listgarten MA. Periodontics in the Tradition of Gottlieb and Orban, 6th ed. St. Louis: CV Mosby Co, 1988:761–768.

2. Grant DA, Stern IB, Listgarten MA. Periodontics in the Tradition of Gottlieb and Orban, 6th ed. St. Louis: CV Mosby Co, 1988:770–774.
3. Newman MG, Takei HH, Carranza FA. Carranza's Clinical Periodontology, 9th ed. Philadelphia: WB Saunders, 2002:749–753.
4. Rateitschak KH, ed. Color Atlas of Dental Medicine, Vol 1. Periodontology, 2nd ed. New York: Thieme Medical Publishers, 1989:274–277.
5. Butler RT, Kalkwarf KL, Kaldahl WB. Drug-induced gingival hyperplasia: phenytoin, cyclosporine and nifedipine. J Am Dent Assoc 1987;114:56–60.
6. Fedi PF, Vernino AR, Gray JL. The Periodontal Syllabus, 4th ed. Philadelphia: Lippincott Williams & Wilkins, 2000:136–144.
7. Carranza FA, Newman MG. Clinical Periodontology, 8th ed. Philadelphia: WB Saunders, 1966: 588–590.

8. Prichard J. Advanced Periodontal Disease/Surgical and Prosthetic Management, 2nd ed. Philadelphia: WB Saunders, 1972:419–436.

9. Babcock JR. Incidence of gingival hyperplasia associated with Dilantin therapy in a hospital population. J Am Dent Assoc 1963;71:1447–1458.

10. Marakoglu I, Gursoy UK, Cakmak H, Marakoglu K. Phenytoin-induced gingival overgrowth in uncooperative epilepsy patients. Yonsei Med J 2004; 45:337–340.

11. King GN, Fullinfaw R, Higgins TJ, Walker RG, Francis DM, Wiesenfeld D. Gingival hyperplasia in renal allograft recipients receiving cyclosporin-A and calcium antagonists. J Clin Periodontol 1993; 20:286–293.

12. Seymore RA, Smith DG. The effect of a plaque control programme on the incidence and severity of cyclosporine-induced gingival changes. J Clin Periodontol 1991;18:107–110.

13. Westbrook P, Bednarczyk EM, Carlson M, Sheehan H, Bissada NF. Regression of nifedipine-induced gingival hyperplasia following switch to a same class calcium channel blocker isradipine. J Periodontol 1997;68:645–650.

14. Allen EP. Surgical crown lengthening for function and esthetics. Dent Clin North Am 1993;37: 163–179.

15. Levine RA, McGuire M. The diagnosis and treatment of the gummy smile. Compend Contin Educ Dental 1997;18:757–762.

16. Dolt AH 3rd, Robbins JW. Altered passive eruption: an etiology of short clinical crowns. Quintessence Int 1997;28:363–372.

17. Casavecchia P, Uzel MI, Kantarci A, Hasturk H, Dibart S, Hart TC, Trackman PC, Van Dyke TE. Hereditary gingival fibromatosis associated with generalized aggressive periodontitis: a case report. J Periodontol 2004, 75:770–778.

18. Davis RK, Baer PN, Palmer JH. A preliminary report on a new therapy for Dilantin gingival hyperplasia. J Periodontol 1963;34:17–22.

19. Babcock JR. The successful use of a new therapy for Dilantin gingival hyperplasia. Periodontics 1965;3: 196–199.

20. Nyman S, Lindhe J, Rosling B. Periodontal surgery in plaque-infected dentitions. J Clin Periodontol 1977;4:240–249.

21. Goldman HM. Gingivectomy. Oral Surg Oral Med Oral Pathol 1951;4:1136–1157.

22. Sanz M, Newman MG, Anderson L, Matoska W, Otomo-Corgel J, Saltini C. Clinical enhancement of post-periodontal surgical therapy by a 0.12% chlorhexidine gluconate mouthrinse. J Periodontol 1989;60:570–576.

23. Vaughan ME, Garnick JJ. The effect of a 0.125% chlorhexidine rinse on inflammation after periodontal surgery. J Periodontol 1989;60:704–708.

24. Westfelt E, Nyman S, Lindhe J, Socransky S. Use of chlorhexidine as a plaque control measure following surgical treatment of periodontal disease. J Clin Periodontol 1983;10:22–36.

25. Heitz F, Heitz-Mayfield LJ, Lang NP. Effect of post-surgical cleaning protocols on early plaque control in periodontal and/or implant wound healing. J Clin Periodontol 2004;31:1012–1018.

26. Walker CR Jr, Tomich CE, Hutton CE. Treatment of phenytoin-induced gingival hyperplasia by electrosurgery. Oral Surg 1980;38:306–311.

27. Coleton S. Lasers in surgical periodontics and oral medicine. Dent Clin North Am 2004;48:937–962.

28. Pick RM, Colvard MD. Current status of lasers in soft tissue dental surgery. J Periodontol 1993;64: 589–602.

29. Bader HI. Use of lasers in periodontics. Dent Clin North Am 2000;44:779–791.

30. Malkoc S, Buyukyilmos T, Gelgor I, Gursel M. Comparison of two different gingivectomy techniques for gingival cleft treatment. Angle Orthod 2004;74:375–380.

31. Wilhelmsen NR, Ramfjord SP, Blankenship JR. Effects of electrosurgery on the gingival attachment in rhesus monkeys. J Periodontol 1976;47:160–170.

32. Azzi R, Kenney FB, Tsao TF, Carranza FA Jr. The effect of electrosurgery upon alveolar bone. J Periodontol 1983;54:96–100.

33. Glickman I, Imber IR. Comparison of gingival resection with electrosurgery and periodontal knives: a biometric and histologic study. J Periodontol 1970;41:142–148.

34. Fisher SF, Frame JW, Browne RM, Tranter RM. A comparative histologic study of wound healing following $CO_2$ laser and conventional surgical excision of the buccal mucosa. Arch Oral Biol 1983;28: 287–291.

35. The American Academy of Periodontology Statement Regarding Lasers in Periodontics. J Periodontol 2002;73:1231–1239.

36. Yukna RA, Bowers GM, Lawrence JJ, et al. A clinical study of healing in humans following the excisional new attachment procedure. J Periodontol 1976;47:696–700.

37. Yukna RA, Lawrence JJ. Gingival surgery for soft tissue new attachment. Dent Clin North Am 1980; 24:705–718.

38. Carranza FA. A technique for reattachment. J Periodontol 1954;25:272–278.

39. Halik FJ. The role of subgingival curettage to periodontal therapy. Dent Clin North Am 1969;13:19–32.

40. The American Academy of Periodontology Statement Regarding Gingival Curettage. J Periodontol 2002;73:1229–1230.

41. Caton J, Nyman S, Zander H. Histometric evaluation of periodontal surgery. II. Connective tissue attachment levels after four regenerative procedures. J Clin Periodontol 1980;7:224–231.

42. Yukna RA. A clinical and histologic study of healing following the excisional new attachment procedure in rhesus monkeys. J Periodontol 1976;47:701–709.

43. Litch JM, O'Leary TJ, Kafrawy AH. Pocket epithelium removal via crestal and subcrestal scalloped internal bevel incisions. J Periodontol 1984; 55: 142–148.

44. Yukna RA, Williams JE Jr. Five year evaluation of the excisional new attachment procedure. J Periodontol 1980;51:382–385.
45. D'Archivio D, Di Placido G, Tumini V, Del Giglio Matarazzo A, Tritapepe R, Paolantonio M. A comparative evaluation of the efficacy of the excisional new attachment procedure (ENAP) relative to root planing in the etiological phase of periodontal therapy. Minerva Stomatol 1999;48:439–45.
46. Robinson RE. The distal wedge operation. Periodontics 1966;4:256–264.
47. Saadoun AP. Surgical management of the maxillary tuberosity area. Cont Educ 1984;5:34–53.
48. Kramer GM, Schwartz MS. A technique to obtain primary intention healing in pocket elimination adjacent to an edentulous area. Periodontics 1964; 2:252–257.
49. Grant DA, Stern IB, Listgarten MA. Periodontics in the Tradition of Gottlieb and Orban, 6th ed. St. Louis: CV Mosby Co, 1988:796–801.

## CHAPTER 14
## REVIEW QUESTIONS

1. Gingivoplasty and gingivectomy have several similar goals. Which of the following is a goal of gingivectomy but not gingivoplasty?
   a. To reduce gingival enlargement
   b. To create more normal gingival contours
   c. To eliminate suprabony pockets
   d. To make plaque control easier for the patient

2. Gingivectomy cannot be used to treat which one of the following conditions?
   a. Gingival enlargement from medications
   b. Periodontal abscesses
   c. Delayed passive eruption
   d. Hereditary gingivofibromatosis

3. Phenytoin-induced gingival enlargement is best treated by an internal beveled gingival flap instead of an external beveled gingivectomy because:
   a. The patient has less postoperative pain and discomfort
   b. Recurrence of gingival enlargement is delayed
   c. The internal beveled gingival flap is easier to perform
   d. There is no difference between the two surgical techniques

4. The most successful treatment to delay recurrent gingival enlargement is to:
   a. Perform a gingivectomy with postsurgical gingival massage
   b. Perform an internal beveled gingival flap with postsurgical gingival massage
   c. Perform gingivoplasty with postsurgical gingival massage
   d. Perform a gingivectomy and make a positive-pressure appliance

5. The purpose of the Orban Nos. 1 and 2 instruments used in a gingivectomy is to:
   a. Make bleeding points before gingivectomy
   b. Make the externally beveled, initial incision
   c. Make the externally beveled, interproximal incision
   d. Debride the exposed root surfaces

6. The initial incisions for a gingivectomy are guided by bleeding points at the levels of the bases of the pockets. How many bleeding points are marked for each tooth both buccally and lingually?
   a. 1
   b. 2
   c. 4
   d. 6

7. Once initiated, epithelium covers a wound at the rate of 0.5 mm/day. At that rate, how many days would it take for epithelium to cover a gingivectomy wound 5 mm in width?
   a. 11 days
   b. 10 days
   c. 9 days
   d. 8 days

8. The gingival flap is basically similar to:
   a. The modified Widman flap
   b. The replaced flap
   c. The excisional new attachment procedure (ENAP)
   d. The apically positioned flap

9. Which one of the following conditions would be an indication for the gingival flap?
   a. An inadequate zone of keratinized tissue
   b. A wide zone of gingival tissue with moderate pocket depths
   c. Osseous defects are present that need correction
   d. Pseudopockets are present that need correcting

10. Which of the following statements about the gingival flap is the most accurate?
    a. The gingival flap is never reflected away from alveolar bone.
    b. The gingival flap is always reflected away from alveolar bone.
    c. To achieve better flap approximation, the gingival flap is reflected from alveolar bone past the mucogingival junction.
    d. To achieve better flap approximation, the gingival flap is reflected from alveolar bone, but not past the mucogingival junction.

# Management of Soft Tissue: Flaps for Pocket Management

Raymond A. Yukna

## BASIC CONCEPTS AND CONSIDERATIONS

### Objectives of Flaps

Periodontal flap procedures are designed to accomplish one or more of the following:

1. Provide access for root surface detoxification
2. Reduce probing depths including those that extend to or beyond the mucogingival junction
3. Preserve or create an adequate zone of attached gingiva
4. Permit access to underlying bone for treatment of osseous defects
5. Facilitate regenerative procedures

## CLASSIFICATION OF FLAPS

A flap is defined as that portion of the gingiva, alveolar mucosa, or periosteum that retains its blood supply when it is elevated or dissected from the tooth and alveolar bone.

Flaps may be classified on the basis of tissue components and the positioning of these components at the completion of surgery. The following section is a classification and description of the more popular flap techniques for pocket management.

## CLASSIFICATION BASED ON TISSUE CONTENTS

### Full-Thickness (Mucoperiosteal) Flap (FTF)

A full-thickness (mucoperiosteal) flap contains gingiva, mucosa, submucosa, and periosteum. It is prepared by bluntly dissecting the soft tissue from the bone as follows[1–3]:

1. A scalloped, internally bevelled incision is made from the gingival margin to the crest of the alveolar bone, preserving as much keratinized gingiva as possible. Scalpel blades numbers 11, 12b, 15, or 15c are commonly used to make this primary incision. The number 11 or 15c blade in a modified handle works well on the lingual or palatal surfaces (Fig. 15-1, A and B). The primary incision should extend around the necks of the teeth and interproximally, to include the height of the interproximal papilla for primary wound closure.
2. Flap reflection is best begun in the papillae with a small elevator such as a plastic instrument. Further flap elevation is performed by bluntly separating the midfacial and midlingual tissue from the bone with a periosteal elevator or chisel to obtain sufficient flap reflection and mobility and adequate access to the underlying structures (crestal bone, osseous defects, contaminated root surfaces; Fig. 15-1C).
3. A second, sulcular incision is made around each tooth to the bone crest or coronal aspect of the periodontal ligament with the scalpel blade or sharp chisels (Ochsenbein or Fedi chisels). This secondary incision severs the supracrestal gingival fibers from the tooth (Fig. 15-1D).
4. The scalpel blade or gingivectomy knives are then used to sever the remaining collar of soft tissue by cutting horizontally at the crest of the bone (Fig. 15-1E). This frees the collar of pocket tissue and allows for its easy removal.
5. The granulomatous tissue is debrided from the crest of the bone and from any osseous defects.
6. The exposed root surfaces are cleaned of calculus and plaque with ultrasonic, sonic, rotary, or

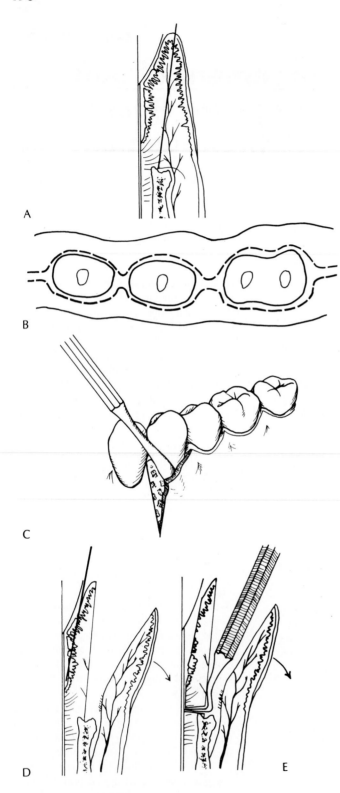

A

B

C

D                                             E

*Figure 15.1* ●

hand instruments. The involved root surfaces are planed until smooth and hard to remove embedded bacteria and endotoxins. Remember that the healthy connective tissue fibers attached at the very apical portion of the exposed root surfaces should be left attached (0.5 to 1 mm coronal to the crest of the alveolar bone).[4,5] Only the root surfaces that have been exposed to the environment of the pocket (using probing depth as a guide) need to be planed.

7. The surgical site should be irrigated with sterile saline and examined for any residual debris on the root or soft tissue tags.

8. Chemical agents (such as citric acid, tetracycline solution, EDTA) may be applied to attempt to further improve biologic compatibility of the root surface for soft tissue attachment.[6–8] These chemicals should only be used on those areas of the root surface that will be covered with the flaps at the conclusion of surgery.

9. Depending on their severity and configuration, bony defects may be treated by osseous resection, debridement, grafting, or guided tissue regeneration as desired (see Chapters 16, 17, and 18).

10. Depending on the surgical objective, the flaps can be replaced near their original position or can be apically positioned at various levels and sutured (see below).

11. Periodontal dressing (chemical cured or light cured) may be applied if desired for surgical site protection. The clinician may desire to apply a topical antibiotic ointment to prevent wedging of the dressing beneath the flap and to prevent the dressing from binding to the sutures. Appropriate postoperative and oral hygiene instructions are provided.

12. Dressing and sutures are usually removed after 7 to 10 days. The area is gently debrided and polished. Proper mechanical or chemical plaque control instructions are provided. Patients are seen again at about 20 and 30 days, then a proper supportive periodontal therapy schedule is arranged.

## Partial-Thickness (Mucosal) Flap (PTF)

The partial-thickness (mucosal) flap is composed of gingiva, mucosa, or submucosa, but not the periosteum. The partial-thickness flap is prepared by sharp dissection close to the alveolar bone, with the intent of leaving the periosteum and some connective tissue attached to and covering the bone.[9,10]

The technique for performing a partial-thickness flap is the same as the technique for performing a full-thickness flap except for the initial dissections and method of flap reflection.

1. A scalloped, internally beveled incision is made with a scalpel starting at the gingival margin parallel to and close to the outer surface of the bone, leaving about a 0.5- to 1-mm thickness of soft tissue attached to the bone. The incision is carried past the mucogingival junction. Scalpel blade numbers 11, 12b, 15, or 15c are commonly used (Fig. 15-2).

2. Sharp dissection with the scalpel rather than blunt dissection with an elevator is used. This often results in increased bleeding during surgery. Steps 3 through 12 are essentially the same as for the full-thickness flap.

## Comparison of Full-Thickness and Partial-Thickness Flaps

There are differences of opinion regarding the indications for use of either a full-thickness or a partial-thickness flap. Some clinicians believe that surgical bone loss is less likely to be permanent if partial-thickness flaps are used. Others have shown that full-thickness flaps actually result in less bone loss. Advocates of full-thickness flaps point out that there is greater likelihood of necrosis of wound edges of the partial-thickness flap because of the possibility of compromising the blood supply. Also, surgical perforation is more likely with the partial-thickness flap. These complications could result in loss of tissue and delayed healing.[11–13]

In actual practice, partial-thickness flaps are more difficult to perform and true indications for their use are infrequent. Although this technique may seem to be indicated in areas of thin gingival or mucosal tissue (e.g., prominent roots), the thinness of the tissue presents technical problems at incision and there is an increased possibility that the blood supply will be compromised.

## CLASSIFICATION BASED ON POSITIONING

The flap placements most frequently used in periodontal surgery for pocket reduction are the replaced flap and the apically positioned flap. Facial and lingual aspects of a surgical site may involve any combination of flap positioning, depending on therapeutic goals. Both full-thickness and partial-thickness flaps can be used, but in clinical practice partial-thickness flaps are usually not used when the tissues are going to be replaced.

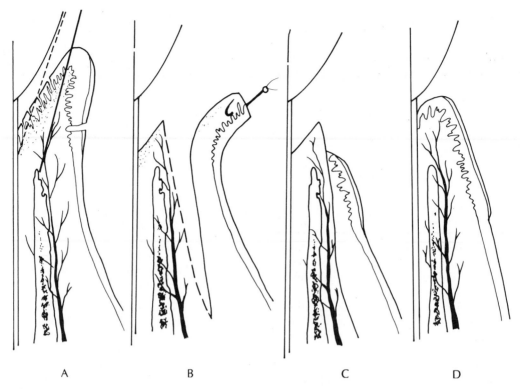

A                          B                                      C                          D

*Figure 15.2* ●

## Replaced Flap (RF)

Indications: A replaced flap (also called repositioned flap and modified Widman flap) is one that is repositioned in or near its original location (Fig. 15-3, A and B).[1] A replaced flap is used to:

1. Gain access to root surfaces for detoxification
2. Allow access to and management of bone defects
3. Achieve primary wound closure at the conclusion of the procedure

4. Reduce pockets by establishing a new epithelial or connective tissue attachment at a more coronal level
5. Provide soft tissue closure over regenerative procedures
6. Minimize postsurgical recession

The replaced flap is contraindicated if there is an inadequate zone of keratinized gingiva. In this instance, the apically positioned flap is used, not

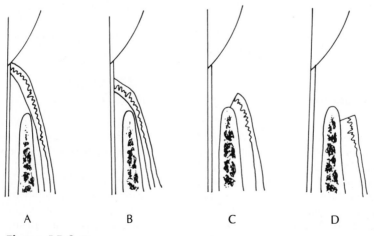

A                          B                                      C                          D

*Figure 15.3* ●

only to increase the width of the gingiva, but also to dissipate the pull of the connective tissue and muscle fibers.

Technique: In the replaced flap procedure, a full-thickness flap is used for access to the diseased root surface and adjacent alveolar bone. At the completion of root preparation and osseous treatment, the flaps are replaced near their original position and are sutured (interrupted or vertical mattress sutures) interproximally. Every attempt must be made to approximate wound edges, create a seal around the tooth, and to obtain primary wound closure, particularly interdentally.[1,14,15]

## Apically Positioned Flap (APF)

Indications: An apically positioned flap is one that is placed apical to its original height at the completion of the surgical procedure.[16] In addition to the access indications of the replaced flap, the apically positioned flap is also used to:

1. Reduce pockets by moving the gingival tissue margin apically[17]
2. Increase the zone of keratinized and attached gingiva[18]
3. Expose additional root structure for restorative dentistry

If some alveolar bone is left exposed, fibroblasts from the periodontal ligament and any retained connective tissue on the bone will form new connective tissue fibers coronal to the margin of the apically positioned gingiva. When mature, this new tissue will function as additional attached gingiva. The final position of the flap margin will depend on clinical conditions and the desired results of surgery.

The degree of apical positioning can vary, and the final flap position may be:

1. On the tooth root 1 to 2 mm coronal to the alveolar crest (APF-T; Fig. 15-4B).
2. At the alveolar bone crest (APF-C; Fig. 15-4C).
3. Apical to the alveolar bone crest (subcrestal; APF-SC; Fig. 15-4D).

Technique: The apically positioned flap procedure may involve the use of either a full-thickness or partial-thickness flap (Figs. 15-1 and 15-3). The following technique modifications and suggestions should be considered.

1. Because the interproximal apposition of wound edges is not a surgical goal, it is not critical to retain all of the papilla in the flaps. A slightly scalloped incision or straight-line incision can be used as long as the maximum amount of keratinized gingiva is retained on the wound edge.[19]

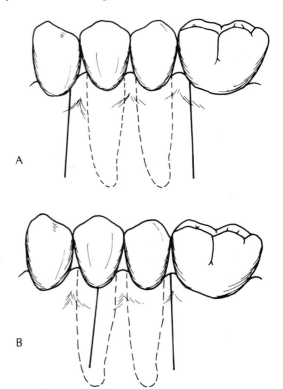

A

B

**Figure 15.4** ●

2. A combination full-thickness and partial-thickness flap is often used. It is common to begin the flap procedure by performing a full-thickness flap in the gingiva and then to change to a partial-thickness flap in the mucosa to achieve flap mobility.
3. Because more root surface will be exposed postsurgically, aggressive mechanical or chemical root treatment may be contraindicated to reduce postsurgical sensitivity.
4. Flap margins are sutured so that they rest at the desired level on the alveolar process (APF-T, APF-C, and APF-SC). The most common error in suturing an apically positioned flap is to suture too tightly, pulling the flap coronally and defeating the purpose of the procedure. Most commonly, sling type suturing is used for apically positioned flaps.[20,21]

## SPECIAL CONSIDERATIONS
### Vertical Releasing Incisions

Vertical releasing incisions may be used when increased access and visibility are needed. The convex nature of the anatomy on the facial surface stretches the flap during reflection, often resulting in tears and perforations. For that reason, vertical releasing incisions are most commonly used on the facial surface of the jaws. They should be made at line angles to preserve the interdental papillae for suturing and to prevent necrosis of the wound edge (Fig. 15-2A).

Under no circumstances should vertical incisions be made over the midfacial (radicular) surface of roots (Fig. 15-2B). Vertical releasing incisions should not be performed indiscriminately, and careful attention must be paid to vital structures, especially on the mandibular lingual and palate.[22]

## Palatal Flaps

On the palate, the tightly bound masticatory mucosa does not allow for the apical movement of the tissue. Any apical displacement of the margin must be accomplished by surgical reduction of the tissue height. The initial incision is begun somewhat apical to the free gingival margin and is aimed at a point slightly apical to the alveolar crest. The level of this incision is based on the probing depth (about one-half of the proximal probing depth), the level of the palatal osseous tissues, and the shape of the palatal vault (the shallower the palatal vault, the closer to the gingival margin the incision needs to be made). This type of incision results in a wedge of tissue (secondary flap) remaining between the outer (primary) flap and the tooth. The removal of this wedge of tissue with curets or chisels and the position of the initial incision determine the marginal height of the palatal tissues postsurgically. If necessary, further trimming of the gingival margin can be accomplished with a fresh scalpel blade or sharp scissors.[3,10]

Special care must be taken when performing a palatal flap owing to several anatomic structures.

1. The greater palatine artery and nerve may be damaged if flap reflection is extensive. Generally, this artery and associated nerve run in a bony channel about halfway between the crest of the alveolar bone and the midpalatal suture. Severing this vessel may lead to extensive bleeding that requires special management.
2. About one-third of the time, palatal exostoses will be present in the molar region.[23] The presence of these bony nodules creates thin tissue in the region and makes atraumatic flap reflection and proper flap margin placement difficult. Generally, these exostoses need to be removed during surgery.
3. The incisive papilla is often in the incision line of a flap procedure in the anterior palate. There appear to be no detrimental effects to surgical removal of this structure at the time of the initial incision. Additionally, its removal may avoid an excess bulk of tissue between the central incisors.
4. The presence of palatal rugae at or near the flap margin may create poor gingival margin contours postsurgically. Generally, it is preferable to trim these rugae before flap reflection or suturing to obtain an even, thin, confluent flap margin against the teeth.

## REFERENCES

1. Ramfjord SP, Nissle R. The modified Widman flap. J Periodontol 1974;45:601–618.
2. Caton J, Nyman S. Histometric evaluation of periodontal surgery. I. The modified Widman flap procedures. J Clin Periodontol 1980;7:212–223.
3. Johnson RH. Basic flap management. Dent Clin North Am 1976;20:3–21.
4. Levine HL, Stahl SS. Repair following flap surgery with retention of gingival fibers. J Periodontol 1972;43:99–103.
5. Dello Russo NM. Use of the fiber retention procedure in treating the maxillary anterior region. J Periodontol 1981;52:208–213.
6. Zaman KU, Sugaya T, Hongo O, Kato H. A study of attached and oriented human periodontal ligament cells to periodontally diseased cementum and dentin after demineralising with neutral and low pH etching solution. J Periodontol 2000;71:1094–1099.
7. Nyman S, Lindhe J, Karring T. Healing following surgical treatment and root demineralization in monkeys with periodontal disease. J Clin Periodontol 1981;8:249–258.
8. Cole RT, Crigger M, Bogle G, Egelberg J, Selvig KA. Connective tissue regeneration to periodontally diseased teeth. A histological study. J Periodontal Res 1980;15:1–9.
9. Staffileno H, Levy S, Gargiulo A. Histologic study of cellular mobilization and repair following a periosteal retention operation via split-thickness mucogingival flap surgery. J Periodontol 1966;37:117–131.
10. Staffileno H. Palatal flap surgery: mucosal flap (split thickness) and its advantages over the mucoperiosteal flaps. J Periodontol 1969;40:547–552.
11. Staffileno H. Significant differences and advantages between the full thickness and split thickness flaps. J Periodontol 1974;45:421–425.
12. Wood DL, Hoag PM, Donnenfeld DW, Rosenfeld LD. Alveolar crest reduction following full and partial thickness flaps. J Periodontol 1972;43:141–144.
13. Tisot RJ, Sullivan HC. Evaluation of survival of partial thickness and full thickness flaps. J Dent Res IADR 1971;170 (Abstract 470).
14. Steiner SS, Crigger M, Egelberg J. Connective tissue regeneration to periodontally diseased teeth II. Histologic observations of cases following replaced flap surgery. J Periodontal Res 1981;16:109–116.

15. Caffesse RG, Castelli WA, Nasjleti CE. Vascular response to modified Widman flap surgery in monkeys. J Periodontol 1981;52:1–7.

16. Donnenfeld OW, Mark RM, Glickman I, et al. The apically repositioned flap: A clinical study. J Periodontol 1964;35: 381–387.

17. Ammons WF Jr, Smith DH. Flap curettage: rationale, technique, and expectations. Dent Clin North Am 1976;20:215–226.

18. Carnio J, Miller PD. Increasing the amount of attached gingiva using a modified apically repositioned flap. J Periodontol 1999;70:1110–1117.

19. Cattermole AE, Wade AB. A comparison of the scalloped and linear incisions as used in the reverse bevel technique. J Clin Periodontol 1978; 5:41–49.

20. Holmes CH, Strem BE. Location of flap margin after suturing. J Periodontol 1976;47:674–675.

21. Machtei E, Ben-Yehouda A. The effect of post-surgical flap placement on probing depth and attachment level: a 2–year longitudinal study. J Periodontol 1994;65:855–858.

22. Kon S, Caffesse RG, Castelli WA, Nasjleti CE. Vertical releasing incisions for flap design: clinical and histological study in monkeys. Int J Periodontics Restorative Dent 1984;4:48–57.

23. Nery EB, Corn H, Eisenstein IL. Palatal exostosis in the molar region. J Periodontol 1977;48:663–666.

## CHAPTER 15
## REVIEW QUESTIONS

1. Periodontal flap procedures are designed to accomplish all of the following except:
   a. Close class III furcations
   b. Facilitate regenerative procedures
   c. Preserve or create an adequate zone of attached gingiva
   d. Reduce probing depths

2. Full-thickness flaps involve:
   (1) Incisions near the gingival margin
   (2) Blunt dissection from the bone
   (3) Complete root surface detoxification of periodontally involved root surfaces
      a. 1 and 2
      b. 1 and 3
      c. 2 and 3
      d. 1, 2, and 3

3. Partial-thickness flaps differ from full-thickness flaps primarily in that with partial-thickness flaps:
   (1) Blunt dissection from the bone is used
   (2) Sharp dissection leaves periosteum and connective tissue covering the bone
   (3) The entire periodontally involved root surfaces are mechanically and clinically detoxified
   (4) Mechanical and chemical root detoxification needs to be limited to the root surfaces near the bone
      a. 1 and 3
      b. 1 and 4
      c. 2 and 3
      d. 2 and 4

4. Some of the potential drawbacks of a partial-thickness flap include all of the following except:
   a. Increased postsurgical bone loss
   b. Necrosis of the flap margins because of compromised vascularity
   c. Surgical perforation of the flaps
   d. All of the above

5. Replaced flaps are used to accomplish all of the following except:
   a. Gain access to diseased root surfaces
   b. Provide access to bony defects
   c. Increase attached gingiva
   d. Minimize recession

6. Apically positioned flaps are indicated to accomplish which of the following:
   (1) Increase the zone of keratinized and attached gingiva

   (2) Expose additional root structure for restorative dentistry
   (3) Provide tissue coverage over bony defects
      a. 1 and 2
      b. 1 and 3
      c. 2 and 3
      d. 1, 2, and 3
      e. None of the above

7. When an apically positioned flap is positioned at the alveolar bone crest, it is termed an:
   a. APC-T
   b. APC-C
   c. APC-SC
   d. RF

8. Vertical releasing incisions should not be made in which locations?
   (1) Line angles of teeth to include the papilla
   (2) Mandibular lingual molar area
   (3) Mid-root of teeth
      a. 1 and 2
      b. 1 and 3
      c. 2 and 3
      d. 1, 2, and 3

9. Anatomic structures that are of significant concern during flap reflection on the palate include:
   (1) Bone exostoses
   (2) Greater palatine artery and nerve
   (3) Incisive papilla containing blood vessels and nerves
      a. 1 and 2
      b. 1 and 3
      c. 2 and 3
      d. 1, 2, and 3
      e. None of the above

10. A partial-thickness flap is composed of all of the following except:
    a. Gingiva
    b. Mucosa
    c. Submucosa
    d. Periosteum
    e. None of the above, all are components

11. The level of incision in palatal flaps is based on which of the following:
    (1) Probing depth
    (2) Level of palatal osseous tissue
    (3) Shape of palatal vault
       a. 1 and 2
       b. 1 and 3
       c. 1, 2, and 3
       d. None of the above

## CHAPTER 16

# Management of Soft Tissue: Mucogingival Procedures

John Rapley

## MUCOGINGIVAL CORRECTIVE SURGERY

### Indications

Gingival recession (atrophy) is an abnormality of the mucogingival complex. Areas of recession may be the result of problems with a frenum or the attached gingiva. Exposed root surfaces associated with recession may be unesthetic or sensitive. The determination and correction of etiologic factors (such as prominent tooth position, frena, toothbrushing technique, restoration margins or contours, and factitious habits) are important in overall treatment success.

### Objectives

1. Establish an adequate width and thickness of keratinized and attached gingiva.
2. Eliminate tension on the free gingival margin by frena or muscle attachments.
3. Correct areas of gingival recession.
4. Establish new gingival attachment at a more coronal level.

Mucogingival corrective procedures involve pedicle flaps and free soft tissue grafts. Pedicle flap procedures include the laterally positioned flap and the coronally positioned flap. Free soft tissue grafts include the free gingival or subepithelial connective tissue grafts. Additionally, materials such as allogeneic freeze-dried skin or barrier membranes (GTR), have also been used in gingival augmentation procedures as a substitute for the host donor graft tissue.

### Techniques

#### Laterally Positioned Flap

The laterally positioned flap is used to reposition gingiva from an adjacent tooth or edentulous area to a prepared adjacent recipient site.[1,2] This procedure requires that only one or two teeth require therapy and that sufficient width and thickness of donor tissue is available in adjacent areas. Also, adequate vestibular depth is necessary for a laterally positioned flap to be performed correctly. When adjacent tooth sites are to be used as donor areas, care must be exercised that the healthy donor gingival tissue is thick, wide, and keratinized with no underlying bony fenestrations or dehiscences.

Indications: The laterally positioned flap is used to:

1. Increase the zone of keratinized attached gingiva
2. Cover isolated areas of recession where the adjacent proximal gingival height is more coronal

Either a full-thickness or a partial-thickness flap can be used. Both types of flaps result in satisfactory clinical healing, but studies of root coverage suggest that full-thickness, laterally positioned flaps result in more connective tissue attachment. Partial-thickness flaps may be indicated when protection of the donor area (especially thin bone over radicular surfaces) is desired. Clinical root coverage of about 70% of the original recession area can be routinely expected. Similarly, about 1 mm of recession at the donor site usually occurs.

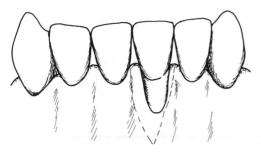

**Figure 16.1** ●

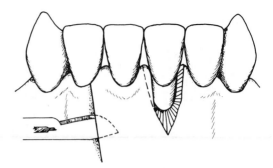

**Figure 16.3** ●

The surgical technique for the laterally positioned flap is as follows[1,2]:

1. After local anesthesia, make a V-shaped incision with a suitable scalpel blade (Nos. 15 or 15c are the most commonly used) and create a beveled wound edge around the recipient site (Figs. 16-1, 16-2). The wound edge to be sutured must be over bone.
2. Remove the incised tissue with a curet, and root plane the cementum until it is smooth and hard.
3. Make a vertical incision at a distance of at least one and a half times the measurement of the recipient site. This incision should be angled slightly toward the recipient site (Fig. 16-2).
4. Perform either a full-thickness or partial-thickness dissection (Fig. 16-3) to free the donor flap tissue from its bed, being careful to maintain its base and blood supply. A useful modification is to perform a partial-thickness dissection in the gingiva and to shift to a full-thickness dissection in the alveolar mucosa. Enough vestibular depth and mobility of the donor pedicle must be present to allow the unstrained, relaxed positioning of the flap at the recipient site.
5. Position the flap at the recipient site to completely cover the defect. If there is tension on the flap as the lip or cheek is extended, further dissection and elevation at the base may be performed (Fig. 16-4).

6. Suture the flap to ensure that the desired coverage of the denuded root surface is maintained (Fig. 16-5). Place interrupted sutures (5-0 suture material is preferred), beginning apically and working coronally. No more than two or three sutures are usually necessary. A sling suture is carried around the tooth and is tied on the facial side to prevent the graft from slipping apically. Particular attention must be paid to the suturing of the apical area to immobilize the entire length of the flap to the bed at both the mesial and distal corners.
7. Apply gentle but firm pressure to the flap for 2 to 3 minutes with cotton-free gauze moistened with sterile water or saline solution.
8. Cover the surgical site with an appropriate dressing to protect the flap from displacement. The dressing must not displace the flap or impinge on its base. An improperly placed dressing may impede the blood supply to the coronal part of the flap and result in necrosis and failure.
9. Remove the dressing and sutures after 7 to 10 days. Debride the area and instruct the patient in plaque control. The area should not be probed for at least 3 months.

When properly performed, the laterally positioned flap is a predictable surgical procedure for increasing the zone of keratinized attached gingiva

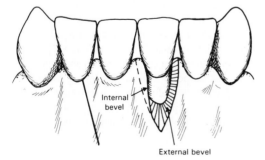

**Figure 16.2** ●

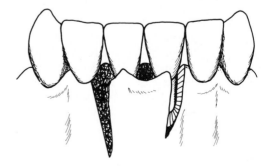

**Figure 16.4** ●

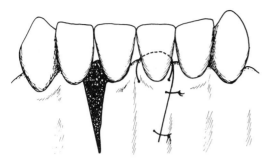

**Figure 16.5** ●

or repair of gingival clefts when there is sufficient width of keratinized gingiva at the donor site.

## Double Papillae Flap

### Indications

The double papillae flap[3] is a modification of the laterally positioned flap.

It can be used to repair narrow gingival clefts when there is an adequate amount of healthy interproximal tissue adjacent to the recipient site and minimal keratinized gingiva over the radicular surfaces. Clinical situations favoring this procedure are few, because many recession areas are too wide to use the adjacent papillae. In practice, many clinicians have had limited success with the double papillae flap because the suture line is usually over the avascular root surface.

## Free Gingival Graft (Free Soft Tissue Autograft)

### Indications

The free soft tissue autograft[4] is an extremely versatile and highly predictable technique. It is used to:

1. Increase the zone of keratinized attached gingiva
2. Eliminate aberrant frena or muscle attachments
3. Deepen the vestibule
4. Repair *minimal* gingival clefts

Wound-healing studies have demonstrated the effectiveness of the technique in the treatment of the first three aforementioned problems. These same studies, however, indicate that the free soft tissue autograft can also repair narrow clefts, but may not adequately bridge deep, wide gingival clefts.

The technique for performing the free soft tissue autograft is as follows:

1. **After local anesthesia,** an internally beveled incision is made using an appropriate scalpel blade, 1 mm coronal to the mucogingival junction.
2. Sharply dissect the connective tissue proximate to the bone, leaving a thin nonmobile connective tissue bed attached to bone. Extend the incision to include the involved teeth. Prepare the bed by removing excess connective tissue with iris scissors or tissue nippers. All muscle fibers must be removed (Fig. 16-6). Exposure of bone does not jeopardize the results.
3. Optional: Make a periosteal fenestration by exposing a small horizontal strip of bone near the apical border of the recipient site (Fig. 16-6B). The mucosal flap on the lip or cheek side may be sutured to the reflected periosteum apical to the fenestration with small resorbable sutures.
4. Prepare a template of the recipient site by using the sterile wrapper of the sterile surgical blade or suture material.
5. Take the template to the donor site (edentulous ridge or hard palate) and superficially outline with a blade slightly larger than the template. If the palate is used, care must be taken to avoid incorporating rugae in the graft or encroaching on the major palatal blood vessels.
6. Remove the donor tissue with a scalpel blade or one of the special instruments designed to

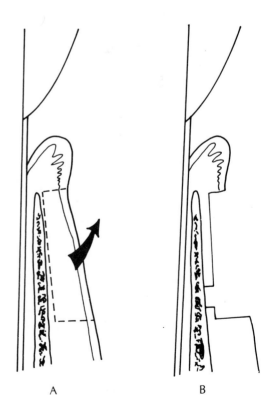

A                                    B

**Figure 16.6** ●

remove thin sections of tissue. The graft should be between 1.0 and 1.5 mm in thickness and should be wide enough to cover the recipient site. Achieve hemostasis of the donor site wound. A protective surgical stent in combination with hemostatic agents is beneficial in this regard.

7. If the donor tissue is removed from the palate, some tissue may need to be removed from the inner surface to obtain uniform graft thickness.

8. Rinse the undersurface of the graft and the recipient site with **sterile water or saline** solution to remove clots and debris. Clot formation will prevent initial nutrition of the graft by diffusion and will result in necrosis of the graft before revascularization can occur.

9. Suture the graft at the coronal margin to ensure immobilization (Figs. 16-7, 16-8). In addition, vertical external compression sutures may be used for better graft adaptation to an irregular surface.

10. Apply gentle but firm pressure for 2 to 3 minutes with gauze moistened with sterile water or saline solution to assist in initial fibrin clot formation and an effective union between the graft and the recipient site (Fig. 16-8).

11. Carefully apply an appropriate protective dressing to the surgical site. Do not displace the graft while placing the dressing.

12. Remove the dressing and sutures after 7 to 10 days. Polish the area and instruct the patient in plaque control procedures. Inform the patient about the "dead" appearance of the surface of the graft at the end of the first postoperative week and caution the patient against disturbing the graft until clinical healing is complete. The area should not be probed for at least 3 months. Healing of the recipient site is usually uneventful. A **grayish-white,** sloughing epithelial layer is present after 1 week, and

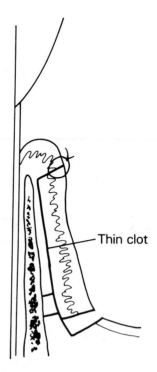

**Figure 16.8** ●

the graft is essentially united to the bed in this time frame. Healing of the palatal donor site is usually more of a problem for the patient as the large denuded area is slow to granulate and epithelialize. Dressing retention is difficult on the palate, and many clinicians fabricate an acrylic stent to protect the area during healing.

A progressive coronal shift (up to 1 mm) of the gingival tissue after an adequate band of keratinized attached gingiva has been established is common within the first year. This phenomenon is called "creeping attachment" and may result in complete or partial coverage of an exposed root surface.

## Coronally Positioned Flaps

The coronally positioned flap[5] is another alternative to correct areas of recession. This procedure is often preceded by a free soft tissue autograft to increase the amount of keratinized tissue available at the local site. There appears to be a similar rate of successful root coverage with this procedure as there is with the laterally positioned flap procedure (Fig. 16-9).

### Technique

1. A free soft tissue autograft is performed apical to the area of recession. The graft is allowed to heal for 6 to 8 weeks.

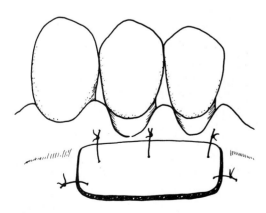

**Figure 16.7** ●

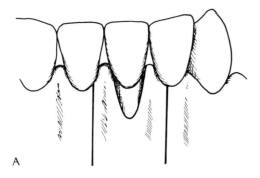

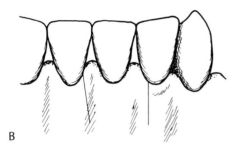

**Figure 16.9 ●**

2. After local anesthesia, a full-thickness flap is reflected, with vertical incisions at its lateral boundaries (to release the tissue and to allow the flap to be passively positioned and secured at a more coronal level; Fig. 16-9).
3. Root detoxification is performed with curets.
4. Suture the flap passively in its new coronal position to cover the prepared roots.
5. Apply gentle but firm pressure for 2 to 3 minutes to achieve hemostasis and to minimize the size of the blood clot.
6. Apply an appropriate protective dressing if indicated.
7. Remove the dressing and sutures after 7 to 10 days. Debride the area and instruct the patient in home care.

## Other Considerations in Root Coverage

Other factors that may influence the results of mucogingival procedures should be mentioned, which relate primarily to root coverage attempts. The first involves the treatment of endodontically treated teeth. Conflicting reports and clinical impressions abound, but several research reports seem to indicate that root coverage attempts are as successful on endodontically treated teeth as on vital teeth. Another factor influencing the success of root coverage is root preparation. Generally,

cementum and dentin exposed to the oral cavity absorb endotoxins and other substances that have an adverse influence on fibroblasts and epithelial cells. As a general rule, aggressive scaling and root planing (and at times, minimal odontoplasty of the root) are recommended to remove enough root structure to eliminate these toxic substances, as well as to reduce the prominence of the root. Additionally, the majority of investigators have concluded that patients who smoke have less root coverage with mucogingival procedures because of the long-term effects of smoking on the tissue.

## MANAGEMENT OF OTHER SOFT TISSUE PROBLEMS

### Aberrant Frena (Frenectomy)

Aberrant frena can be treated by incising the frenum at its insertion, allowing it to retract into the lip or cheek, and allowing healing of that mucosal wound with or without placement of a free soft tissue graft. Occasionally a frenum, especially a maxillary labial or mandibular lingual frenum, is so large that it should be totally excised and the wound should be sutured. This procedure is termed a frenectomy.

One technique for frenectomy is as follows:

1. After local anesthesia, grasp the frenum with a slightly curved hemostat at its base. Cut the tissue with scissors above the hemostat and then below it, until the hemostat is free (Fig. 16-10, A and B).
2. Use scissors to remove any dense fibers that may be observed in the wound (Fig. 16-10C). Extend the lip and check to determine whether there is still pull on the periosteum.
3. Suture the edges of the diamond-shaped wound together (Fig. 16-10D). This will reduce postoperative discomfort and help promote healing.
4. Remove sutures after 7 to 10 days.

Another technique for treating aberrant frena is to perform a free soft tissue autograft in the area where the frenum is causing a problem. This technique not only removes the aberrant frena but also increases the amount of keratinized attached gingiva and, therefore, helps preclude a return of the aberrant frena.

### Subperiosteal Connective Tissue Grafts

The subepithelial connective tissue graft is a successful technique for root coverage, which is attributed to a double blood supply from both the

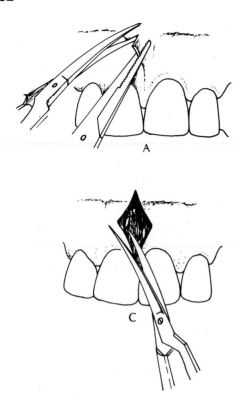

**Figure 16.10** ●

underlying connective tissue bed and the overlying flap. The technique is indicated for isolated or multiple areas of gingival recession.[6]

The technique for the connective tissue graft is as follows:

1. After local anesthesia, a split-thickness flap with vertical incisions is reflected and should be one-half tooth wider mesial-distally than the area of recession. The interproximal papillae are left intact, and the flap must be reflected past the mucogingival junction so that it may be coronally positioned (Figs. 16-11, 16-12).
2. The root is thoroughly débrided, and pronounced convexities may be reduced.

3. The donor tissue is removed from the palate, and the ideal site is palatal to the bicuspids owing to its increased thickness (Figs. 16-13, 16-14). Two parallel horizontal incisions are made in an anterior–posterior direction and are continued toward the palatal bone so that a connective tissue wedge can be removed. The donor site can be sutured with or without the addition of a hemostatic agent (Fig. 16-15).

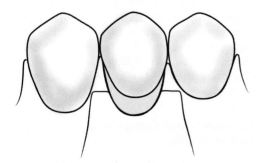

**Figure 16.11** ●

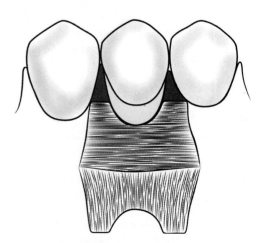

**Figure 16.12** ●

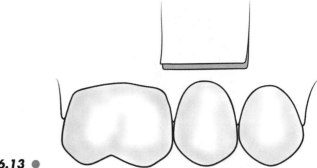

**Figure 16.13** ●

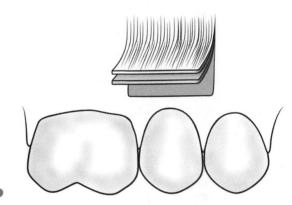

**Figure 16.14** ●

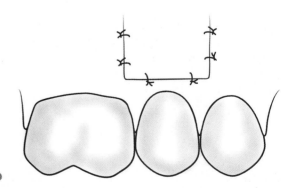

**Figure 16.15** ●

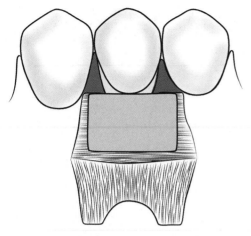

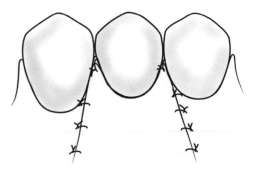

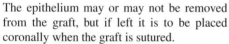

**Figure 16.17** ●

**Figure 16.16** ●

time. A future gingivoplasty may be indicated to recontour the graft but is usually not needed.

## REFERENCES

The epithelium may or may not be removed from the graft, but if left it is to be placed coronally when the graft is sutured.

4. The graft is placed over the denuded roots and sutured to the recipient tissue bed (Figs. 16-16, 16-17). The overlying tissue flap is coronally positioned over the graft to cover as much of the graft as possible and then sutured.
5. Gentle pressure is applied to form a fibrin clot, and an appropriate dressing is applied to the surgical site.
6. Remove the dressing and sutures after 7 to 10 days. The graft may appear thick during the healing period but may lessen considerably with

1. Grupe HE, Warren RE. Repair of gingival defects by a sliding flap operation. J Periodontol 1956;27: 92–95.
2. De Wall H, Kon S, Ruben M. The laterally positioned flap. Dent Clin North Am 1988;32:267–282.
3. Cohen DW, Ross SE. The double papilla repositioned flap in periodontal therapy. J Periodontol 1968;39: 65–70.
4. Sullivan HC, Atkins JH. Free autogenous gingival grafts. I. Principles of successful grafting. Periodontics 1968;6:121–129.
5. Maynard JG. Coronal positioning of a previously placed autogenous gingival graft. J Periodontol 1977; 48:151–155.
6. Langer B, Langer L. Subepithelial connective tissue graft technique for root coverage. J Periodontol 1985; 56:715–720.

# Management of Osseous Defects: Bone Replacement Grafts

Raymond A. Yukna

For many years, researchers and clinicians alike have attempted to regenerate lost periodontal attachment apparatus by promoting regeneration of bone and its ligamentous attachment to the tooth with various osseous stimulators. Autogenous, allogeneic, xenogeneic, and alloplastic (synthetic) materials have been tried with varied success. Clinical, radiographic, and histologic evidence of successful regeneration has been found with all types. New grafting materials are constantly being developed, and combinations of different types are often used.

## INDICATIONS FOR BONE GRAFTING

### Patient Selection

Patient selection is of critical importance when considering bone replacement graft procedures. The factors causing the inflammatory periodontal disease must be controlled before regenerative procedures are attempted. The patient must demonstrate effective oral hygiene; have no compromising physical or medical problems, mental conditions, or social habits (especially smoking); have a positive attitude toward therapy; and be amenable to a long-term posttherapy maintenance program.[1,2]

### Defect Selection

The morphology of the osseous defect to be grafted is as important as patient selection. Realistic expectations of success are directly proportional to the number of vascular osseous walls surrounding the defect and are inversely related to the number of avascular tooth root walls. A narrow (less than 2 mm) three-wall defect, confined to a single tooth surface, has great inherent osseous regenerative potential even without the use of bone replacement

grafts. A wide (more than 2 mm) three-wall defect, confined to one or more surfaces of the tooth root; a two-wall or one-wall defect; or combinations of the foregoing have progressively less inherent osseous regenerative potential, and bone replacement grafts may help regenerate only limited amounts of the lost tooth support. The least predictable situations for new bone formation are furcation defects and supracrestal regeneration of bone.[3–7]

The basic functions of all osseous grafting materials are one or more of the following:

1. *Osteogenesis.* The cells and matrix of the graft actually produce new bone. Only autogenous bone is osteogenic.
2. *Osteoinduction.* The graft acts to stimulate or to induce new bone formation by undifferentiated cells in the wound. Demineralized freeze-dried bone has shown osteoinductive properties in animals.
3. *Osteoconduction.* The graft acts as a template or trellis to assist in bone formation and deposition. Osteoblasts are comfortable depositing bone on the graft material. Almost all bone replacement graft materials act in this manner.

## TYPES OF BONE REPLACEMENT GRAFTS

### Autografts

Osseous autografts contain cortical, cancellous, or a combination of cortical and cancellous bone and can be obtained from extraoral or intraoral sites. Clinical experience suggests that cancellous bone affords greater opportunity for success because of its less dense composition, but it is often more difficult to obtain and often only in limited amounts. Consequently, the majority of defects are filled with a combination of cortical and cancellous bone, with the higher percentage usually being cortical bone particles.

Studies have consistently shown that autogenous cancellous bone and marrow grafts have extremely high regenerative potential because they contain numerous viable pluripotential cells, which may differentiate, proliferate, and actually participate in bone formation (osteogenesis).

Extraoral sources of autogenous bone and marrow are almost never used for periodontal defects, so this section focuses on the use of intraoral bone.

## Osseous Coagulum

Bone that is removed during osteoplasty or ostectomy is an excellent source of donor material. The size of the chips may vary from fairly large fragments (diameter in millimeters) to very small particles (diameter in micrometers) depending on how the bone removal is performed. If rotary instruments are used, the particle size is small (200 to 400 μm). There is evidence that the small particles of donor bone may more actively induce regeneration in osseous defects. Small particles offer the advantage (compared with large fragments) of a greater surface area for resorption and replacement by new host bone.[8–11]

A suggested technique uses a large (No. 8 or 10) round carbide bur, revolving at 25,000 to 30,000 rpm or more, to reduce bone to small particle size during osteoplasty or ostectomy. The donor bone particles are gathered by placing a large, bladed elevator in position to catch the bone particles as they come off the bone surface. A surprising amount of bone can be obtained from cortical bone shavings obtained when performing osteoplasty and ostectomy procedures or reducing the bulk of nonsupporting bone or tori. Hand instruments that are also useful for this purpose are Ochsenbein, Wedelstaedt, Chigo, or Fedi chisels.

## Healing Sockets

Bone may also be obtained from a healing socket 6 to 12 weeks after an extraction. A flap is reflected to expose the socket area, the cancellous bone or marrow slush is harvested from the socket with rongeurs or large curets, and the donor material is placed in the periodontal osseous defect. The immature bone and cells appear to offer excellent healing and reparative potential.[12–14]

## Other Sources

Donor bone can also be obtained from maxillary tuberosities, edentulous ridges, or retromolar areas. Usually, a window is made in the outer cortical bone for access to the cancellous areas. Rongeurs, trephines, or large curets can then be used to harvest the bone. Cancellous bone in the tuberosities once contained hemopoietic marrow, but in the adult the hemopoietic content is minimal. Limited visual and mechanical access, together with the frequent occurrence of an alveolar extension of the maxillary sinus in the tuberosity, severely reduces the availability of graft material in this region.

## Allografts

An allograft (allogeneic bone) is tissue transplanted between persons of the same species. Although allografts may possess some osteoinductive capacity, they may initiate adverse tissue responses and graft rejection by the host unless specially processed. The most commonly used and safest form of allografts are those processed by freeze-drying (lyophilization) or specific chemical washing protocols. Most commonly, this type of tissue is obtained from tissue banks.

The bone tissue is procured under rigidly controlled conditions from carefully selected donor cadavers and must be tested to ensure it is an aseptic donation of tissue that is free of any transmissible pathologic conditions.[15] Considerable research on the use of freeze-dried bone (FDBA) and demineralized freeze-dried bone (DFDBA) in periodontal osseous defects has been conducted during the past 30 years.[16] Considerable testing has demonstrated this form of allograft to be nonantigenic. Some freeze-dried bone allograft materials are decalcified with the intent of exposing bone morphogenic protein, thereby theoretically increasing regenerative potential. However, clinical research suggests that the nondemineralized and demineralized forms yield equal results in periodontal defects.[17] The advantage of using allografts compared with autografts is that there is no need to create an additional surgical wound to procure donor material and still maintain comparable osseous repair potential. There is some evidence that combining four parts of freeze-dried bone allograft with one part of tetracycline powder may improve bone repair.[18]

## Xenografts

Xenografts (xenogeneic grafts) are materials obtained from a different species, usually cows (bovine) or pigs (porcine) for human use. Particulate bovine natural hydroxylapatite grafts are produced by chemical processing (Bio-Oss) or high-heat processing (OsteoGraf/N) to remove the organic material. This leaves a natural hydroxylapatite skeleton that mimics the macroporous and microporous structure of human bone, and the particles appear to be slowly resorbed while bone is deposited in juxtaposition to them. Some of these have peptides (PepGen P-15) or collagen added to them to improve cell attachment and bone repair.[19,20]

A different form of xenograft is Emdogain, a group of enamel matrix proteins obtained from pigs. This material appears to encourage the initial formation of cementum that is then followed by associated bone deposition. Clinically detectable results take longer to become evident with this gel-like material than with other grafts.[21,22]

## Alloplastic Grafts

Alloplastic grafts are synthetic substances, and several are available for periodontal use. Currently available synthetic bone replacement graft materials include the following:

1. Porous, resorbable α- and β-tricalcium phosphate (Synthograft, Peri-Oss, CeraSorb, and others)
2. Dense, nonresorbable hydroxylapatite (Calcitite, OsteoGraf/D, and others)
3. Porous, nonresorbable hydroxylapatite (Interpore)
4. Calcium carbonate (coral; Biocoral)
5. Polymers (Bioplant HTR)
6. Plaster of Paris (Capset, SurgiPlast, and others)
7. "Resorbable" hydroxyapatite (Osteogen, OsteoGraf/LD)
8. Bioactive (silica-based) glasses (PerioGlas, Biogran)
9. Algae-derived (C-graft, Algipore)

Histologic evidence suggests that these substances are essentially biocompatible fillers, with limited evidence of bone or attachment apparatus regeneration. Clinical results indicate that these materials may effectively fill the defect and may encourage bone deposition on their surface, and thus help maintain bone and soft tissue height.[2,23–25]

## Composite Grafts

Composite grafts are usually combinations of autogenous bone and an allograft, xenograft, or alloplast. Even though autogenous bone is the preferred graft material, at times the amount available is insufficient to meet therapeutic needs. An expander, in the form of an allograft, xenograft, or alloplast, is used to increase the usable amount of bone replacement graft material. There is some evidence to indicate that the composite grafts form more new bone than either of their components used independently.[26]

## Results With Bone Replacement Grafts

A large number of clinical studies and limited human histologic evidence suggest that there is no one type of bone replacement graft material that is superior to the others. There is no material preferable to or that yields better results than autogenous bone. However, there is often a limited amount of the patient's bone conveniently available in the oral cavity, so allografts, xenografts, or alloplasts may be indicated instead. Evaluation of research reports suggests that all types of bone replacement grafts yield essentially similar clinical results. These results demonstrate fill of the original intrabony defect of about 50 to 70%.[20,27–29]

## SURGICAL PROCEDURES

The technique for preparation of the osseous defect recipient site is the same regardless of what donor material is used.[1,2] The replaced flap technique usually used is explained in Chapter 15.

1. Make a scalloped, internally bevelled incision around the necks of the teeth to remove the sulcular epithelium and the inner soft tissue wall of the pocket associated with the defect. Preserve as much gingival tissue as possible to enhance primary closure of the wound.
2. Elevate a full-thickness (mucoperiosteal) flap to expose the root and bony defect. Occasionally, one or more vertical releasing incisions may be needed to provide better access, especially for deep defects.
3. Remove the granulomatous tissue from within and around the osseous defect. The entire inner surface of the bony defect should be vigorously debrided and free of soft tissue.
4. Mechanically detoxify the root surface with ultrasonic, sonic, or hand instruments until it is smooth and hard. Chemical conditioning agents may also be used if desired.
5. Intramarrow penetrations with a sharp instrument or a No. 1/2 round bur may be performed. The compact bone that lines the defect is perforated to allow rapid ingress of new blood vessels and bone-forming cells into the defect from the surrounding marrow spaces.
6. Place the bone replacement graft material into the defect in increments, pack gently but

firmly, and fill to a level at or only slightly coronal to the existing bony defect walls.

7. Replace the flap over the graft and suture. Be sure to approximate the wound edges interproximally to ensure primary flap closure, containment of the graft material, and a circumferential soft tissue seal against the root surface.

8. Place a suitable periodontal dressing over the surgical area.

9. Provide written and oral postoperative instructions to the patient to minimize postsurgical sequelae (Chapter 13). Appropriate prescriptions to control swelling, infection, and pain should be provided.

10. Remove dressing and sutures after 7 to 10 days, debride the wound, and remove plaque from the involved teeth. Redress if necessary.

11. After final dressing removal, instruct the patient in mechanical and chemical plaque control. Biweekly professional plaque debridement for several months after surgery enhances the final results. Do not probe the graft sites for at least 3 months.[30]

NOTE: An antibiotic regimen is usually prescribed for the first 10 to 14 days of healing (tetracycline hydrochloride, 250 mg every 6 hours, or its equivalent is preferred). Studies have shown that results are enhanced if therapeutic levels of tetracycline are maintained for plaque reduction and collagenase suppression during the first week or two of healing.[1,2]

# REFERENCES

1. Mellonig JT. Periodontal bone graft technique. Int J Periodontics Restorative Dent 1990;10:288–299.

2. Yukna RA. Synthetic bone grafts in periodontics. Periodontology 2000 1993;1:92–99.

3. Tonetti MS, Pini Prato G, Cortellini P. Periodontal regeneration of human intrabony defects. IV. Determinants of healing response. J Periodontol 1993;64:934–940.

4. Laurell L, Gottlow J, Zybutz M, Persson R. Treatment of intrabony defects by different surgical procedures. A literature review. J Periodontol 1998; 69:303–313.

5. Renvert S, Garrett S, Nilveus R, et al. Healing after treatment of periodontal intraosseous defects. VI. Factors influencing the healing response. J Clin Periodontol 1985;12:707–715.

6. Nielsen IM, Glavind L, Karring T. Interproximal periodontal intrabony defects: Prevalence, localization, and etiologic factors. J Clin Periodontol 1980; 7:187–198.

7. Vrotsos J, Parashis A, Theofanatos D, Smulow J. Prevalence and distribution of bone defects in moderate and advanced adult periodontitis. J Clin Periodontol 1999;26:44–48.

8. Froum SJ, Ortiz M, Witkin RT, Thaler R, Scopp IW, Stahl SS. Osseous autografts. III. Comparison of osseous coagulum-bone blend implants with open curettage. J Periodontol 1976;47:287–294.

9. Nabers C. Long-term results of autogenous bone grafts. Int J Periodontics Restorative Dent 1984;4: 51–67.

10. Robinson RE. Osseous coagulum for bone induction. J Periodontol 1969;40:503–510.

11. Zaner DJ, Yukna RA. Particle size of periodontal bone grafting materials. J Periodontol 1984;55: 406–409.

12. Amler MH. The time sequence of tissue regeneration in human extraction wounds. Oral Surg Oral Med Oral Pathol 1969;27:309–318.

13. Passanezi E, Jansen W, Nahas D, Campos A Jr. Newly forming bone autografts to treat periodontal infrabony defects: clinical and histological events. Int J Periodontics Restorative Dent 1989;9:140–153.

14. Soehren SE, Van Swol RL. The healing extraction site: a donor area for periodontal grafting material. J Periodontol 1979;50:128–133.

15. Mellonig JT, Prewett AB, Moyer MP. HIV inactivation in a bone allograft. J Periodontol 1992;63: 979–983.

16. Mellonig JT. Decalcified freeze-dried bone allograft as an implant material in human periodontal defects. Int J Periodontics Restorative Dent 1984;4:41–55.

17. Reynolds M, Bowers G. Fate of demineralized freeze-dried bone allografts in human infrabony defects. J Periodontol 1996;67:150–157.

18. Mabry T, Yukna RA, Sepe WW. Freeze-dried bone allografts combined with tetracycline in the treatment of juvenile periodontitis. J Periodontol 1985; 56:74–81.

19. Richardson CR, Mellonig JT, Brunsvold MA, McDonnell HT, Cochran DL. Clinical evaluation of Bio-Oss: a bovine-derived xenograft for the treatment of periodontal osseous defects in humans. J Clin Periodontol 1999;26:421–428.

20. Yukna RA, Callan DP, Krauser JT, Evans GH, Aichelmann-Reidy ME, Moore K, Cruz R, Scott JB. Multi-center clinical evaluation of combination anorganic bovine-derived hydroxyapatite matrix (ABM)/cell binding peptide (P-15) as a bone replacement graft material in human periodontal osseous defects. 6-month results. J Periodontol 1998; 69:655–663.

21. Froum SJ, Weinberg MA, Rosenberg E, Tarnow D. A comparative study utilizing open flap debridement with and without enamel matrix derivative in the treatment of periodontal intrabony defects: a 12-month re-entry study. J Periodontol 2001;72:25–34.

22. Tonetti MS, Lang NP, Cotellini P, Suvan JE, Adriaens P, Dubravec D, Fonzar A, Fourmousis I, Mayfield L, Rossi R, Silvestri M, Tiedemann C, Topoll H, Vangsted T, Wallkamm B. Enamel matrix proteins in the regenerative therapy of deep intrabony defects. J Clin Periodontol 2002;29:317–325.

23. Yukna RA. Osseous defect responses to hydroxylapatite grafting versus open flap debridement. J Clin Periodontol 1989;16:398–402.

24. Froum SJ, Weinberg MA, Tarnow D. Comparison of bioactive glass synthetic bone graft particles and open debridement in the treatment of human periodontal defects. A clinical study. J Periodontol 1998; 69:698–709.

25. Aichelmann-Reidy ME, Yukna RA. Bone replacement grafts. The bone substitutes. Dent Clin North Am 1998;42:491–503.

26. Sanders JJ, Sepe WW, Bowers GM, Koch RW, Williams JE, Lekas JS, Mellonig JT, Pelleu GB Jr, Gambill V. Clinical evaluation of freeze-dried bone allografts in periodontol osseous defects. Part III. J Periodontol 1983;54:1–8.

27. Bowen JA, Mellonig JT, Gray JL, Towle HT. Comparison of decalcified freeze-dried bone allograft and porous particulate hydroxyapatite human periodontal osseous defects. J Periodontol 1989;60: 647–654.

28. Rummelhart JM, Mellonig, JJ, Gray JL, Towle HJ. A comparison of freeze-dried bone allograft and demineralized freeze-dried bone allograft in human periodontal osseous defects. J Periodontol 1989;60: 655–663.

29. Bowers GM, Schallhorn RG, Mellonig JT. Histologic evaluation of new attachment in human intrabony defects. A literature review. J Periodontol 1982;53:509–514.

30. Rosling B, Nyman S, Lindhe J. The effect of systematic plaque control on bone regeneration in infrabony pockets. J Clin Periodontol 1976;3:38–53.

# CHAPTER 18
## REVIEW QUESTIONS

1. Bone for grafting to another site may optimally be obtained from a healthy healing socket _____ weeks after an extraction.
   a. 2–4
   b. 4–8
   c. 6–12
   d. 24–30
2. Sources of intraoral donor bone include:
   a. Maxillary tuberosity
   b. Edentulous ridge
   c. Retromolar area
   d. All of the above
   e. None of the above
3. Clinical research on the use of nondemineralized and demineralized freeze-dried bone allografts suggests that demineralized bone allografts yield _____ results compared with nondemineralized bone allografts in periodontal defects.
   a. Better
   b. Worse
   c. Equal
4. _____ is a group of enamel matrix proteins obtained from pigs that appears to encourage the initial formation of cementum followed by associated bone deposition.
   a. Bio-Oss
   b. Emdogain
   c. OsteoGraf/N
   d. Algipore
5. Currently available synthetic bone replacement graft materials include all of the following except:
   a. Bioactive glass
   b. Bio-Oss
   c. Calcium carbonate
   d. Plaster of Paris
   e. None of the above, all are synthetic
6. The technique for preparation of the osseous defect recipient site varies depending on the type of donor material used.
   a. True
   b. False
7. After final dressing removal, a bone graft site should not be probed for at least _____ months.
   a. 1
   b. 3
   c. 6
   d. 12
8. The type of bony defect that has the best regenerative potential is a _____ defect.
   a. One-wall
   b. Two-wall
   c. Three-wall
   d. Furcation
   e. All of the above are equal

9. When a bone replacement graft material acts to stimulate new bone formation by undifferentiated mesenchymal cells, it is called:
   a. Osteogenesis
   b. Osteoinduction
   c. Osteoconduction
10. Which type of bone replacement graft is obtained from a different species?
    a. Autograft
    b. Allograft
    c. Xenograft
    d. Synthetic graft
11. When small bone chips are collected during bone reshaping procedures, the material is called:
    a. Block graft
    b. Freeze-dried bone
    c. Osseous coagulum
12. The most commonly used allografts are:
    (1) Demineralized freeze-dried bone
    (2) Fresh cadaver bone
    (3) Mineralized freeze-dried bone
       a. 1 and 2
       b. 1 and 3
       c. 2 and 3
       d. 1, 2, and 3
       e. None of the above are allografts
13. Which of the following is not an alloplastic bone replacement graft material?
    a. Bioactive glass
    b. Emdogain
    c. Plaster of Paris
    d. Polymers
    e. Porous hydroxylapatite
14. Overall results with bone replacement grafts demonstrate fill of the original bony defect of about:
    a. 10–29%
    b. 30–49%
    c. 50–69%
    d. 70–89%
    e. 100%
15. When placing a bone replacement graft into a defect, the amount used should:
    a. Fill the defect about 50% full
    b. Fill the defect level with the existing bony defect walls
    c. Overfill the defect to rebuild the normal height and contour for the area
16. Which of the following is (are) an important patient selection factor(s) when considering bone replacement graft treatment?
    a. Effective oral hygiene
    b. No significant medical problems
    c. Smoking
    d. Amenable to long-term maintenance
    e. All of the above

# Management of Osseous Defects: Furcation Involvement Treatment Considerations

Arthur Vernino

## PHILOSOPHY

Treatment of teeth with furcation involvement complicates periodontal treatment. A furcation involvement may be defined as a pathologic condition that has destroyed the periodontium in the intra-radicular area of a multirooted tooth. Treatment of these teeth has varied from conservative (nonsurgical) maintenance to extraction. Recently, the trend has been toward retaining these teeth, especially if they are of strategic importance in the overall treatment plan. Nevertheless, the dentist is cautioned to avoid unnecessary heroics in attempting to salvage seriously involved, multirooted teeth by means of "interesting" techniques. Before attempting extensive therapy, the dentist should ask the following questions.

1. Can a morphologic environment be established that can be adequately maintained by the patient?
2. Will retention of this tooth preserve arch integrity and obviate prosthetic replacement?
3. Will retention permit better prosthetic design?
4. Is the tooth vital to an existing prosthesis?
5. Can the proposed therapeutic effort be considered realistic therapy?
6. Is there a more predictable alternative to retaining this tooth?

## DIAGNOSIS

The anatomic characteristics of multirooted teeth predispose to furcation diseases.[1] The features that make these teeth susceptible to periodontal disease include (a) bacterial plaque accumulation in difficult access areas, (b) root morphology, (c) accessory canals, and (d) length of root trunk and location of the root separation relative to root trunk.[2–8]

Pathologic conditions in this area are diagnosed by the use of a periodontal probe, a pigtail or cowhorn explorer, a Nabors probe, and radiography. The use of radiography must be related to the clinical examination. For example, radiographic examinations may reveal evidence of a furcation involvement, whereas probing reveals that the soft tissue attachment is still intact, with no entrance into the furcation area. Obviously, the clinical examination is the critical evaluation in this instance.

Maxillary molars, with extensive pocket depths (5 mm or more) on the mesial, distal, or midfacial aspect, should automatically be suspected of having furcation involvement. In mandibular molars, extensive midfacial or midlingual pocket formation strongly suggests an intra-radicular pathologic process, regardless of the radiographic evidence.

Probing and positive identification of maxillary furcation involvement can be especially difficult.[9–11] Occasionally, local anesthesia must be used to permit adequate diagnosis. The mesial entry in the furca is best accomplished from the palatal aspect. The distal entry may be accomplished from either the palatal or the facial aspect. Although careful presurgical diagnosis can minimize the possibility of an unexpected, surprise furcation problem, final, positive evidence is often found only at the time of surgery.

## CLASSIFICATION

Classification of furcation pathology can be divided into four grades[12]:

1. Grade I (incipient defects)
2. Grade II (moderate involvement)
3. Grade III
4. Grade IV

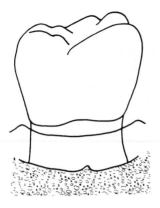

*Figure 19.1* ●

The classification may be defined in greater detail as follows[13]:

Grade I. A soft tissue lesion extending to the furcation level but with minimal osseous destruction. The probe will just enter the furcation area (less than 1 mm). Radiography of these incipient lesions reveals little, if any, evidence of a pathologic condition (Fig. 19-1).

Grade II. A soft tissue lesion combined with bone loss that permits a probe or explorer to enter the furcation from one aspect but not to pass completely through the furcation. Grade II is further subdivided as follows:

Degree 1. Greater than 1 mm and less than 3 mm of horizontal bone loss in the furcation. The probe or explorer enters the furcation more than 1 mm and less than 3 mm.

Degree 2. Horizontal loss of bone of 3 mm or greater, but not through-and-through involvement. The probe or explorer enters the furcation more than 3 mm but does not go through and through (Fig. 19-2).

Grade III. A lesion with extensive osseous destruction that permits through-and-through communication but the furcation is still covered by soft tissue (Fig. 19-3).

Grade IV. A through-and-through furcation involvement that is clinically exposed and open. There is complete visualization through the furcation (Fig. 19-4).

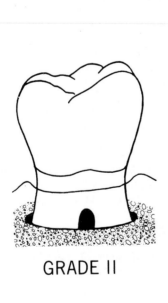

GRADE II

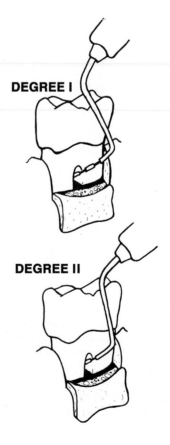

DEGREE I

DEGREE II

*Figure 19.2* ●

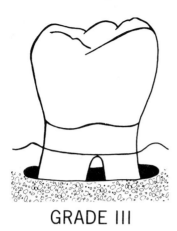

## GRADE III

*Figure 19.3* ●

## PROGNOSIS

The prognosis of teeth with a furcation involvement depends on the following factors[14]:

1. Extent of horizontal and vertical bone destruction in the intra-radicular space
2. Number of roots, their morphology, and furcal roof morphology
3. Morphology of the intra-radicular space (width, depth, and so forth)
4. Health status of the periodontal ligament (determined by tooth mobility, percussive response, and so forth)
5. Access for surgical correction
6. Access for plaque control by the patient after surgical correction

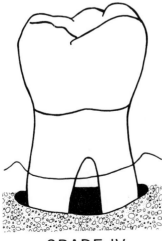

## GRADE IV

*Figure 19.4* ●

7. Pulpal status and prospects for successful endodontics therapy and root removal procedures
8. Ability to control occlusal factors
9. History of caries

When the foregoing factors are equal, mandibular first molars, generally, have the best prognosis, followed by mandibular second molars and maxillary first molars. The prognosis of maxillary premolars is considered poor, even when there is only moderate furcation involvement. Anatomically, premolar teeth do not lend themselves to satisfactory plaque control or to root amputation.

The possibility of new attachment in the furcation area, with or without osseous grafting, is not a highly predictable procedure. There is some evidence that guided tissue regenerative procedures may be more successful in treating furcation involvements.

## PULPAL–PERIODONTAL RELATIONSHIPS

The relationship between pulpal disease and periodontal disease has been increasingly appreciated. It is apparent that there are many direct communications between pulpal tissues and the periodontal ligament. Dentists cannot consider these areas as separate and unrelated environments. Therefore, in diagnostic terms, a pulpal evaluation should be a part of every periodontal examination.[15]

Pulpal–periodontal interaction is especially important in intra-radicular areas. Because of the potential accessory foramina in the furcation areas, grade II and grade III furcation lesions are sometimes associated with pulpal disease. It has been demonstrated that the intra-radicular periodontal apparatus is especially sensitive to excessive occlusal stress. Thus, the combination of pulpal disease, periodontal traumatism, and inflammatory periodontitis might reasonably be expected to produce extensive destruction in the furcation area.

The potential for pulpal–periodontal interrelationships provides continual diagnostic challenges to the therapist. The clinician must be highly suspicious of pulpal disease, especially when the following conditions exist:

1. Periodontal pockets near or leading to the furcation area or apex
2. Sinus tract of uncertain origin
3. Discolored teeth
4. Chronic drainage from the sulcus
5. History of acute or chronic pulpal insult (periodontal traumatism, extensive restorative dentistry, and so forth)

6. Prolonged hypersensitivity
7. Evidence of slow or inadequate healing of periodontal lesions

## THERAPY
### Grade I Involvement

Treatment for incipient furcation lesions is essentially the same for an uncomplicated soft tissue pocket. If the width of attached gingiva is adequate (see Chapters 1 and 14), gingivoplasty or odontoplasty may be used, together with thorough debridement and root preparation. The surgery is accomplished to permit access to the furcation for both the therapist and patient.

1. Careful attention should be given to the character of the cervical crown area. Inadequate class IV restorations, cervical caries, and poor crown contours may be predisposing factors that should be corrected.
2. Projections of enamel into the furcation area may influence the spread of gingival inflammation. This anomaly occurs on the buccal aspect of about 25% of all molars. Although the importance of such projections is not clear, the therapist should be aware of them. Removal of the enamel projections by odontoplasty may be indicated, especially if new attachment is anticipated. On the other hand, if the furcation is left permanently exposed, removal of these anomalies may cause unnecessary tooth sensitivity.[16]

### Grade II Involvement

The prognosis and treatment approach are related to the severity of the grade II furcation involvement.

#### Grade II, Degree 1

The prognosis for maintaining a furcation with this severity of involvement is good. Therapy will vary from conservative (nonsurgical) root preparation to surgical access of the furcal area for osseous surgery. Furcation plasty may be necessary for maintenance of oral hygiene by the patient.

#### Grade II, Degree 2

The prognosis for maintaining a furca with degree 2 severity of involvement is less favorable than a degree 1 involved tooth. Therapy will include, in addition to the procedures for the degree 1 furcation, more aggressive approaches, such as guided tissue regeneration, root resection, or hemisection.

## Grades III and IV Involvement

There are several categories of therapy for grade III and grade IV furcation involvement. These involve:

1. Increasing the furcation opening to facilitate plaque control
2. Eliminating the furcation by various root removal procedures
3. Extracting the tooth

Attempts to reestablish total furcation integrity (new bone, periodontal attachment apparatus, and dentogingival relationship) by bone grafting continue to represent an unpredictable form of treatment.

### Furcation Plasty

Enlargement of an existing class III furcation defect may facilitate plaque control and permit retention of the tooth. Enlargement may be at the expense of the tooth structure, the bone, or both. This approach, however, is generally limited to mandibular molars. Occasionally, a trifurcation area can be opened widely, but adequate plaque removal is difficult. Even after successful treatment of the class III furcation involvement, caries in the furcation area is a constant threat. Caries control is essential for success in the treatment of all furcation involved teeth. The use of the various topical fluorides is recommended.

### Root Resection

Root amputation is a predictable procedure for grade III trifurcation involved teeth. The root with the greatest overall bone loss is the logical candidate for amputation.[17] If there is no marked difference, then the distobuccal (DB) root is the root most likely chosen for removal. The mesiobuccal (MB) root is the most desirable for retention because of favorable root size and position in alveolar bone (Fig. 19-5) (PAL = palatal; RT = root trunk). There are several points to consider before root resection is attempted.

1. The therapist should review root and furcation anatomy on extracted molars.
2. Occlusion should be checked and corrected. The occlusal table should be narrowed, and lateral occlusal forces should be removed (Fig. 19-6).
3. The need for splinting should be established.
4. The strategic importance of teeth indicated for root resection should be thoroughly evaluated.
5. The maxillary sinus should be located and avoided.

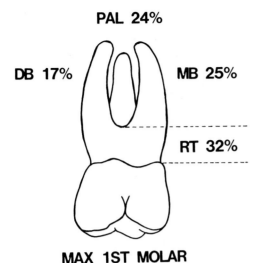

PAL 24%

DB 17%          MB 25%

RT 32%

MAX 1ST MOLAR

**Figure 19.5** ●

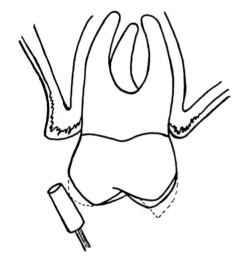

**Figure 19.6** ●

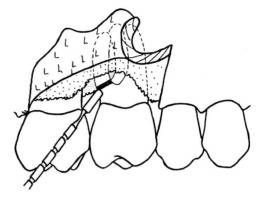

**Figure 19.8** ●

## Technique

1. Elevate a mucoperiosteal (full-thickness) flap to expose the defect (Fig. 19-7). Relaxing incisions may be required for adequate access and tissue placement.
2. Make the initial cut on the root, with an appropriate bur, apical to the cementoenamel junction, beginning in the furcation area. Amputation should be at the expense of the root rather than of the crown (Fig. 19-8).
3. Remove the severed root, with appropriate instruments.
4. Contour the resected root stump. The root surface must be tapered and gently curving to permit complete access by the patient for plaque control (Fig. 19-9).
5. Suture the flap (Fig. 19-10) and cover with a suitable periodontal dressing.
6. Remove sutures in 1 week and recheck the contour.
7. Polish the stump with a fluoride-containing polishing agent.

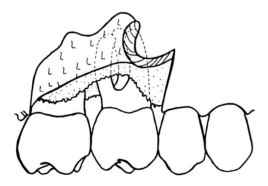

**Figure 19.7** ●

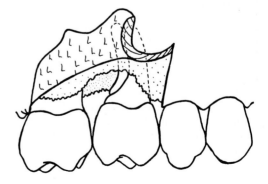

**Figure 19.9** ●

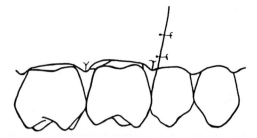

*Figure 19.10* ●

8. Teach the patient proper plaque control techniques.
9. Accomplish endodontic therapy before or soon after (within 2 weeks) root amputation.

## Hemisection

Hemisection involves the removal of one-half of the tooth. The same technique is used as was described for root resection. This procedure is most often performed on the mandibular molars, and the retained root can often serve as a suitable abutment for a fixed prosthesis or fixed splinting. Special attention must be given to the restoration of these periodontally weakened teeth.[18]

## Guided Tissue Regeneration

Guided tissue regenerative procedures show some promise for successfully reestablishing the periodontium in the grade II and grade III involved teeth.[19,20] The procedure has shown predictability for connective tissue attachment in grade II furcation involvements, with bone regeneration less predictable. The guided tissue procedures have not shown reliability in managing the grade III furcations.

## REFERENCES

1. Gher M, Vernino A. Root morphology—clinical significance in pathogenesis and treatment of periodontal disease. J Am Dent Assoc 1980;101:627–633.
2. DeSanctis M, Murphy K. The role of resective periodontal surgery in the treatment of furcation defects. Periodontol 2000 2000;22:154–168.
3. Bower R. Furcation morphology relative to periodontal treatment—furcation entrance architecture. J Periodontol 1979;50:23–37.
4. Villaca JH, Rodrigues DC, Novaes AB Jr, Taba M Jr, Souza SL, Grisi MF. Root trunk concavities as a risk factor for regenerative procedures of class II furcation lesions in humans. J Periodontol 2004;75: 1493–1499.
5. Kerns DG, Greenwell H, Wittwer JW, Drisko C, Williams JN, Kerns LL. Root trunk dimensions of 5 different tooth types. Int J Periodontics Restorative Dent 1999;19:82–91.
6. Gutmann JL. Prevalence, location, and patency of accessory canals in the furcation region of permanent molars. J Periodontol 1978;49:21–26.
7. Ward C, Greenwell H, Wittwer JW, Drisko C. Furcation depth and inter root separation dimensions for 5 different tooth types. Int J Periodontics Restorative Dent 1999;19:251–257.
8. Hermann DW, Gher ME Jr, Dunlap RM, Pelleu GB Jr. The potential attachment area of the maxillary first molars. J Periodontol 1983;54:431–434.
9. Svardstrom, G Wennstrom JL. Periodontal treatment decisions for molars: an analysis of influencing factors and long-term outcome. J Periodontol 2000;71: 579–585.
10. Mealey BL, Neubauer MF, Butzin CA, Waldrop TC. Use of furcal bone sounding to improve accuracy of furcation diagnosis. J Periodontol 1994;65: 649–657.
11. Abdallah F, Kon S, Ruben M. The furcation problem: etiology, diagnosis, therapy and prognosis. J West Soc Periodontol 1987;35:129–141.
12. Glickkman I. Clinical Periodontology, 2nd ed. Philadelphia: WB Saunders, 1958:694–896.
13. Hamp S, Nyman S, Lindhe I. Periodontal treatment of multirooted teeth. Results after 5 years. J Clin Periodontol 1975;2:126–135.
14. Blomlof L, Jansson L, Appelgren R, Ehnevid H, Lindskog S. Prognosis and mortality of root resected molars. Int J Periodontics Restorative Dent 1997;17: 191–201.
15. Chen S, Wang H, Glickman G. The influence of endodontic treatment upon periodontal wound healing J Clin Periodontol 1997;24:449–456.
16. Masters, Hoskins S. Projections of cervical enamel into molar furcations. J Periodontol 1964;33:49–53.
17. Ross I, Thompson R. A long tern study of root retention in the treatment of maxillary molars with furcation involvement. J Periodontol 1978;49:238–244.
18. Shillingburg H, Hobo S, Whitsett L, Jacobi R, Brackett S. Preparations for periodontally weakened teeth. In: Fundamentals of Fixed Prosthodontics, 3rd ed. Chicago: Quintessence, 1997:211–223.
19. Pontoriero R, Lindhe J. Guided tissue regeneration in the treatment of degree II furcations in maxillary molars. J Clin Periodontol 1995;22:756–763.
20. Pontoriero R, Lindhe J. Guided tissue regeneration in the treatment of degree III furcations in maxillary molars. J Clin Periodontol 1995;22:810–812.

# CHAPTER 19
# REVIEW QUESTIONS

1. When considering extensive therapy for the tooth with furcation involvement, the dentist should consider all of the following except:
   a. Whether a morphologic environment can be established that can be adequately maintained by the patient
   b. Whether all teeth with furcation involvements can be adequately treated
   c. Whether the proposed therapeutic effort can be considered realistic therapy
   d. Whether there is a more predicable alternative to retaining this tooth

2. The potential accessory foramina in the furcation areas of grade II and grade III furcation lesions are sometimes associated with:
   a. Pulpal disease
   b. Occlusal traumatism
   c. Adfaction lesions
   d. None of the above

3. A lesion with extensive osseous destruction that permits through-and-through communication but the furcation is still covered by soft tissue is classified as:
   a. Grade I
   b. Grade II, degree 2
   c. Grade III
   d. Grade II, degree 1

4. The prognosis of teeth with a furcation involvement depends on the following factors except:
   a. Extent of horizontal and vertical bone destruction in the intra-radicular space
   b. Age of patient
   c. Number of roots and their morphology
   d. Furcal roof morphology

5. The following points should be considered before root resection is attempted:
   a. Root and furcation anatomy
   b. Occlusion checked and corrected
   c. Location of the maxillary sinus
   d. All the above

6. Considering the maxillary first molar, the most desirable root for retention because of favorable root size and position in the alveolar bone is:
   a. Palatal
   b. Mesiobuccal
   c. Distobuccal
   d. No preference

7. The therapies for grades III and IV involvement of furcations can involve:
   a. Increasing the furcation opening to facilitate plaque control
   b. Eliminating the furcation by various root removal procedures
   c. Extracting the tooth
   d. All the above

8. The procedure of enlargement of an existing class III furcation defect in mandibular molars to facilitate plaque control and permit retention of the tooth is referred to as:
   a. Osteoplasty
   b. Furcation plasty
   c. Odontoplasty
   d. Gingival plasty

9. The procedure that involves the removal of one-half of the tooth is:
   a. Hemisection
   b. Root resection
   c. Furcation plasty
   d. Odontoplasty

10. Which of the following statements is true regarding guided tissue regenerative procedures in the grade II and grade III involved teeth?
    a. Guided tissue regenerative procedures have shown bone regeneration predictability in grade II furcations.
    b. Guided tissue regenerative procedures have shown connective tissue attachment predictability in the grade II furcations.
    c. Guided tissue regenerative procedures have shown reliability in managing the grade III furcations.
    d. Guided tissue regenerative procedures do not show any promise in treatment of furcation lesions.

# Management of Osseous Defects: Additional Techniques and Summary

John Rapley

## FLAP CURETTAGE, FLAP DEBRIDEMENT, AND OPEN DEBRIDEMENT

Several reports have suggested that complete surgical debridement of osseous defects and adjacent pathologic root surfaces may result in partial bony defect fill.[1–3] Full-thickness (mucoperiosteal) flaps with osseous defect debridement for osseous regeneration appears to be most effective in narrow three-wall defects, with less favorable results achieved in other types of defects.[1] Thorough and frequent professional and personal plaque control after surgery is critical to maximizing the bony regeneration.[4] Almost every clinical research evaluation comparing flap curettage with bone replacement grafts has demonstrated better clinical results when using graft material as part of the treatment of the defect.

## GUIDED TISSUE REGENERATION

Extensive animal and clinical research has established the principle of guided tissue regeneration for treatment of some types of periodontal defects.[5–9] Most intrabony defects, grade II furcations, and some dehiscences have been shown to respond well to this type of therapy.

Guided tissue regeneration is based on the following principles:

1. Create a biologically acceptable wound repair area by debridement of the osseous defect or furcation and root detoxification (mechanical).
2. Place a barrier or membrane between the external tissues (gingival connective tissue and epithelium) and the internal tissues (bone, periodontal ligament, root surface).
3. Create and maintain a space between the barrier and the tooth for clot stabilization. This

will create conditions for bone, cementum, and periodontal ligament regeneration.
4. Position and suture the flap to cover the barrier and stabilize the wound.
5. Monitor closely during the 6-week postsurgical period.
6. Nonresorbable barriers will need to be surgically removed at about 6 weeks in a second surgical procedure. Resorbable barriers do not need to be removed and have been shown to have the same efficacy as the nonresorbable barriers.

Although an expanded polytetrafluoroethylene (e-PTFE) nonresorbable barrier was the first commercially available product, multiple nonresorbable and resorbable types are currently used. Depending on the type of osseous defect that is being treated, results with all of them are generally favorable. However, in some types of defects as in interproximal bone loss, the use of a barrier by itself or in combination with a bone replacement graft has not shown an advantage compared with the results of using only a bone replacement graft or flap curettage.[10,11] Patient and defect selection are very important when considering the extra time and expense involved in using guided tissue regeneration for periodontal defects.

## SELECTIVE EXTRACTION

Selective extraction (strategic extraction) of some periodontally involved teeth can significantly improve the prognosis of adjacent teeth.[12–14] For example, in Figure 20-1, severe periodontal involvement of this vital first premolar has also resulted in bone loss on the adjacent teeth. The tooth exhibits grade III mobility and its prognosis is poor. If it is extracted, the socket will fill approximately to the most coronal level of the alveolar

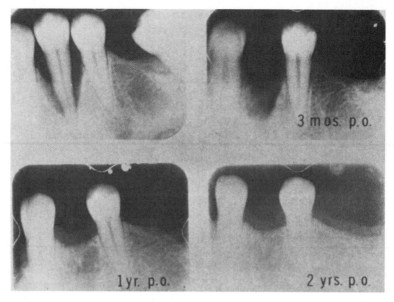

3 mos. p.o.

1 yr. p.o.

2 yrs. p.o.

**Figure 20.1** ●

crest on the adjacent teeth, as shown in Figure 20-1. Consequently, there is an improved prognosis for the adjacent teeth. Selective extraction can be a predictable method of case management.[15]

## MINOR TOOTH MOVEMENT

Orthodontic tooth movement can create favorable alterations of gingival form and osseous morphology.[16] These changes often modify the extent of or eliminate the need for pocket elimination or reduction surgery. Teeth can be moved into a vertical bony defect to narrow the osseous lesion and improve the chances for success with regenerative techniques. Teeth can also be moved away from the osseous defect (such as in molar-uprighting techniques), thereby leveling the bone and modifying or eliminating the bony defects. Similarly, forced eruption can be used to modify the osseous topography. Some corrective osseous surgery is frequently needed after the forced eruption to finalize the hard and soft tissue contours. In all cases, inflammation control must be accomplished before beginning orthodontic therapy.

## SUMMARY OF TREATMENT OF OSSEOUS DEFECTS

The prognosis for successful resolution of infrabony pockets is influenced by the:

1. Number of remaining osseous walls
2. Size of the osseous defect (wide or narrow)
3. Number of root surfaces involved

4. Extent of bony destruction (severity)
5. Presence or absence of furcation involvement
6. Ability to effectively detoxify and debride the defect and tooth

As a general rule, the greater the number of osseous walls and the narrower the defect, the better the prognosis for regeneration. (This is with no furcation involvement).

The type of therapy chosen for the defects found at the time of surgery will depend on the osseous morphology and location of the defects as well as the clinician's experience, knowledge, and skill. Osseous resection, flap curettage, and bone replacement grafts have all been used for each type of bony defect.

Some guidelines for treating various osseous defects follow:

1. Broad interproximal ledges—consider osteoplasty
2. Interproximal irregularities of bone—consider osteoplasty
3. Exostoses that interfere with pocket reduction or proper flap closure—consider osteoplasty
4. Three-wall defect
   a. Narrow—consider
      (1) Bone replacement graft
      (2) Flap curettage
   b. Broad defect—consider
      (1) Bone graft replacement
      (2) Guided tissue regeneration depending on the location of the defect
      (3) Flap curettage
5. Two-wall defect

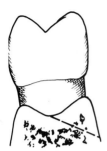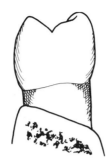

**Figure 20.2** •

a. Shallow crater—consider
  (1) Osteoplasty or ostectomy (Fig. 20-2)
  (2) Flap curettage
b. Deep crater—consider
  (1) Bone replacement graft
  (2) Flap curettage
  (3) Combined procedures including defect debridement, osteoplasty or ostectomy, with or without bone replacement graft, with or without guided tissue regeneration
6. One-wall defect
  a. Shallow—consider
    (1) Osteoplasty or ostectomy (if adjacent teeth are not jeopardized)
    (2) Bone replacement graft
    (3) Orthodontic extrusion
  b. Deep—consider
    (1) Bone replacement graft
    (2) Guided tissue regeneration (limited success)
    (3) Combined procedures
7. Combination defects—consider combination procedures
8. Grade I furcation involvement—consider
  a. Scaling and root planing
  b. Osteoplasty or ostectomy plus odontoplasty
  c. Apically positioned flap
9. Grade II furcation involvement—consider
  a. Osteoplasty or ostectomy and odontoplasty
  b. Root resection or hemisection
  c. Bone replacement graft
  d. Guided tissue regeneration
  e. Combination procedures
  f. Extraction depending on severity of furcation involvement
10. Grade III and grade IV furcation—consider
  a. Root resection or hemisection
  b. Osteoplasty or ostectomy with odontoplasty (tunneling) and apically positioned flap to create through-and-through furcation for plaque control
  c. Extraction

## REFERENCES

1. Froum SJ, Coran M, Thaller B, Kushner L, Scopp IW, Stahl SS. Periodontal healing following open debridement flap procedures. I. Clinical assessment of soft tissue and osseous repair. J Periodontol 1982;53:8–14.
2. Grassi M, Tellenbach R, Lang NP. Periodontal conditions of teeth adjacent to extraction sites. J Clin Periodontol 1987;14:334–339.
3. VanVenrooy JR, Yukna RA. Orthodontic extrusion of single-rooted teeth affected with advanced periodontal disease. Am J Orthod Dentofacial Orthop 1985;87:67.
4. Polson AM, Heijl LC. Osseous repair in infrabony periodontal defects. J Clin Periodontol 1978;5:13–23.
5. Page RC. Animal models in reconstructive periodontal therapy. J Periodontol 1994;65:1142.
6. Selvig KA. Discussion: animal models in reconstructive therapy. J Periodontol 1994;65:1169–1172.
7. Pontoriero R, Nyman S, Ericsson I, Lindhe J. Guided tissue regeneration in surgically-produced furcation defects. An experimental study in the beagle dog. J Clin Periodontol 1992;19:159–163.
8. Gottlow J, Nyman S, Lindhe J, Karring T, Wennstrom J. New attachment formation in the human periodontium by guided tissue regeneration. Case reports. J Clin Periodontol 1986;13:604–616.
9. Cortellini P, Pini Prato G, Baldi C, Clauser C. Guided tissue regeneration with different materials. Int J Periodontics Restorative Dent 1990;10: 136–151.
10. Schallhorn RG, McClain PK. Combined osseous composite grafting, root conditioning, and guided tissue regeneration. Int J Periodontics Restorative Dent 1988;8:9–32.
11. Anderegg CR, Martin SJ, Gray JL, Mellonig JT, Gher ME. Clinical evaluation of the use of decalcified freeze-dried bone allograft with guided tissue regeneration in the treatment of molar furcation invasions. J Periodontol 1991;62:264–268.
12. Yukna RA. Clinical human comparison of expanded polytetrafluoroethylene barrier membrane and freeze-dried dura mater allografts for guided tissue regeneration of lost periodontal support. I. Mandibular molar class II furcations. J Periodontol 1992;63:431–442.
13. Saadoun AP. Periodontal and restorative considerations in strategic extractions. Compend Cont Educ Dent 1981;2:48.
14. Machtei EE, Zubrey Y, Ben Yehuda A, Soskolne WA. Proximal bone loss adjacent to periodontally "hopeless" teeth with and without extraction. J Periodontol 1989;60:512–515.
15. DeVore CH, Beck FM, Horton JE. Retained "hopeless" teeth; effects on the proximal periodontium of adjacent teeth. J Periodontol 1988;59:647–651.
16. Kozlovsky A, Tal H, Lieberman M. Forced eruption combined with gingival fiberotomy. A technique for clinical crown lengthening. J Clin Periodontol 1988;15:534–538.

## CHAPTER 20
## REVIEW QUESTIONS

1. Guided tissue regeneration (GTR) is based on the principle of initial exclusion of what tissue type:
   a. Bone
   b. Cementum
   c. Epithelium
   d. Connective

2. The type of GTR membrane that has produced the best efficacy is:
   a. Resorbable
   b. Nonresorbable
   c. Neither, both have the same efficacy

3. GTR has been shown to be of little added benefit with:
   a. Three-wall defects
   b. Interproximal bone loss
   c. Class II maxillary molar furcation defects

4. A three-wall narrow defect is best treated by:
   a. Extraction
   b. Flap debridement
   c. Bone replacement graft
   d. Guided tissue regeneration

5. A two-wall osseous defect is termed a:
   a. Crater
   b. Hemiseptum
   c. Suprabony defect

6. A grade III furcation is best treated by:
   a. Osteoplasty
   b. Odontoplasty
   c. Bone replacement graft
   d. Root resection or hemisection

7. A grade I furcation is best treated by:
   a. Tunnel procedure
   b. Bone replacement graft
   c. Apically positioned flap
   d. Hemisection or root resection

8. The prognosis for successful resolution of infrabony pockets is influenced by the number of remaining osseous walls. It is also affected by the presence or absence of a furcation involvement.
   a. Both statements are true.
   b. Both statements are false.
   c. The first statement is true and the second statement is false.
   d. The first statement is false and the second statement is true.

9. In treating osseous defects, the best therapy for broad interproximal ledges is osteoplasty. Also, the best therapy for a three-wall defect is minor tooth movement.
   a. Both statements are true.
   b. Both statements are false.
   c. The first statement is true and the second statement is false.
   d. The first statement is false and the second statement is true.

10. A full-thickness flap is also called a mucoperiosteal flap. The full-thickness flap is the most commonly used periodontal flap.
    a. Both statements are true.
    b. Both statements are false.
    c. The first statement is true and the second statement is false.
    d. The first statement is false and the second statement is true.

# Dental Implants

Donald Callan

## INTRODUCTION

Currently, dental implant therapy and prosthodontic reconstruction are routine treatments for the partially and fully edentulous patient. Dental implants have become a predictable treatment alternative for the replacement of missing teeth in partially or completely edentulous patients. It is estimated the U.S. market for dental implants is in excess of $243.3 million with a growth of 16.4% a year.[1] As with any innovative advances, there are inherent problems that develop in effectively communicating with patients, dentists, dental laboratories, physicians, other health professionals, and insurance companies. Most dentists already possess the necessary skills and abilities, which can be maximized, to include some aspect of implant therapy into their practice. However, the surgical placement of dental implants with or without augmentation procedures requires additional commitment and training beyond the experience received in the undergraduate dental experience. Dentists getting started in implant dentistry must realize a greater commitment is required than just a refresher course in oral surgery. The surgical, restorative dentist and the dental laboratory must have a good understanding of bone physiology, soft tissue physiology, wound healing, occlusion, anatomy, implant designs, advanced prosthodontic designs, pharmacology, and advanced surgical skills. The practice of implant dentistry is a building block learning process.

## PATIENT SELECTION AND CONSIDERATIONS

The goal of implant dentistry is to prevent or rescue the dental-challenged patient by restoring oral health, function, and esthetics, regardless of existing dental deterioration, that a patient can and will maintain. Therefore, the selection of an appropriate dental implant for a patient must be determined by evaluating a variety of oral, systemic, and economic factors. Not every edentulous or semiedentulous area is a site for a dental implant. Dental implants, like any other implants, are merely artificial replacements for lost or traumatized natural structures; therefore, implants cannot exceed or last longer than the original dentition.

The past and present state of oral repair is of paramount importance with regard to a favorable long-range prognosis. If a patient's mouth is in a poor state of repair or in need of periodontal and endodontic therapy, as well as removal of decay and temporization, education must be a primary goal to prevent the seeding of pathogenic bacteria about the newly placed dental implants.[2] If the individual lost his or her teeth as a result of decay or periodontal disease, an accurate pretreatment index of their ability to care for the remaining teeth and dental implants must be achieved. Those individuals who cannot demonstrate acceptable oral home care are either poor risk or contraindicated for implant reconstruction surgery. Implant maintenance will be presented in Chapter 22.

The quantity and quality of the horizontal and vertical bone structure and the proximity of the adjacent vital structures, such as the maxillary sinus, inferior alveolar canal, and the mental foramen, will help in treatment planning for implant therapy. The presence or absence of keratinized gingival tissues, unfavorable muscle attachment, decreased vertical dimension, and freeway space, along with class II or class III maxillomandibular relationships, may also influence the treatment plan. The presence of hard or soft tissue disease, in addition to the presence of intraoral plates, screws, or wires, in the area of anticipated implant placement must be eliminated preoperatively.

It is recommended that the desires and expectations of the patient are verbalized and documented. If these desires and expectations are realistic and obtainable, the treatment plan process can proceed. The treatment objective is to provide the patient a positive result. The goal in implant dentistry is "to restore the patient's mouth to a condition that the patient can and will maintain." The following indications should be met to obtain this goal.

## IMPLANT INDICATIONS

1. Restore function
2. Improve esthetics
3. Decrease gag reflex
4. Preserve teeth
5. Preserve bone
6. Improve speech problems
7. Improve psychological state

After the dental evaluation and examination, a medical evaluation is needed. The medical history will determine the degree of presurgical workup required. Because patient selection influences the success rate, the patient must be carefully screened for potential medical, dental, and psychological contraindications. The purpose of a medical evaluation is to assess whether a patient is a candidate for dental implants and what alterations in the treatment plan may be required to account for existing medical conditions. As a general rule, those individuals who have undergone primary or secondary radiation of the head and neck region, chemotherapy, or brittle diabetics, and individuals with connective tissue disorders (i.e., pemphigus, pemphigoid, lupus erythematosus, etc.) are either poor risk or contraindicated for implant reconstruction surgery. In addition, the categories of patients who have undergone or are presently under active psychiatric therapy are also poor implant candidates. If a patient has undergone other implant procedures, such as total hip, total knee, prosthetic valves, or artificial vascular grafts, a thorough consultation with the vascular or orthopedic surgeon is indicated. If in doubt concerning any medical condition, consult with the physician.

## IMPLANT CLASSIFICATIONS

Generally speaking, the design of the implants would fit into four major classifications.

1. Subperiosteal (over the bone)
2. Transosseous (staple; through the bone)
3. Epithelial (mucosal; soft tissue)
4. Endosseous (into the bone)
   a. Ramus frame
   b. Endodontic stabilizer
   c. Blade
   d. Sinus ("S")
   e. Basket
   f. Root form (most used today)
   g. Mini (used as transitional implants)

The remainder of this chapter will focus on the root form implant.

## IMPLANT MATERIAL

The chemical makeup of the implant system, grafting material, and regeneration material should be biocompatible to the host at the hard and soft tissue interface. Without biocompatibility, the host tissue has a potential for damage and rejection. Titanium and titanium alloy appear to be the materials of choice, although other materials show biocompatibility. Numerous articles have been published documenting the biocompatibility of titanium for the use of dental implants[3] and orthopedic implants. Anchorage of bone to the titanium dental implant is mechanical in nature and is called "osseointegration."[4,5]

In recent years there have been applications of inorganic biocompatible coatings to metal implants. Hydroxylapatite coating (HA) appears to be the coating most often used on dental implants. Bone can bond directly to the HA coating, with a faster rate of bone formation and five to eight times more interfacial strength.[6,7] The direct bonding of bone to HA is called "biointegration," and it can occur as early as 8 weeks and may demonstrate more bone to the implant surface than non–HA-coated implants. Greater bone density and less fibrous tissue encapsulation of HA-coated implants have also been reported with HA-coated implants.[8,9]

The HA-coated implants appear to have the following advantages[4–10]:

1. Biointegration (bone bonding)
2. Greater bone–implant surface
3. Earlier and stronger implant–bone interface
4. No metal ion release from the metal part of the implant
5. Faster integration
6. Applied to all implant modalities and systems
7. Bridge bone deficiencies
8. Increased success with type IV bone

Although the implant may be biocompatible, its surface must be acceptable to the host tissue. Different manufacturers are claiming different success and accelerated healing time with various types of surfaces. These claims have not been proven histologically. Integration to bone involves

## TABLE 21.1

### Approximate Surface Area Root Form Implants (mm$^2$)

| Length (mm) | 3.25D Cylinder | 3.25D Threaded | 3.8D Cylinder | 3.8D Threaded | 4.5D Threaded |
|---|---|---|---|---|---|
| 8 | 90 | 118 | 140 | 140 | 164 |
| 10 | 110 | 149 | 175 | 175 | 206 |
| 12 | 130 | 180 | 211 | 211 | 284 |
| 14 | 150 | 210 | 247 | 247 | 291 |
| 16 | 170 | 241 | 283 | 283 | 333 |
| 18 | 190 | 271 | 319 | 319 | 376 |

more than biocompatibility of the dental implant material.

Packaging and sterilization of the implant before insertion must be considered. Once the implant package is open, the surface of the implant must be kept sterile before insertion. It is best not to resterilize implants. If in doubt, contact the implant manufacturer for instructions.

Although charts list the surface area for tooth roots and implants, a direct one-to-one correlation cannot be made. The information listed below is intended to be used for reference purposes only. There are no hard and fast rules for the surface area of an implant required for replacing a given tooth. Common sense dictates the total surface area of the implants being used come as close to the surface area of the teeth being replaced as possible. The surface areas of dental implants shown in Tables 21-1 and 21-2 do not include any factors such as surface design (screw design, surface texture, cylinder design, and so forth) or surface roughness of the implant. Surface area of a rough coating may be as much as six times the area of a similar smooth implant. Length, surface roughness, surface design, diameter, and coating are only a few factors that must be considered when determining the load-bearing area of an implant.

Factors to consider for implant selection will include:

1. Size (length, diameter)
2. Cylinder versus thread type
3. Neck design (implant abutment microgap size)
4. Neck height
5. Surface texture (rough, smooth)
6. Surface activity (HA, non-HA)
7. Material mechanical limits
8. Hard tissue compatibility (implant material)
9. Soft tissue compatibility (smooth neck)
10. Abutment attachment mechanism

## PROSTHODONTICS

The long-term success of an implant depends on treatment planning, proper selection, prosthodontic fabrication, existing occlusion, and hygiene maintenance of the prosthodontic device. The choice may be narrowed by the preference of the patient and hygiene history, anatomy of the available bone, soft tissue quality, and existing dentition. The implant team members are encouraged to refer to current published literature for current prosthodontic principles. The occlusion principles of natural teeth can be applied to implant prosthodontics. This may require a wax model of the proposed result. In most

## TABLE 21.2

### Approximate Surface Area of Natural Dentition (mm$^2$)[11]

| Tooth | Central Incisor | Lateral Incisor | Cuspid | First Bicuspid | Second Bicuspid | First Molar | Second Molar |
|---|---|---|---|---|---|---|---|
| Maxilla | 204 | 179 | 273 | 234 | 220 | 443 | 431 |
| Mandible | 154 | 168 | 268 | 180 | 207 | 431 | 426 |

cases it is best to review a full wax model before starting the treatment plan. The case type and the retention must also be considered before the start of any dental treatment. *The case selection for presurgical treatment planning must start with the vision of the final result.* A more detail discussion will follow within this chapter.

## CASE TYPES

1. Single unit
2. Three-unit bridge
3. Multiple units
4. Full replacement
5. Ball-supported denture
6. Bar-supported denture
7. Partial denture

## RETAINMENT

1. Fixed prosthesis (prosthesis cemented to abutment)
2. Fixed-removable prosthesis (screw-retained prosthesis)
3. Patient-removable prosthesis (ball- or bar-supported denture)

## IMPLANT SITE PREPARATION

It is far beyond the scope of this text to discuss site preparation in detail. What follows is a brief review of current procedures and materials.

Previously, surgeons placed implants where there was available bone. Today, that is an unacceptably restrictive approach to implant placement. The current philosophy calls for the surgeon to regenerate hard and soft tissues, thereby creating a site that is suitable for placing implants in an ideal location (Fig. 21-1).

## SOCKET PRESERVATION

The simplest type of site preparation involves careful tooth removal with minimal trauma (so-called atraumatic extraction) and placement of an osseous graft or barrier before wound closure. Most clinicians use both a graft and a membrane, and wait 2 to 3 months before implant placement (Fig. 21-2).

## GUIDED BONE REGENERATION

Regeneration of lost bone usually involves osseous grafting in either a horizontal or vertical dimension, or both. These procedures are known as "guided bone regeneration (GBR)." In most patients, the buccal or labial cortical plate resorbs soon after tooth loss. In some cases, the tooth removal itself is the cause of bone loss. Vertical bone loss also occurs in some patients. Generally speaking, regeneration of the buccal or lingual cortical plates is more predictable than regeneration of vertical bone loss.

Guided bone regeneration resembles guided tissue regeneration procedures (see Chapter 18). Available graft materials include:

1. Autogenous bone (blocks or particulate)
2. Allografts (FDBA)
3. Xenografts—bovine bone
4. Alloplasts—bioactive glasses, plaster of Paris

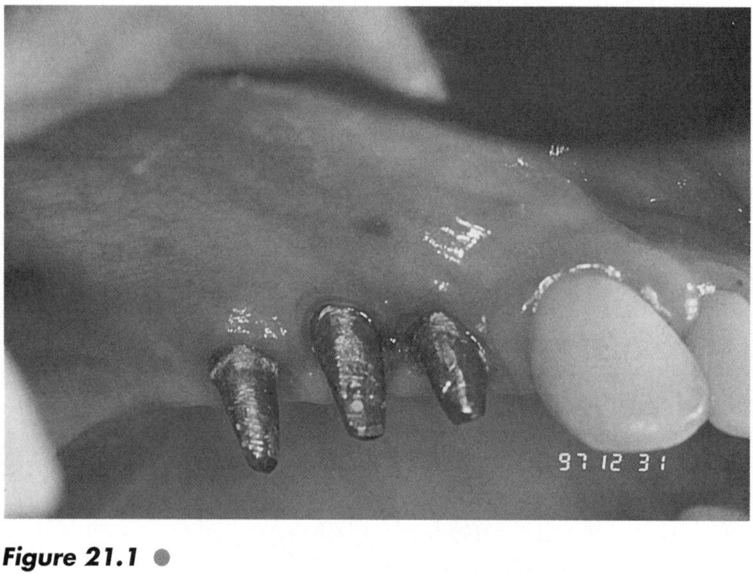


***Figure 21.1*** ●

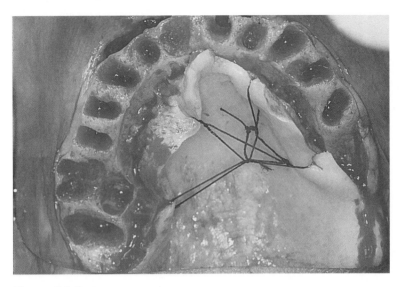

**Figure 21.2** ●

The most frequently used barriers are either collagen, expanded polytetrafluoroethylene (e-PTFE), or resorbable polylactic acid barriers, and they are generally secured with tacks or screws to prevent movement. Screws may also be used to serve as "tent poles," thereby maintaining space for the graft material and healing cells beneath the membrane. Autogenous grafts are one of the best procedures to obtain regeneration in a vertical dimension. In general terms, one harvests the graft either from the chin or the ramus. The osseous graft is secured onto the donor site with screws, and a particulate graft is placed around the periphery as necessary. Autogenous grafts may also be used as a particulate graft either as a stand-alone graft or with a block graft. The other graft materials listed above can be used at the discretion of the surgeon. Often the most difficult aspect of guided bone regeneration is soft tissue closure over the graft. If the graft site cannot be closed completely and without tension, the prognosis for regeneration is greatly reduced. Incision designs intended to extend the soft tissue flap over the graft have been developed for these purposes. Also, it is possible to place incisions through the periosteum to extend the flap. It is usually the buccal or facial flaps that are extended. One problem that results is an inadequate gingival zone around the implant after lingual or palatal advancement of the flaps. This situation can be corrected after the implants have been placed.

## SINUS AUGMENTATION

In some cases, there is insufficient bone adjacent to the maxillary sinus to permit implant placement. In these situations, there are two options: lateral sinus augmentation (sinus lift) or an osteotome approach. The lateral approach involves reflecting a flap to expose the osseous wall lateral to the sinus. A "window" is created in the osseous wall, exposing an intact sinus membrane. An osseous graft material is used to fill the space inferior to the sinus membrane. Implants can be placed simultaneously, or the area can be closed for 4 to 6 months for later implant placement.

The osteotome technique requires a minimum of 5 mm of bone between the sinus floor and the crest of the ridge. An osteotomy is prepared with twist drills, and an instrument known as an osteotome is used to gently elevate the sinus floor and back fill the area with graft material. The implant is then placed.

## IMPLANT FAILURE

The rate of implant failures is low, although it is higher among smokers and patients who lost their teeth because of periodontal disease. Most implants that are lost have inflammatory problems; the second most common cause of implant complications is prosthodontic failure. So-called ailing or failing implants with peri-implantitis (inflammation around the implant associated with bone loss) are usually treated surgically. Attempts at guided tissue regeneration are the most common modality of treatment, although outcomes are unpredictable (Fig. 21-1).

## BONE GRAFTING APPLICATIONS

1. Extraction sockets (Fig. 21-2)
2. Osseous defects (Fig. 21-3)

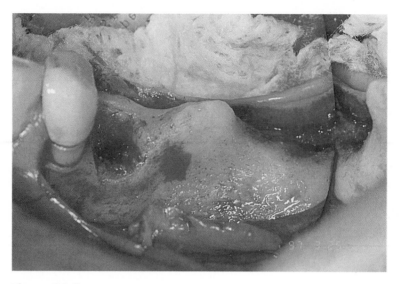

*Figure 21.3* ●

3. Ridge enlargement (Fig. 21-4)
4. Sinus lifts (Fig. 21-5)
5. Implant repair (caution!) (Fig.21-6)

## IMPLANT PLACEMENT

### Treatment Planning Options

One- Versus Two-Stage Implant Placement

1. One-stage procedure: After implant placement, an appropriate healing abutment is attached. The soft tissue flap is adapted around the healing abutment and sutured. This elimi-

nates the need for a second surgical procedure to expose the implant fixture for restoration.
2. Two-stage procedure: The implant is placed and covered by the soft tissue flap. A second surgical procedure is necessary to expose the fixture for restoration.

Immediate Versus Delayed
Implant Placement

1. Immediate: The implant fixtures are placed immediately after tooth removal with the osteotomy site extended beyond the extraction

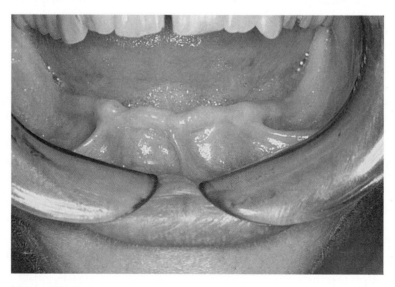

*Figure 21.4* ●

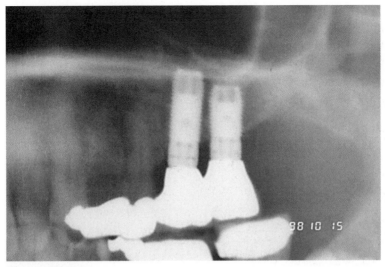

**Figure 21.5** ●

socket. This usually requires a longer implant to obtain immediate stabilization.

2. Delayed: The placement of the implant fixture is delayed 2 to 3 months to achieve either soft tissue or hard tissue healing. If the site of future implant placement receives an osseous graft, the date of implant placement might be delayed for 4 to 9 months for complete healing to take place.

### Immediate Versus Delayed Temporization

1. Immediate temporization: A temporary restoration is placed on the fixture immediately after implant placement. This restoration is usually not in occlusion.
2. Delayed temporization: The temporary restoration is placed after healing of the surgical site.

### Immediate Load Versus Delayed Load

1. Immediate load: The implant fixture receives the permanent restoration at the time of implant placement.
2. Delayed restoration: The implant fixture is loaded after the implants have integrated.

## SURGICAL GUIDES

Many designs of surgical guides have been developed. It is best to have a surgical guide with well-defined cementoenamel junctions. The guide is fabricated by the restorative dentist and used by the surgeon as a positional guide for implant placement, and is best made from a diagnostic

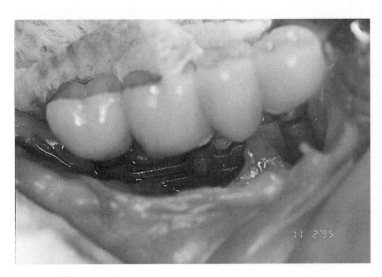

**Figure 21.6** ●

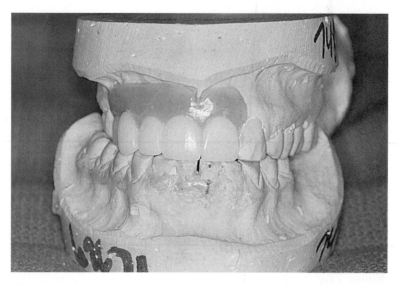

*Figure 21.7* ●

wax-up that has been approved by the patient. The guide will aid the surgical dentist to obtain the ideal mesiodistal, buccolingual, and long-axis orientation of the implant(s), the best emergence profile, and the proper axial direction of the occlusal forces. If there is insufficient bone or anatomic structures preventing ideal placement, secondary sites may be chosen as predetermined in the alternative treatment plan. If the required number, location, or axial orientation of the implants cannot be achieved, the surgeon may elect to place no implants. The surgical dentist may need to proceed with hard tissue grafting to obtain the best result. The surgical guide may also be an aid in formulating a comprehensive treatment plan and fee estimate. To fabricate the surgical guide, the implant laboratory may assist the surgical and the restorative dentist as well as provide suggestions. It is best to start with a diagnostic wax-up for an ideal end result (Fig. 21-7). From this wax-up, the surgical guide is fabricated in a hard, clear acrylic material (Fig. 21-8). The restorative dentist should place holes in the center of each tooth to be supported by the dental implant. The surgical guide is then delivered to the surgical dentist.

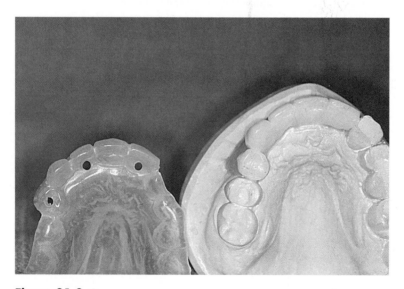

*Figure 21.8* ●

## IMPLANT PRESURGICAL CHECKLIST

1. Current radiographs or computerized images
2. Mounted study cast
3. Surgical guides
4. Medical clearance or health history review
5. Consent form signed
6. Agreement among all team members (treatment plan)
7. Alternative treatment plans
8. Financial arrangements
9. Postoperative medications
10. Preoperative and postoperative written instructions
11. Implants ordered and received
12. Communication and understanding with the patient about the procedure
13. Follow-up appointment for suture removal and evaluation

## THE IMPLANT SURGICAL PROCEDURE

As with any surgery, the implant procedure should be performed under aseptic conditions using local anesthesia, with or without sedation. A mesiodistal incision is made along the alveolar crest through the mucoperiosteum and attached gingiva to the bone. The incision should be long enough to permit adequate reflection without tearing the tissue and to provide a broad field of view. Vertical incisions may be used, if necessary. Using a periosteal elevator, carefully lift the periosteum to expose enough of the alveolar bone as necessary to provide an adequate surgical working area (Fig. 21-9). Place retraction sutures as needed. Remove bony irregularities using a bur or rongeurs to create as flat a bone plateau as possible. Keep bone removal to a minimum. Insufficient bone width and abnormal defects or contours not previously detected may now contraindicate placement of the implant. Ridge width should allow at least 2 mm of bone to remain buccal and lingual to the implant after placement. Maintain proper spacing as previously determined with the surgical guide (Fig. 21-10). The surgical guide is placed over the surgical site to verify proper location of the implant(s) (Fig, 21-11). Bone-cutting procedures must be performed with a low-speed, high-torque, and internally irrigated handpiece to prevent damage to the remaining bone. This will minimize excessive heat generation and preserve the vitality of the bone that is in contact with the implant.[12,13] The implants must also be placed with a minimum gap between the bone and implant to ensure maximum integration of the implant to bone.[14] After placing the implants, approximate the mucoperiosteal flaps over the surgical site. The tissue is now sutured together with 4-0 plain gut followed with 4-0 Monocryl suture. Written postoperative instructions are provided to the patient. Postoperative prescriptions are written for postoperative discomfort.

The technique of implant placement will vary depending on the system being used. The surgical dentist must follow the guidelines as set forth by the manufacturer. If the guidelines are not followed, the final result may be compromised or the manufacturer may not provide support. The initial

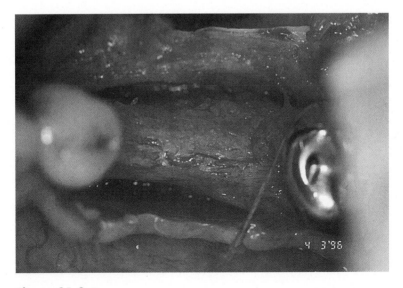

*Figure 21.9* ●

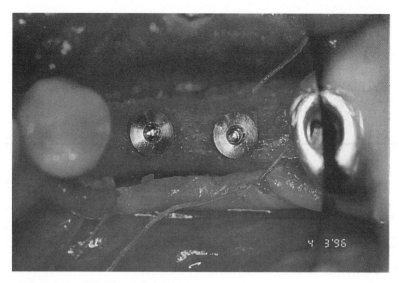

*Figure 21.10* ●

placement responsibility is with the surgical dentist. However, the exact placement location of the
implant is the responsibility of the restorative dentist, based on the implant location transferred from
the surgical guide.

## POSTOPERATIVE CARE

The patient is instructed to follow a postsurgery regimen including cold packs to the surgical site for the
initial 24 hours. Heat packs may be applied the
second day after surgery to reduce any swelling.

An antibiotic of choice may be prescribed if the clinician feels the need to do so. Sutures may be
removed after 10 days. Do not use silk sutures
because they tend to wick oral fluids and possibly
bacteria into the healing site. In cases in which a
prosthodontic appliance is to be worn during the
healing phase, the prosthesis is relieved and relined
with a soft liner to prevent premature loading and
micromovement of the implants. Patients are
recalled to evaluate soft tissue health, to review the
condition of the reline materials, and to confirm that
the implants are not being loaded by the prosthesis.

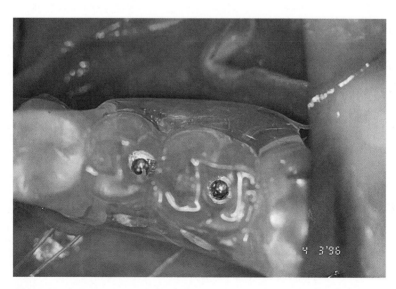

*Figure 21.11* ●

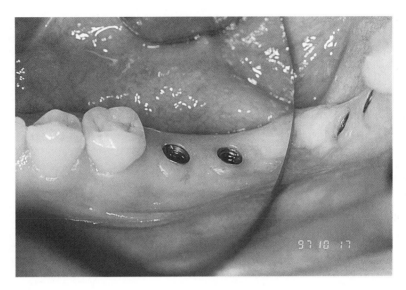

**Figure 21.12** ●

## SUMMARY OF POSTOPERATIVE CARE

1. Educate patients on postoperative care (written instructions)
2. Review with patient on the healing time required based on the procedure
3. Be available for postoperative care
4. Prescribe the needed postoperative medications
5. Plan postoperative visits for suture removal and evaluations

Figures 21-12, 21-13, and 21-14 are photographs of a completed case following the proper protocol.

## PROSTHODONTIC FACTORS (DETERMINED BEFORE SURGERY)

1. Occlusion (location) (nut cracker effect)
2. Position and implant inclination
3. Surface area (length, thread, cylinder, diameter)
4. Spacing to distribute occlusal load and esthetics
5. Occlusal table
6. Opposing occlusion
7. Muscle mass
8. Progressive loading
9. Spacing (rim to rim) determined by tooth being replaced

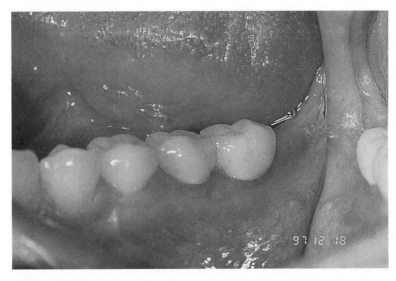

**Figure 21.13** ●

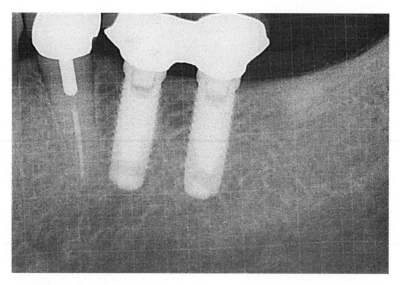

**Figure 21.14** ●

10. Type of restoration (screw- or cement-retained)
11. Parafunctional habits
12. Amount of bone loss (crown-to-root ratio)
13. Arch form
14. Bone quality
15. Implant surface material
16. Tooth being replaced (diameter)
17. Length of edentulous span
18. Replacing roots of teeth
19. Self-cleansing
20. Open embrasures
21. Good accessibility for maintenance
22. Patient's ability to maintain
23. Esthetics
24. Functional

## RESTORATIVE OPTIONS

1. Fixed crown and bridge (cement-retained prosthesis)
2. Fixed-removable crown and bridge (screw-retained prosthesis)
3. Implant-supported bar-overdenture
4. Patient-removal overdenture (ball or bar)
5. Fixed-removable denture (screw-retained prosthesis)
6. Milled bar overdenture

## FIXED CROWN AND BRIDGE (CEMENT-RETAINED PROSTHESIS)

Fixed-implant restorations are similar, but not identical, to conventional crown and bridge restorations. The restoration is cemented to a prepared abutment, which is attached to the implant. The use of provisional cement makes it easier to remove the prosthesis, if necessary. However, the provisional cement can be a problem as it may result in unplanned prosthesis loss.

## FIXED-REMOVABLE CROWN AND BRIDGE (SCREW-RETAINED PROSTHESIS)

Fixed-removable restorations are retained by a coping screw that enters through the occlusal or cingulum of the restoration. The coping screw passes through the crown and threads either into an abutment or directly into the implant. The restoration is removed by the dentist. This type of restoration is usually used with a limited amount of interocclusal distance. Screw loosening and breakage can be a problem.

## IMPLANT-SUPPORTED OVERDENTURE

An implant-supported overdenture is a conventional acrylic denture retained by attachments (e.g., clips and bar, O-rings) to the implants. The denture can be either tissue- and implant-supported (resilient) or all implant-supported (rigid). The retention type denture considerations are primarily related to patient manual dexterity, patient desires, occlusion, bone type, and arch form. The design of the bar is determined by the number, length, and location of the implants, and the quality and quantity of the supporting bone. Currently, the ball-supported overdenture seems to be the better of the two methods. The ball, Delrin, allows for easy hygiene by the patient, low maintenance of the attachments, lower cost of the abutments, improved esthetics, and better retention of the denture. Implants are also placed as distal stops in posterior edentulous ridges for both complete and partial dentures.

## FIXED-REMOVABLE IMPLANT-SUPPORTED DENTURE (SCREW-RETAINED PROSTHESIS)

A fixed-removable denture incorporates a conventional denture attachment as seen with a screw-retained bridge. Denture teeth are processed to a metal framework, which is attached directly to the implants or to the abutments on the implants. An attachment-retained overdenture is an implant- or tissue-supported conventional overdenture retained by attachments, which are fixed directly into the implants. This method only allows the dentist to remove the denture. Home care of the prostheses is a problem for the patient and may limit the long-term success of the implants because of limited hygiene procedures of the dental implants.

## MILLED BAR OVERDENTURE

A milled bar overdenture is a precision-milled, attachment-retained, double-bar restoration. The cast and milled, implant-supported, primary bar supports a removable prosthesis, which is processed to a secondary (telescoping) cast framework. Stability and retention of the prosthesis are gained through the precision fit and use of attachments. This is an excellent prosthesis for a severely resorbed maxilla reconstruction. Again, home care hygiene procedures may be a problem for the patient.

## REFERENCES

1. Millennium Research Group; Toronto, ON, Canada; 2003.
2. Quirynen M, Listgarten MA. The distribution of bacterial morphotypes around natural teeth and titanium implants, ad modum Bränemark. Clin Oral Implants Res 1990;1:8–12.
3. Davies JE. Mechanisms of endosseous integration. Int J Prosthodont 1998;11:391–401.
4. Brånemark PI, Hansson BO, Adell R, Breine U, Lindstrom J, Hallen O, Ohman A. Osseointegrated implants in the treatment of edentulous jaw. Experience from a 10 year period. Scand J Plast Reconstr Surg 1977;16:1–132.
5. Hansson H-A, Albertsson T, Brånemark PI. Structural aspects of the interface between tissue and titanium implants. J Prosthet Dent 1983;50:108–113.
6. Denissen H, de Groot K. Immediate dental root implants from synthetic dense calcium hydroxylapatite. J Prosthet Dent 1979;42:551–556.
7. Ogiso M, Aikawa S, Tabata T, Inoue M. Two-step apatite implant: animal experiment and clinical application. Transactions 11th Annual Meeting, Society for Biomaterials, 1985;8:166.
8. Akagawa Y, Satiomi K, Kikai H, Tsuru H. Initial interface between submerged hydroxyapatite-coated titanium alloy implant and mandibular bone after nontapping and tapping insertions in monkeys. J Prostht Dent 1990;63:559–564.
9. Jansen JA, Van de Walden J, Wolke J, de Groot K. Histologic evaluation of osseous adaptation to titanium and hydroxylapatite-coated titanium implants. J Biomed Mat Res 1991;25:973–989.
10. Block M, Kent J, Kay J. Evaluation of hydroxylapatite-coated titanium dental implants in dogs. J Oral Maxillofac Surg 1987;45:601–607.
11. Jepsen A. Root surface measurement and a method for x-ray determination of root surface area. Acta Odontol Scand 1963;21:35–46.
12. Eriksson L, Albertsson T, Grane B, McQueen D. Thermal injury to bone: a vital microscopic description of heat effects. Int J Oral Surg 1982;11: 115–121.
13. Eriksson L, Albertsson T. Temperature threshold levels for heat induced bone injury: a vital microscopic study in the rabbit. J Prosthet Dent 1983;50:101–107.
14. Carlsson l, Rostlund T, Albertsson BMP, Albertsson T. Implant fixation improved by close fit. Cylindrical implant-bone interface studied in rabbits. Acta Orthop Scand 1988;59:272–275.

## CHAPTER 21
## REVIEW QUESTIONS

1. With titanium or titanium alloy implants, the anchorage is primarily:
   a. Mechanical
   b. Chemical
   c. Biologic
   d. None of the above

2. Hydroxylapatite-coated implants and titanium implants have the same attachment mechanism to bone.
   a. True
   b. False

3. Bone attachment of the hydroxylapatite implants is termed:
   a. Biointegration
   b. Osseointegration
   c. Mechanical integration
   d. None of the above

4. Replacement of teeth with dental implants should approximate the root surface area of the tooth being replaced measured in:
   a. Square millimeters
   b. Length
   c. Diameter
   d. Cubic meters

5. Before dental implant placement, bone regeneration is:
   a. Sometimes needed
   b. Never needed
   c. Best evaluated by radiographs
   d. Best determined before any implant treatment

6. In preparation for a surgical guide, it is best to start with:
   a. A mental picture
   b. Questions to the patient
   c. A wax-up from the laboratory
   d. Surgical guide is usually not needed

7. During the site preparation of the dental implant, it is best to allow the drill to:
   a. Turn as fast as possible
   b. Irrigate the drill with water
   c. Perform at low speed with internally irrigated drills
   d. It makes no difference

8. If a site has been grafted before implant placement, one should wait 4 to 9 _____ for complete healing.
   a. Days
   b. Weeks
   c. Months
   d. Years

9. The type of restoration of the dental implant depends on the:
   a. Restorative dentist
   b. Surgical dentist
   c. Laboratory
   d. Objective of the tooth being replaced

10. Placement of an implant followed by burial is called:
    a. A single-stage procedure
    b. A two-stage procedure
    c. Early loading
    d. Delayed loading

11. Immediate implants usually require a longer implant.
    a. True
    b. False

12. It is best for the surgical dentist to place the dental implants and then refer the implant patient back to the restorative dentist for the restorative procedures without a surgical guide.
    a. True
    b. False.

# Implant Maintenance

John Rapley

Periodontal maintenance is an essential part of total periodontal therapy, and is regarded as the major factor in therapeutic success. Long-term studies have demonstrated that regular periodontal maintenance can maintain the periodontal attachment. Similarly, the importance of long-term implant maintenance cannot be underestimated.

A basic understanding of implant maintenance entails knowledge about the peri-implant attachment apparatus, its susceptibility to disease, possibility of reinfection, and specific microbiology. Clinical parameters of implant health are evaluated at each maintenance appointment and consist of clinical probing, use of radiographs, tissue evaluation, and mobility assessment. Clinical instruments and materials, both for patient's home care and therapist's use in implant debridement, may differ from periodontal maintenance and need to be understood.

## PERI-IMPLANT ATTACHMENT APPARATUS AND DISEASE SUSCEPTIBILITY

Researchers have consistently found in all various types of implants an epithelial attachment in the peri-implant tissues mediated by hemidesmosomes, which is identical to the epithelial attachment found in periodontal tissues. However, the connective tissue component is significantly different, for instead of having the insertion of perpendicular connective tissue fibers into the cementum as is found in the periodontal attachment, there is a peri-implant connective tissue cuff that surrounds the implant.[1] This cuff has predominantly a parallel fiber orientation without any insertion to the implant. Research has illustrated the increased susceptibility of the peri-implant tissue to plaque-induced disease, which may be related to a combination of the lack of a connective tissue attachment, the absence of a periodontal ligament, a decreased vascularity in the peri-implant tissues, or a combination of these.[2–5]

## REINFECTION

The phenomenon of reinfection from diseased sites to nondiseased sites has been shown to occur in the periodontal patient, and the same phenomenon has been demonstrated in the partially edentulous implant patient.[6] This possibility of reinfection from diseased periodontal sites to implant sites necessitates the completion of any needed periodontal therapy for control of the existing periodontal disease before implant placement and should be an integral part of treatment planning.[7] Therefore, concurrent periodontal and implant maintenance is vital in the partially edentulous implant patient, for ongoing periodontal disease can significantly influence implant health.

## MICROBIOLOGY

Implant and periodontal microbiology are similar in that a stable healthy implant has the same microflora as a healthy tooth (i.e., mainly Gram-positive, nonmotile, aerobic, and mainly cocci). The ailing implant has the similar microflora as a periodontally involved tooth (i.e., Gram-negative, motile, anaerobic).[8,9] The pathogens in periodontitis, *Paragnathus intermedius* and *Porphyromonas gingivalis,* are the same pathogens found in peri-implantitis.[10] Implant plaque formation is identical, with comparable time frames and succession as seen in periodontal disease with the progression from cocci to filamentous forms, and then to pathogens with spirochetes. As in the periodontal tissues, there is also a positive correlation between increased implant plaque accumulation with peri-implant inflammation.[8] Therefore, the importance of the prevention and removal of plaque is key in both the periodontal and peri-implant tissues. Tests using microbial monitoring may be reliable indicators or predictors of implant health in the future.

## CLINICAL PARAMETERS

Clinical parameters are evaluated at both periodontal and implant maintenance appointments. Parameters include probing depth, bleeding on probing, radiographs, tissue health, and mobility.

## PROBING

There is some controversy regarding implant probing in that some therapists feel that it may be an invasive procedure, i.e., the probe penetrates into the connective or bone zone owing to the lack of inserting connective tissue fibers, thus wounding the tissue or seeding bacteria deep into the tissue.[11] Others believe it is a valuable parameter if the change of probing depth is evaluated and monitored.[12] The probing depth is influenced by many variables, such as force of probing, angulation of the probe, state of tissue inflammation, probe diameter, type of probe, and implant access. It must be emphasized that there is no clear numerical value of a "healthy probing depth" as is associated with the dentate individual. Additional factors that influence the peri-implant probing depth, such as the thickness of the tissue, position of the implant, or the amount of countersinking, that do not affect the probing depths of the dentate individual must also be considered.

Several studies have correlated bleeding on probing to disease activity in the dentate patient, and it may also be of value in the implant patient.[13] The bleeding status may provide knowledge of the health of the tissue, but also may be related to probing force and tissue woundability.

## RADIOGRAPHS

The most reliable parameter for monitoring implant health is the dental radiograph.[14] An accurate radiograph is exposed at 65 to 70 kV(p) with a long cone paralleling technique with adequate exposure time to distinguish any vents or implant fixture landmarks. Two periapical radiographs at 6 to 12 degrees of variation on the horizontal plane may enhance the evaluation of the interproximal bone. A disposable grid overlay on the radiographs

may aid in the assessment of implant bone levels by eliminating magnification errors.

Radiographic inaccuracies can result from magnification error or a nonparallel technique. Image magnification on periapical radiographs range from 2 to 5%, and a panoramic radiograph may have as high as 15 to 25% magnification depending on the manufacturer. Even with the best technique, a parallel image-to-film may not be possible because of implant angulation or anatomic limitations for film placement as in resorbed maxilla or mandibles, which cause a poor implant-to-film relationship.[15]

It is recommended that radiographs be taken at the following times[16]:

1. At the second-stage implant uncovering, or at the end of the healing period for a one-stage implant immediately before initiating the restoration as a baseline radiograph
2. After the prosthesis is seated or cemented
3. One year after prosthetic loading
4. Yearly or more often as needed during maintenance

## TISSUE HEALTH

The peri-implant tissues are evaluated for changes in color, contour, and consistency during maintenance. Some studies report no disease correlation with the presence or absence of keratinized tissue adjacent to the implant, although others show less attachment loss with keratinized tissue with plaque-induced inflammation. Others feel that mobile connective tissue associated with nonkeratinized tissue adversely affects the epithelial seal.[17–19] Augmentation of keratinized tissue would be indicated if patient discomfort during normal oral hygiene procedures for the dental implant is caused by the presence of alveolar mucosa that may not be able to withstand normal oral hygiene techniques. The overall conclusion is that the type of peri-implant tissue may not be crucial on implant health in the presence of good oral hygiene.[20]

## MOBILITY OR OCCLUSION

Mobility of an implant fixture is a very negative finding and indicates that the implant has failed.[14] However, it is difficult to determine slight mobility of a single implant, or to assess individual implant mobility when they are connected to adjacent teeth or other implants. Occlusion should be evaluated at each maintenance appointment and abnormalities adjusted immediately. Untreated occlusal overload can lead to rapid and substantial peri-implant bone loss. It is also recommended to periodically remove the prosthesis to assess the individual mobility of each fixture.

## GINGIVAL CREVICULAR FLUID MONITORING

Various investigators have explored the monitoring of enzymes in the gingival crevicular fluid to assess the status of an implant. Enzymes that have been investigated include neutral protease, arylsulfatase, elastase, myeloperoxidase, β-glucuronidase, and aspartate aminotransferase.[21]

## PATIENT'S HOME CARE

There are several home care aids for the implant patient that are used for plaque removal:

1. The primary aid is the soft toothbrush, which includes both the manual and the powered toothbrush. Patients may find that the smaller head toothbrushes are superior in accessing the lingual and palatal aspects of a prosthesis.
2. Interproximal plaque removal can be achieved using normal floss, yarn, nylon "floss," or other products that can also be threaded beneath the prosthesis and around the abutments.
3. Gauze can be used to debride the distal aspects of implants, and is especially convenient to use for cantilever areas.
4. Antimicrobial mouth rinses can decrease supragingival plaque formation.
5. Water-irrigation systems, adjusted at low power, may aid in removing food debris beneath and around the prosthesis.
6. The interdental brushes with a plastic-coated wire core are very effective techniques in areas with poor or minimal access.

All of these home care aids do not alter the implant abutment surface and are safe for the patient to use.[22] However, it must be noted that oral hygiene may be more difficult or uncomfortable for the implant patient because of poor access to the dental implant caused by a prosthesis or anatomic factors.

## THERAPIST INSTRUMENTATION

Recommended instruments for implant debridement include plastic, nylon, or special alloy scaler-type instruments that do not create any adverse surface alterations to the implant surface. Many of the instruments available have the problem of lacking a working surface "edge" to effectively and easily remove calculus. A rubber cup, with or

without flour of pumice, is also a useful adjunct and may actually improve the abutment surface.[22]

Instruments not recommended include metal hand scalers, ultrasonic scalers, and sonic scalers because of the danger of significant alteration of the implant surface.[22] Some sonic scalers are available with plastic sleeves for the tips, which have shown to be both effective and safe.[23] There is still some debate on the air-powder abrasive because it may remove the protective oxide layer and increase corrosion.

## ADJUNCTIVE THERAPY

Evidence is available that subgingival irrigation can be a benefit to temporarily reduce peri-implant inflammation. The use of various local drug delivery systems into the peri-implant pocket may be a useful option in the temporary treatment of peri-implant inflammation and works mainly as a detoxifying agent with minimal long-term effects. If a systemic antimicrobial is needed, the first drug of choice would be tetracycline or doxycycline because it is concentrated in the gingival crevicular fluid.

## REFERENCES

1. Listgarten MA, Lang NP, Schroeder HE, Schroeder A. Periodontal tissues and their counterparts around endosseous implants. Clin Oral Implants Res 1991; 2:1–19.
2. Berglundh T, Lindhe J, Ericsson I, Marinello CP, Liljenberg B, Thomsen P. The soft tissue barrier at implants and teeth. Clin Oral Implants Res 1991;2: 81–90.
3. Berglundh T, Lindhe J, Jonsson K, Ericsson I. The topography of the vascular systems in the periodontal and peri-implant tissues in the dog. J Clin Periodontol 1994;21:189–193.
4. Lindhe J, Berglundh T, Ericsson I, Liljenberg B, Marinello C. Experimental breakdown of peri-implant and periodontal tissues. Clin Oral Implants Res 1992;3:9–16.
5. Berglundh T, Lindhe J, Marinello C, Ericsson I, Liljenberg B. Soft tissue reaction to de novo plaque formation on implants and teeth. An experimental study in the dog. Clin Oral Implants Res 1992;3:1–8.
6. Quirynen M, Listgarten M. The distribution of bacterial morphotypes around natural teeth and titanium implants ad modum Branemark. Clin Oral Implants Res 1990;1:8–12.
7. Bragger U, Burgin WB, Hammerle CH, Lang NP. Associations between clinical parameters assessed around implants and teeth. Clin Oral Implants Res 1997;8:412–421.
8. Lekholm U, Ericsson I, Adell R, Slots J. The condition of the soft tissues at the tooth and fixture abutment supporting fixed bridges. J Clin Periodontol 1986;13:558–562.

9. Mombelli A, Buser D, Lang NP. Colonization of osseointegrated titanium implants in edentulous patients. Early results. Oral Microbiol Immunol 1988; 3:133–120.

10. Becker W, Becker BE, Newman MG, Nyman S. Clinical and microbiological findings that may contribute to dental implant failure. Int J Oral Maxillofac Implants 1990;5:31–38.

11. Lang NP, Wetzel AC, Stich H, Caffesse RG. Histologic probe penetration in healthy and inflamed peri-implant tissues. Clin Oral Implants Res 1994;5:191–201.

12. Quirynen M, van Steenberghe D, Jacobs R, Schotte A, Darius P. The reliability of pocket probing around screw-type implants. Clin Oral Implants Res 1991;2:186–192.

13. Lekholm U, Adell R, Lindhe J, Branemark PI, Eriksson B, Rockler B, Lindvall AM, Yoneyama T. Marginal tissue reactions at osseointegrated titanium fixtures (II). A cross-sectional study. Int J Oral Maxillofac Surg 1986;15:53–61.

14. Schnitman P, Shulman L, eds. Dental Implants: Benefit and Risk. NIH-Harvard Consensus Development Conference. NIH Publication No. 81-1531, 1978.

15. Cox JF. Radiographic evaluation of tissue-integrated prostheses. In: van Steenberghe D, Albrektsson T, Branemark P-I, et al., eds. Tissue-integration in Oral and Maxillo-facial Reconstruction. Amsterdam: Excerpta Medica, 1978;278–286.

16. Albrektsson T, Zarb G, Worthington P, Eriksson AR. The long term efficacy of currently used dental implants: a review and proposed criteria of success. Int J Oral Maxillofac Implants 1986;1:11–25.

17. Hanisch O, Cortella CA, Boskovic MM, James RA, Slots J, Wikesjo UM. Experimental peri-implant tissue breakdown around hydroxyapatite-coated implants. J Periodontol 1997;68:59–66.

18. Warrer K, Buser D, Lang NP, Karring T. Plaque-induced peri-implantitis in the presence or absence of keratinized mucosa. An experimental study in monkeys. Clin Oral Implants Res 1995;6:131–138.

19. Wennstrom J, Bengazi F, Leukhom U. The influence of the masticatory mucosa on the peri-implant soft tissue condition. Clin Oral Implants Res 1994; 5:1–8.

20. Bauman GR, Mills M, Rapley JW, Hallmon WW. Plaque-induced inflammation around implants. Int J Oral Maxillofac Implants 1992;7:330–337.

21. Apse P, Ellen RP, Overall CM, Zarb GA. Microbiota and crevicular fluid collagenase activity in the osseointegrated dental implant sulcus: a comparison of sites in edentulous and partially edentulous patients. J Periodontol Res 1989;24:96–105.

22. Rapley J, Swan R, Hallmon W, Mills M. The surface characteristics produced by various oral hygiene instruments and materials on titanium implant abutments. Int J Oral Maxillofac Implants 1990;5: 47–52.

23. Gantes B, Nelveus R. The effects of different hygiene instruments on titanium: SEM observations. Int J Periodontics Restorative Dent 1991;11: 225–239.

# CHAPTER 22
## REVIEW QUESTIONS

1. The connective tissue attachment to an implant in alveolar mucosa consists of:
   a. Parallel fibers with some fiber insertion
   b. Perpendicular fibers with some fiber insertion
   c. Parallel fibers with a cufflike barrier
   d. Perpendicular fibers with a cufflike barrier

2. Problems in obtaining correct angulation with periapical radiographs in implant patients are often compounded by:
   a. A requirement for a grid radiograph
   b. The resorption of the mandible and maxilla
   c. A requirement for the fabrication for a paralleling film holder

3. Many studies have dealt with the advisability of having keratinized tissue around an implant. The current opinion is that:
   a. The presence of alveolar tissue will lead to disease
   b. The presence of keratinized tissue will ensure health
   c. Either of the tissues is acceptable if the area is plaque-free

4. Assuming the same level of plaque and plaque-induced inflammation, what has the greater susceptibility to plaque-induced disease?
   a. Teeth
   b. Implants
   c. Both are identical

5. Systemic antibiotics have been used to treat peri-implantitis. One of the most popular and effective ones that is used first includes:
   a. *Cipro*
   b. Tetracycline
   c. Erythromycin

6. Currently, the most *reliable* clinical parameter to assess implant health is:
   a. Probing depths
   b. Periapical radiographs
   c. Gingival crevicular fluid assays

7. Severe alveolar bone loss surrounding implants circumferentially that occurs rapidly is usually caused by:
   a. Peri-implantitis
   b. An occlusal overload
   c. A loose abutment screw

8. The microflora of a failing implant is primarily:
   a. Gram-positive cocci
   b. Gram-negative cocci
   c. Gram-negative motile rods
   d. Gram-positive nonmotile rods

9. The implant surface should remain as smooth as possible to reduce plaque accumulation. The instruments that the patient may use to debride implants includes all except:
   a. Toothpicks
   b. Nylon floss
   c. Soft toothbrush
   d. Proxabrush with metal hub

10. Instruments that the implant therapist can use to debride the implant without altering the implant surface includes all except the:
    a. Plastic scaler
    b. McCall 17/18 metal scaler
    c. Sonic scaler with a plastic tip
    d. Rubber cup with flour of pumice

# Periodontal Maintenance Therapy

## Henry Greenwell

## INTRODUCTION: MANAGEMENT OF A CHRONIC DISEASE

Periodontitis is a long-term chronic disease. Although treatment can arrest disease progression, it does not provide a cure. Therefore, to understand the benefit of therapy, we must compare the course of treated disease with that of untreated disease.

Treated periodontitis progresses at a mean full mouth rate of about 0.03 mm/yr or 0.3 mm every 10 years; whereas, for untreated disease, the mean rate is about 0.2 mm/yr or 2.0 mm every 10 years.[1–12] Thus, untreated disease progresses about seven times faster than treated disease. As the values given are based on full mouth means, it must be recognized that individual teeth can lose attachment at a much faster rate. This can be particularly damaging around molar teeth that can develop furcation involvements with 3.0 to 5.0 mm of attachment loss.

If destructive periodontitis is recognized at age 35, and appropriate treatment continues for 40 years, the patient will lose only a mean of 1.2 mm of attachment. On the other hand, the same patient, if untreated, would lose a mean of 8 mm of attachment, which means they would lose most of their teeth. Therefore, early recognition, treatment, and maintenance therapy for periodontitis is essential if the teeth are to be preserved in health, comfort, function, and acceptable esthetics throughout the patient's lifetime.

## WHEN TO BEGIN PERIODONTAL MAINTENANCE

One of the most critical questions in periodontal therapy is when to begin the maintenance phase of therapy. It seems obvious that maintenance begins once the active treatment phase is complete. The problem is more complex than attaining a particular point in the treatment sequence: It must be based on achieving specific therapeutic end points. The overriding goal is *complete disease resolution*. This is accomplished by eliminating inflammation, bleeding on probing, suppuration, and disease progression. Active treatment should not be considered finished until there is complete disease resolution independent of any adjunctive therapies. This means that disease resolution occurs as a result of mechanical treatment of the root surface directed at elimination of all plaque biofilm and calculus.

Failure to achieve complete disease resolution by mechanical therapy often means adjunctive agents will be used. Unfortunately, these agents eliminate only soft tissue inflammation and bleeding, the best indicators of areas of residual calculus, thereby preventing identification of areas of unresolved disease. What is really needed is additional mechanical root surface treatment until the specific therapeutic end point of total disease resolution has been achieved. It is essential that active treatment produce a root surface totally free of plaque biofilm and calculus. This will be reflected by the establishment of healthy soft tissue that is free from inflammation, bleeding on probing, suppuration, and disease progression. The fundamental biologic principle observed is that periodontal treatment must be *directed at the root surface*. In general, this means mechanical therapy.

One of the main problems in periodontal therapy is the difficulty of performing ideal mechanical root surface instrumentation. Mechanical root instrumentation may be performed nonsurgically, which relies heavily on tactile skills to detect calculus, or surgically, which affords greater access and visibility.[13–15] It is necessary to produce a *biologically compatible root surface* to establish periodontal health. A biologically compatible root surface is one that is free of all visible calculus along a completely exposed root. This allows the host defense system to work effectively, hence the term biologic compatibility. From a microscopic standpoint all calculus is rarely removed; however, microscopic amounts of calculus are probably clinically insignificant.[16,17]

Using adjunctive agents to temporarily hide inflammation has been termed *disease masking*.[18] Disease masking should be avoided. This occurs when treatment is directed at resolving soft tissue inflammation rather than focusing on the elimination of etiologic agents from the root surface by mechanical treatment. The use of adjunctive agents, such as antimicrobials, antibiotics, or host-modulating agents, to reduce soft tissue inflammation prevents the periodontal therapist from identifying sites that need additional mechanical therapy. Treatment is not provided, and disease progression continues. The effect of adjunctive agents often lasts only while they are in use, or for a limited period after they are discontinued.[19] Disease returns when the agent is removed because the root surface problem was never eliminated. Therefore, the use of adjunctive agents during active periodontal therapy is not recommended.

For maintenance therapy to be effective, periodontal health must be established. *By definition, the purpose of a maintenance program is to maintain health, not disease.* Active treatment that does not produce complete disease resolution is a failure, and the patient should be informed that they are at risk of disease progression. If, in the presence of unresolved disease, adjunctive agents are used to temporarily reduce soft tissue inflammation, this should be considered a continuation of

active therapy. Use of these agents will most likely need to be repeated on a recurring basis. This type of active therapy is termed compromised active therapy because it will not correct deficiencies in root surface treatment. *Adjunctive therapy is aimed at the soft tissue, which is not the therapeutic problem, but is merely a reflection of the failed mechanical root therapy.* These patients are not candidates for maintenance therapy until all disease is resolved.

It is important to distinguish between active therapy, compromised active therapy, and maintenance therapy for both therapeutic and legal reasons. From a therapeutic standpoint, it is critical that the periodontal therapist recognize unresolved disease so that: (1) additional treatment or referral to a periodontist can be recommended; (2) it is clearly understood that additional disease progression is likely, and may lead to tooth loss; and (3) compromised active therapy can be explained as a continuation of failing treatment. From a legal standpoint, the patient has the right to know whether disease was resolved or whether compromised active therapy is being recommended. If a course of compromised active therapy is chosen, the patient should sign an informed consent that emphasizes four points: (1) all disease has not been resolved; (2) *compromised* active therapy is being provided; (3) repeat courses of adjunctive agents may be necessary at periodic intervals to control soft tissue inflammation; and (4) additional disease progression, and tooth loss, is likely because complete disease resolution was never achieved. A decision matrix for when to begin maintenance therapy is illustrated in Figure 23-1.

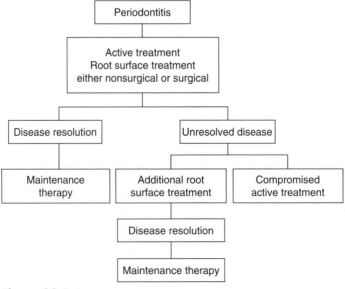

**Figure 23.1** ●

## DISEASE DIAGNOSIS: DETERMINATION OF DISEASE RESOLUTION

The key to successful periodontal maintenance therapy is an accurate diagnosis that is both patient-based and site-specific. The patient-based diagnosis, derived from a single examination, characterizes the aggressiveness of the disease and the amount of destruction.[20] The site-specific diagnosis requires sequential examinations and identifies individual sites of disease progression. Thus, two fundamentally different types of diagnostic information are required for proper management of periodontitis.

Most often, the type of periodontitis present is classified as either chronic or aggressive periodontitis.[20] Aggressive periodontitis tends to have an earlier onset or more rapid progression. In contrast, chronic periodontitis tends to have a later onset and slower progression. The disease is then characterized according to severity, as either slight, moderate, or severe, and by extent, as either localized or generalized. This patient-based diagnosis gives important information about the aggressiveness of the disease. More aggressive forms of periodontitis may require greater vigilance during maintenance therapy.

A complete periodontal examination obtains probing depth and attachment level data for six sites per tooth.[21] Using comparative data from subsequent examinations, disease progression can be detected at individual sites. According to the random disease model, periodontitis progresses randomly and erratically with uncoordinated bone loss at individual sites rather than as a continuous, even, coordinated, full-mouth type of bone destruction.[22] Site-specific data are necessary to detect disease recurrence or to document that destruction has been arrested. Probing data are supplemented with site-based information about bleeding on probing and suppuration.

Maintenance therapy should start only after complete disease resolution has been achieved. This means that the disease is arrested at all sites as verified by the absence of inflammation, bleeding on probing, suppuration, and progressive attachment loss. Placing a patient on maintenance implies that health has been established and that subsequent therapy is designed to maintain health.

## RATIONALE FOR MAINTENANCE

The rationale for maintenance is based on management of subgingival plaque pathogenicity.[23] Disease-associated sites have a pathogenic plaque, whereas, health-associated sites are populated by a nonpathogenic plaque.[24] Because plaque forms naturally in the mouth, it will always be present and must be kept nonpathogenic. Active therapy is designed to establish a health-associated flora before beginning maintenance. The goal of maintenance therapy is to maintain a health-associated flora by removing all pathogenic plaque biofilm, thereby preventing disease progression.

Plaque morphotype studies have shown that coccoid cells and straight rods predominate in health, whereas, motile rods and spirochetes are significantly increased with disease.[24] Mechanical instrumentation of the root will convert the disease-associated plaque to a health-associated plaque. With time, 1 to 3 months, a disease-associated plaque will return and replace the health-associated bacteria.[25] Additional root instrumentation is again needed to convert the disease-associated plaque to a health-associated plaque. Thus, periodontal maintenance therapy is designed to constantly remove potentially pathogenic subgingival plaque.

With time, subgingival plaque forms a complex, interdependent structure and ecosystem. It is this complex ecosystem that is pathogenic. Root instrumentation eliminates the bacterial structure and ecosystem that produces harmful bacteria and bacterial byproducts. On the newly cleaned root surface, the process begins again as health-associated bacteria repopulate.

It has been clearly shown that a 6-month recall interval is inadequate to control the progression of periodontitis.[26] Many studies have demonstrated that a 3-month interval is appropriate and works well for most cases.[27–31] Patients with more aggressive disease may require more frequent maintenance. Thus, the interval has to be tailored to the individual patient's needs.

Disease progression can occur during maintenance as a result of either recurrent or refractory disease.[23] The disease is considered refractory if progression occurs despite excellent patient-performed supragingival plaque control and excellent professional subgingival plaque control.[23] Everything is being done correctly from a therapeutic and compliance standpoint, but the disease continues to progress. Recurrent disease, on the other hand, is attributable to a known cause.[23] It could be compromised patient plaque control or poor compliance with maintenance. The maintenance care might not be optimal. It could also be attributable to local contributing factors such as root grooves, furcations, or other plaque-retentive factors.

When refractory disease is present, systemic disease should be considered as a possible contributing factor. If systemic disease is present, the patient should be referred to a physician for treatment. If no systemic disease is present, then adjunctive agents may be useful in controlling disease progression. For recurrent disease, adjunctive agents may also be helpful. For either refractory or recurrent disease, maintenance appointments more frequent than every 3 months may be indicated.

## Adjuncts to Maintenance

There are numerous agents that are useful in an adjunctive role with mechanical root instrumentation during periodontal maintenance. These include antigingivitis agents, local delivery agents, and systemic agents.[19]

Antigingivitis agents are primarily mouth rinses that work supragingivally to inhibit plaque formation. Gingivitis is reduced through plaque reduction. The main agents used for this purpose are chlorhexidine and phenolic compounds.[19] These are useful during maintenance therapy for patients who have difficulty with good supragingival plaque control.

Local delivery agents are useful when there is localized recurrent disease.[19] These agents may be applied at specific sites that are progressing. It is important that the medication is retained in the site for the period specified. Agents such as tetracycline, doxycycline, minocycline, and chlorhexidine have been used.

When recurrence is more generalized, systemic antibiotics are most appropriate.[19] Mechanical therapy should take place first. A single antibiotic or a combination of antibiotics may be used. Antibiotic selection may be based on a culture and sensitivity test. Antibiotics most often used to control recurrent periodontitis include tetracycline, doxycycline, metronidazole, amoxicillin, amoxicillin and clavulanic acid, azithromycin, and clindamycin, although others may be appropriate. Antibiotic combinations have proved useful, and these include metronidazole plus one of the following antibiotics: amoxicillin, amoxicillin and clavulanic acid, and ciprofloxacin.

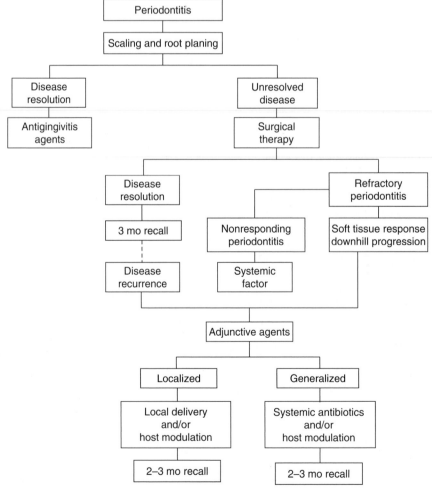

**Figure 23.2** ●

Adjunctive therapy is appropriate in the maintenance phase after successful active therapy that has arrested disease progression. It is not appropriate in the active treatment phase in which it can cause disease masking.

Host-modulating agents can be useful in patients who have recurrent or refractory disease.[19] Nonantibiotic tetracycline-type drugs have been shown to inhibit matrix metalloproteinases and prevent collagen destruction. Nonsteroidal anti-inflammatory drugs (NSAIDs) inhibit the enzyme cyclooxygenase in the arachidonic acid pathway, which reduces prostaglandins that can contribute to the progression of periodontitis. Bisphosphonates inhibit osteoclast activity and may also inhibit matrix metalloproteinases. Triclosan has antimicrobial activity but may also inhibit cyclooxygenase and lipoxygenase, thereby reducing the amount of harmful arachidonic acid metabolites. Tetracyclines to inhibit matrix metalloproteinases are taken systemically, whereas, NSAIDs, bisphosphonates, and triclosan have been tested using topical application. A treatment decision matrix for when to use adjunctive agents is illustrated in Figure 23-2.

## Elements of Maintenance

Successful maintenance care requires careful attention to detail. The first step is to ensure that no patient is placed on maintenance until all disease is arrested by active therapy. The purpose of maintenance is to maintain a state of health.

An oral hygiene index score should be recorded to give an overall indication of the effectiveness of the patient-performed plaque control program. Oral hygiene instruction needs to be reinforced, focusing the patient's efforts on techniques to remove plaque from areas where it has been missed. The color, contour, consistency, and texture of the gingival tissue need to be examined for signs of recurrent inflammation.

Each maintenance appointment must include a thorough periodontal examination. This includes charting recession, probing depth, and attachment level (Fig. 23-3). All sites with bleeding on probing or suppuration should be noted. On the basis of the examination data, areas of disease progression need to be identified. The patient should be informed and the areas retreated.

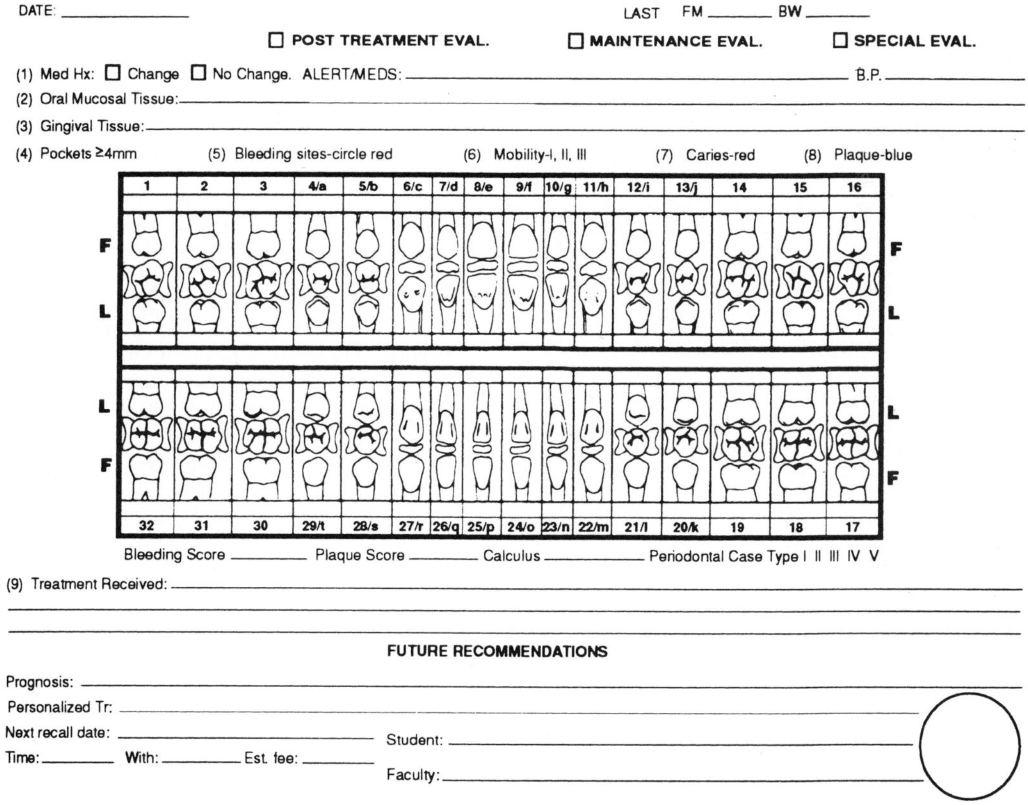
DATE: ____________ LAST FM ______ BW ______

☐ POST TREATMENT EVAL. ☐ MAINTENANCE EVAL. ☐ SPECIAL EVAL.

(1) Med Hx: ☐ Change ☐ No Change. ALERT/MEDS: ____________ B.P. ______

(2) Oral Mucosal Tissue: ____________

(3) Gingival Tissue: ____________

(4) Pockets ≥4mm (5) Bleeding sites-circle red (6) Mobility-I, II, III (7) Caries-red (8) Plaque-blue



Bleeding Score ______ Plaque Score ______ Calculus ______ Periodontal Case Type I II III IV V

(9) Treatment Received: ____________

FUTURE RECOMMENDATIONS

Prognosis: ____________

Personalized Tr: ____________

Next recall date: ____________ Student: ____________

Time: ______ With: ______ Est. fee: ______ Faculty: ____________

***Figure 23.3*** •

The most important part of the maintenance appointment is the thoroughness of the professional subgingival plaque control. It is essential to remove all plaque biofilm and calculus with mechanical instrumentation. *Antibiotics do not penetrate the plaque biofilm, which must be removed mechanically.* Because periodontal maintenance usually occurs every 3 months, the amount of calculus may be minimal. Thus, most of the time will be spent removing subgingival plaque biofilm. The thoroughness of plaque biofilm and calculus removal is critical because the complex ecosystem of the aged plaque must be destroyed, allowing the health-associated bacteria to repopulate the root.

## Compliance With Maintenance

Compliance with maintenance care has been shown to be poor, about a 16% rate of complete compliance.[32] When efforts were increased to motivate patients to comply, the rate increased to about 31%.[33] It is important to inform the patient, before beginning periodontal therapy, that success is dependent on compliance with the maintenance program. Patients who are not willing to accept this are not good candidates for periodontal therapy.

## REFERENCES

1. Wang A, Greenwell H, Chace R Jr, Vance G, Drisko C, Wittwer JW, Yancey J. Rate based analysis of treated disease progression using the periodontitis progression rate index. Periodontal Insights 2000;6:50–56.
2. Westfelt E, Nyman S, Socransky S, Lindhe J. Significance of frequency of professional tooth cleaning for healing following periodontal surgery. J Clin Periodontol 1983;10:148–156.
3. Loe H, Anerud A, Boysen H, Smith M. The natural history of periodontal disease in man. Study design and baseline data. J Periodontal Res 1978;13:550–562.
4. Loe H, Anerud A, Boysen H, Smith M. The natural history of periodontal disease in man. Tooth mortality rates before 40 years of age. J Periodontal Res 1978;13:563–572.
5. Loe H, Anerud A, Boysen H, Smith M. The natural history of periodontal disease in man. The rate of periodontal destruction before 40 years of age. J Periodontol 1978;49:607–620.
6. Loe H, Anerud A, Boysen H, Morrison E. Natural history of periodontal disease in man. Rapid, moderate and no loss of attachment in Sri Lankin laborers 14 to 46 years of age. J Clin Periodontol 1986;13:431–440.
7. Loe H, Anerud A, Boysen H. The natural history of periodontal disease in man: Prevalence, severity, and extent of gingival recession. J Periodontol 1992;63:489–495.
8. Craft G, Greenwell H, Vance G, Wittwer JW, Drisko C, Yancey J. Rate based analysis of untreated disease progression using the periodontitis progression rate index. Periodontal Insights 1999;6:4–9.
9. Axelsson P, Lindhe J. Effect of controlled oral hygiene procedures on caries and periodontal disease in adults. J Clin Periodontol 1978;5:133–151.
10. Axelsson P, Lindhe J. Effect of controlled oral hygiene procedures on caries and periodontal disease in adults. Results after 6 years. J Clin Periodontol 1981;8:239–248.
11. Axelsson P, Lindhe J. The significance of maintenance care in the treatment of periodontal disease. J Clin Periodontol 1981;8:281–294.
12. Machtei EE, Norderyd J, Koch G, Dunford R, Grossi S, Genco RJ. The rate of periodontal attachment loss in subjects with established periodontitis. J Periodontol 1993;64:713–718.
13. Greenwell H, Stovsky DA, Bissada NF. Periodontics in general practice: Perspectives on nonsurgical therapy. J Am Dent Assoc 1987;115:591–595.
14. Greenwell H, Bissada NF, Stovsky DA. Periodontics in general practice: perspectives on surgical therapy. Gen Dent 1989;37:228–233.
15. Wang HL, Greenwell H. Surgical periodontal therapy. Periodontol 2000 2001;25:89–99.
16. Rabbani GM, Ash MM, Caffesse RG. The effectiveness of subgingival scaling and root planing in calculus removal. J Periodontol 1981;52:119–123.
17. Stambaugh RV, Dragoo M, Smith DM, Carasali L. The limits of subgingival scaling. Int J Periodontics Restorative Dent 1982;1:30–41.
18. Greenwell H, Bissada NF, Dodge JR. Disease masking: a hazard of nonsurgical periodontal therapy. Periodontal Insights 1998;5:14–19.
19. Greenwell H, Bissada N. Emerging concepts in periodontal therapy. Drugs 2002;62:2581–2587.
20. Armitage GC. Periodontal diagnoses and classification of periodontal diseases. Periodontol 2000 2004;34:9–21.
21. Greenwell H, Abrams H. Periodontal examination and diagnosis. In: Hardin J, ed. Clark's Clinical Dentistry. Philadelphia: JB Lippincott, 1995.
22. Socransky SS, Haffajee AD, Goodson JM, Lindhe J. New concepts of destructive periodontal disease. J Clin Periodontol 1984;11:21–32.
23. Greenwell H, Abrams H. Rationale for periodontal therapy. In: Hardin J, ed. Clark's Clinical Dentistry. Philadelphia: JB Lippincott, 1991.
24. Listgarten MA, Hellden L. Relative distribution of bacteria at clinically healthy and periodontally diseased sites in humans. J Clin Periodontol 1978;5:115–132.
25. Greenwell H, Bissada NF. Variations in subgingival microflora from healthy and intervention sites using probing depth and bacteriologic identification criteria. J Periodontol 1984;55:391–397.
26. Nyman S, Rosling B, Lindhe J. Effect of professional tooth cleaning on healing after periodontal surgery. J Clin Periodontol 1975;2:80–86.

27. Knowles JW, Burgett FG, Nissle RR, Shick RA, Morrison EC, Ramfjord SP. Results of periodontal treatment related to pocket depth and attachment level. Eight years. J Periodontol 1979;50:225–233.

28. Hill RW, Ramfjord SP, Morrison EC, Appleberry EA, Caffesse RG, Kerry GJ, Nissle RR. Four types of periodontal treatment compared over two years. J Periodontol 1981;52:655–662.

29. Ramfjord SP, Morrison EC, Burgett FG, Nissle RR, Shick RA, Zann GJ, Knowles JW. Oral hygiene and maintenance of periodontal support. J Periodontol 1982;53:26–30.

30. Pihlstrom BL, Ortiz-Campos C, McHugh RB. A randomized four year study of periodontal therapy. J Periodontol 1981;52:227–242.

31. Pihlstrom BL, McHugh RB, Oliphant TH, Ortiz-Campos C. Comparison of surgical and nonsurgical treatment of periodontal disease. A review of current studies and additional results after 6 1/2 years. J Clin Periodontol 1983;10:524–541.

32. Wilson TG, Glover ME, Schoen J, Baus C, Jacobs T. Compliance with maintenance therapy in a private periodontal practice. J Periodontol 1984;55:468–473.

33. Wilson T, Hale S, Temple R. The results of efforts to improve compliance with supportive periodontal treatment in a private periodontal practice. J Periodontal 1993;64:311–314.

# CHAPTER 23
## REVIEW QUESTIONS

1. Active periodontal therapy is complete when all of the following have been eliminated except:
   a. Plaque
   b. Suppuration
   c. Bleeding on probing
   d. Progressive attachment loss
2. A biologically compatible root surface allows _____ to work effectively.
   a. Antibiotics
   b. Host defense system
   c. Chlorhexidine mouthrinse
   d. Matrix metalloproteinases
3. Disease masking can occur with all of the following except:
   a. Antibiotics
   b. Mouth rinses
   c. Host-modulating agents
   d. Scaling and root planing
4. The use of adjunctive agents such as antimicrobials, antibiotics, or host-modulating agents are most appropriate during which of the following?
   a. Active therapy
   b. Nonsurgical therapy
   c. Maintenance therapy
   d. Compromised active therapy
5. Which type of diagnosis is most appropriate to detect disease recurrence?
   a. Full mouth
   b. Site specific

   c. Patient based
   d. Sextant based
6. The rationale for periodontal maintenance is based on proper management of:
   a. Pocket depths
   b. Osseous contours
   c. Plaque pathogenicity
   d. Soft tissue inflammation
7. A recall interval of _____ months has been clearly shown to be inadequate to control the progression of periodontitis.
   a. 2
   b. 3
   c. 4
   d. 6
8. Which of the following morphotypes is part of a disease-associated flora?
   a. Filaments
   b. Spirochetes
   c. Straight rods
   d. Coccoid cells
9. Refractory periodontitis is best characterized by which of the following?
   a. Progressive recession
   b. Stable attachment levels
   c. Excellent plaque control
   d. Poor compliance with maintenance
10. Host-modulating agents may include all of the following except:
    a. Penicillins
    b. Tetracyclines
    c. Bisphosphonates
    d. Nonsteroidal anti-inflammatory drugs (NSAIDs)

# Periodontal Emergencies

Jonathan L. Gray

A periodontal emergency is any circumstance, or a combination of circumstances, that adversely affects the periodontium and requires immediate attention. This definition encompasses a wide variety of conditions that involve the periodontium; however, this chapter will be limited to the emergencies most often encountered, including:

1. Pericoronitis
2. Periodontal and gingival abscesses
3. Chemical and physical injuries
4. Necrotizing periodontal diseases
5. Dentin hypersensitivity
6. Fractured teeth
7. Periodontal and endodontic problems

## VITAL SIGNS: SIGNIFICANCE AND MANAGEMENT

This section deals with clinical findings that are common to most periodontal emergencies, which are usually acute in nature, although they may be chronic. It is essential that the clinician take and record vital signs. At a minimum, patient's blood pressure, pulse, respirations, and body temperature should be recorded. Elevated blood pressure and pulse may indicate underlying cardiovascular disease, anxiety, or the effects of pain. Most dental health professionals are very aware of the significance and management of these vital signs. However, some dental practitioners fail to measure, record, and properly treat elevated body temperature.

In adults, normal oral body temperature is 98.6°F, or 37°C; an oral temperature of 100°F, or 38°C, should be viewed with concern; an oral temperature in excess of 101°F, or 39°C, is an indication of a patient with systemic involvement. Rectal temperatures measure 1°F greater than oral temperatures; axillary temperatures generally measure 1°F less than oral temperatures. Young children, from birth to age 5, often spike fevers in excess of 103°F, 40°C. Although this seems to be an alarming temperature, it is, in fact, not as significant as it would be in an adult.

Patients with an elevated body temperature must be questioned regarding fatigue, chills, and sweating. They must also be examined for the presence of tender lymph nodes (lymphadenopathy) and difficulty breathing, swallowing, and opening or closing the mouth. Patients with positive signs and symptoms have systemic involvement, and are generally treated with systemic antibiotics to isolate the infection and antipyretics such as acetaminophen to reduce the fever.

Antibiotic cultures are always desirable, if possible, and should be taken for patients who fail to respond to the initial choice of antibiotics. The current empiric drugs of choice for most odontogenic infections in adults is amoxicillin (Amoxil), 500 mg, three times per day, or clindamycin (Cleocin), 300 to 450 mg, three to four times per day by mouth for 7 to 10 days. The intravenous dosage is 600 mg every 6 to 7 hours. For patients who are unable to take clindamycin, a combination of amoxicillin/clavulanic acid (Augmentin), 875/125 mg, twice daily, or 500/125 mg, three times daily, by mouth for 7 to 10 days is prescribed. The secondary intravenous drug for patients unable to take clindamycin is cefotetan (Cefotan), 2 g intravenously every 12 hours.[1]

Antibiotics for pediatric patients are as follows. First-line drugs are cefuroxime (Cefizox) or a third-generation cephalosporin. For patients who cannot take either of these, Augmentin or trimethoprim/sulfamethoxazole is recommended. Dosage must be calculated based on age and body weight.[1]

Bacteria that are resistant to β-lactam drugs such as the penicillins and cephalosporins are an increasingly significant problem. These drugs, particularly penicillins, erythromycin, and tetracyclines, are best used after antibiotic culturing, not empirically. In the past, there was concern about pseudomembranous colitis with clindamycin.[2] However, although *Clostridium difficile*–mediated diarrhea does occur, it is rarely serious except in the elderly and immunocompromised patients, and is easily treated by the patient's physician with metronidazole (Flagyl) and intravenous fluids.[3]

For patients who appear to have systemic involvement, it is often wise to obtain a complete blood count and differential. A urinalysis is also useful. At a minimum, the complete blood count and differential will help determine the severity of the infection and dehydration. The urinalysis will also reveal the presence of dehydration. All patients should be encouraged to push fluids. Dehydrated patients may benefit from intravenous fluids in the dental office or the emergency room.

# PERICORONITIS

## Etiology

Pericoronitis is probably the most common periodontal emergency, and the partially erupted or impacted mandibular third molar is the site most frequently involved. The overlying gingival flap is an excellent harbor for the accumulation of debris and an ideal breeding ground for bacteria. Additional insult to the pericoronal flap is often produced by trauma from an opposing tooth.[4,5]

## Signs and Symptoms

The clinical picture is a red, swollen, possibly suppurating lesion that is extremely painful to the touch. Swelling of the cheek at the angle of the jaw, early necrotizing ulcerative gingivitis, partial trismus, lymphadenopathy, and radiating pains to the ear are common findings. The patient may also have systemic complications such as fever, leukocytosis, and general malaise.

## Treatment

The treatment of pericoronitis consists of irrigation of the undersurface of the flap and the surrounding area with warm saline solution or with antimicrobial rinses. A 10-mLsyringe with a blunt 10-gauge needle, bent at an 80-degree angle, is an excellent irrigating instrument. An ultrasonic or sonic instrument can also be used effectively in this region. It

may be necessary to extract the opposing third molar at the first visit if it impinges on the pericoronal flap. The patient is instructed to rinse with warm salt water every 2 hours, and antibiotics are administered if systemic complications are present. Once the acute symptoms have subsided, a careful evaluation is made to determine whether the tooth should be retained and whether further periodontal therapy is indicated to alter the environment.

# PERIODONTAL AND GINGIVAL ABSCESSES

## Gingival Abscess

A gingival abscess is a localized (usually superficial), painful, rapidly expanding lesion that appears suddenly in the marginal gingiva or interdental papilla. The lesion consists of a purulent focus in connective tissue. It is initiated by the forceful embedding, into the gingiva or gingival sulcus, of a foreign body (e.g., a toothbrush bristle or popcorn husk). A gingival abscess may occur in tissue entirely free from periodontal disease.

## Treatment

Treatment consists of drainage to relieve the acute symptoms and removal of the foreign body. If the lesion has become fluctuant, topical anesthesia is first applied to the gingival margin, and the gingival sulcus is gently opened with a curet to permit evacuation of pus. The sulcus is gently instrumented, and copious amounts of warm saline solution are used to flush the area. The patient is advised to rinse with warm salt water every 2 hours. Once the irritant is removed and drainage is established, the tissues usually return to normal with no further treatment.

## Periodontal Abscess

A periodontal abscess is a localized, purulent inflammatory process involving the deeper periodontal structures. Abscess formation is usually associated with infrabony pockets, deep tortuous pockets, and furcation involvement. Conditions that either force material into deep pockets, prevent free drainage, or occlude the orifice of a pocket may result in abscess formation. The latter may occur when patients become conscientious about plaque control and improve the tissue health in the marginal area without treatment of the deeper problem.[6,7]

Periodontal abscesses may be acute or chronic. Acute lesions often subside and persist in the chronic state, whereas chronic lesions may suddenly become acute.

## Signs and Symptoms

The clinical signs of an acute abscess are:

1. Severe pain
2. Swelling of the soft tissues
3. Tenderness to percussion
4. Extrusion of the involved tooth
5. Mobility of the involved tooth

Periodontal destruction in an acute periodontal abscess may be rapid and extensive, and treatment should be instituted promptly.

## Treatment

Treatment of the periodontal abscess is performed in two stages. The first stage involves management of the acute symptoms by drainage. Whenever possible, drainage is established through the lumen of the pocket. If this cannot be done, as is often the case when there is a furcation involvement or a tortuous pocket, drainage is obtained externally by making a "stab" wound through the pointed lesion. The patient is advised to rinse with warm salt water every 2 hours, and antibiotics are prescribed if systemic complications are present. It may be necessary to adjust the occlusion of the involved tooth or teeth.[8]

The second stage of treatment is treatment of the pocket as soon as the acute symptoms have subsided and before the chronic stage is reached.

Treatment may consist of nonsurgical therapy, or careful elevation of a mucoperiosteal flap. All granulomatous tissue is removed, and the root surface is lightly planed. Emphasis is placed on gentle manipulation of the soft tissue. The flap is replaced in its original position (replaced flap) and sutured. A periodontal dressing may be used for 7 to 10 days.

Clinical experience has demonstrated a marked propensity for repair after acute periodontal destruction. For this reason, teeth affected by an acute periodontal abscess should be carefully evaluated before extraction is recommended, and periodontal therapy, if indicated, should be instituted.

## CHEMICAL AND PHYSICAL INJURIES

Injuries caused by toothbrush trauma, chemical burns, cheek and tongue biting, factitious habits, and periodontal dressings are occasionally observed. Emergencies of this type are painful but otherwise of little consequence. Healing usually occurs uneventfully in 10 days to 2 weeks. Treatment is chiefly symptomatic, and patient discomfort is controlled through the use of topical anesthetics or warm saline rinses.

## NECROTIZING PERIODONTAL DISEASES

### Classification

The 1999 International Workshop for a Classification of Periodontal Diseases and Conditions combined the terms necrotizing ulcerative gingivitis (NUG) and necrotizing ulcerative periodontitis (NUP) under the term necrotizing periodontal diseases. It is believed that these diseases represent a spectrum of a single condition. Attachment loss, damage to the periodontal ligament or alveolar bone, is the single distinction between these two conditions.[9]

### Incidence

With the exception of HIV-infected AIDS patients, necrotizing periodontal diseases are much less common than they were several decades ago in developed countries ($<1\%$). However, NUP, rare in the total population, appears to be more common among susceptible, immunosuppressed populations.[10] One possible explanation for the decrease in the incidence of NUG is the increased amount of antibiotics in the food supply.

### Contagion

For many years, NUG was considered a communicable disease, contracted from eating utensils, personal contact, and so forth. There is no evidence to support any pattern of transmission among individuals. The 1966 World Workshop in Periodontics[11] concluded, based on existing evidence, that NUG was not a communicable disease.

### Etiology

The etiology of necrotizing periodontal diseases can be classified as follows:

1. Risk factors
   a. Bacterial plaque, especially spirochetes and fusiformis
   b. Smoking
2. Predisposing factors
   a. Local factors may include calculus, gingival flaps over molar teeth, caries, overhanging margins of restorations, improper tooth contacts, malpositioned teeth, and food impaction
   b. Systemic predisposing factors include diabetes mellitus, HIV or AIDS, other forms of immunosuppression, leukemia, lymphoma, stress, anxiety, heavy alcohol intake, fatigue, and malnutrition

The dramatic response to antibiotics, both topical and systemic, is valid evidence of the role of bacteria in the etiology of NUG. Once antibiotic administration is stopped, the disease usually recurs unless the predisposing factors have been eliminated.

## Diagnosis

NUG can be diagnosed based on clinical findings alone. The onset of the disease is manifested quite suddenly, and patients complain of severe pain about the teeth or gingiva. Often, they cannot determine any one particular area that hurts but say, "My entire mouth hurts," or "All of my gums hurt." The pain is more intense at the sites of ulceration. The second most prominent symptom experienced by the patient is bleeding gums. Bleeding is often spontaneous, and patients may observe blood on their pillows or notice the taste of blood when they awaken. Patients may also experience marked pain and bleeding while brushing their teeth or when eating. Alcoholic beverages, hot or cold liquids, or spicy foods may be intolerable.

The most characteristic and pathognomonic findings of NUG are ulceration and cratering of the interdental papillae (Fig. 24-1). Frequently, the papillae are reduced to punched-out masses of necrotic tissue covered by a gray-white pseudo-membrane. Acute pain and bleeding result from the slightest pressure on the area. Ulcerated areas

spread by contiguity and by contact. The mucosa of the lips, jaws, and palate may be affected, and ulcerated areas may be found on the tongue. The fetid odor of necrosis is usually present, but this distinctive odor is not pathognomonic of NUG, in that the odor may be present in any site of tissue necrosis. There may or may not be a number of systemic findings. Fever, headache, general malaise, loss of appetite, and regional lymphadenopathy may be present. The constitutional symptoms seem to parallel the severity of the disease and are usually more pronounced in younger individuals.

NUP shares the same diagnostic features of NUG with two major exceptions, attachment loss and exposure of alveolar bone. NUP, by definition, results in the destruction of the alveolar bone and periodontal ligament. Unlike NUG, the bone may be exposed as a result of the disease, and the destruction is not limited to the interproximal areas, but may extend 360 degrees around the tooth.

## Differential Diagnosis

A number of diseases produce lesions similar to those of NUG. Lesions most commonly mistaken for NUG include:

1. Acute gingivitis
2. Primary herpetic gingivostomatitis
3. Recurrent aphthous stomatitis
4. Desquamative gingivitis

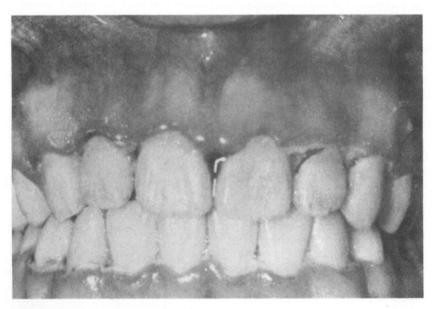

*Figure 24.1* ●

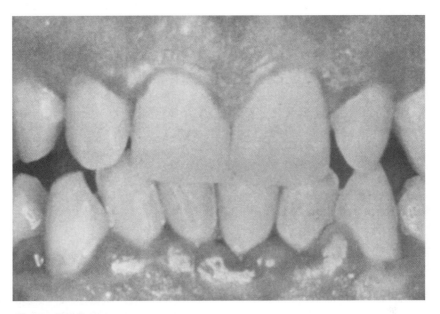

**Figure 24.2** ●

5. Infectious mononucleosis
6. Acute leukemia
7. Agranulocytosis
8. Secondary stage of syphilis

Only NUG, however, produces ulceration and cratering of the interdental papillae. It should be emphasized that NUG can occur in conjunction with any number of systemic debilitating diseases.

1. Acute gingivitis (Fig. 24-2). An intense generalized or even localized acute gingivitis can mimic any of the signs and symptoms of NUG. In gingivitis, pain is not as severe or as persistent, and rarely is there spontaneous bleeding. In many patients with acute gingivitis, the interproximal areas and gingival margins are filled with food, plaque, and materia alba. Once this debris is removed and the interproximal areas can be examined, the lack of necrosis and crater formation will verify the diagnosis of NUG.

2. Primary acute herpetic gingivostomatitis (Fig. 24-3). This disease is characterized by small ulcers with elevated, halolike margins. The lesions are yellowish and cheesy in appearance and bleed less readily on pressure than does NUG. The lips, tongue, buccal mucosa, palate, gingiva, pharynx, and tonsils may be involved. The disease is accompanied by generalized soreness, which interferes with eating or drinking. The typical interdental

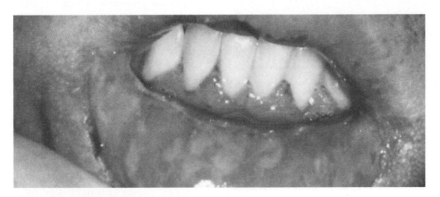

**Figure 24.3** ●

crater of NUG is lacking. Patients usually display rather severe systemic symptoms with typical herpetic lesions, extraorally and intraorally. Diagnosis is based on clinical findings and patient history. Acute herpetic gingivostomatitis usually runs a course of 7 to 10 days. Treatment consists of palliative measures. The patient is placed on a regimen of warm water rinses, soft diet, and forced fluids. Plaque and superficial calculus are removed to reduce gingival inflammation. If the patient experiences pain when eating, a 0.05% solution of dyclonine hydrochloride or viscous Xylocaine may be prescribed for use before meals. It is swished in the mouth for about 2 minutes and then expectorated. Local anesthesia is produced and persists for up to 1 hour. Dyclonine hydrochloride can be used several times daily, without fear of toxicity.

3. Recurrent aphthous stomatitis (canker sores; Fig. 24-4). This condition is characterized by single or multiple epithelial erosions, which can occur on the buccal mucosa, lateral margin of the tongue, floor of the mouth, soft palate, and pharynx. The ulcers are covered by a gray-white membrane with an erythematous

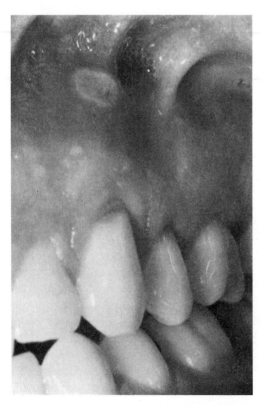

***Figure 24.4*** ●

margin and minimal adjacent erythema. The condition is extremely painful, and one or more oral lesions may be present. Common precipitating factors include mucosal trauma, psychic stress, and endocrine imbalance. In patients who suffer continuously with this condition, a recommended treatment is tetracycline hydrochloride, oral suspension. One teaspoon containing 250 mg is swished around the mouth for 2 minutes and then swallowed. This is done four times a day until the lesions are gone. The mouth rinse is followed by a topical application of a steroid. Begin the treatment as soon as the prodromal signs are recognized. This treatment is not recommended for those individuals who experience only the occasional aphthae or who should not take tetracyclines.

4. Chronic desquamative gingivitis. This gingival condition is probably a clinical syndrome rather than a disease entity. The etiology is not known; however, the condition is probably an oral manifestation of a bullous dermatologic disease, such as benign mucous membrane pemphigoid or lichen planus. Desquamative gingivitis is most commonly observed in women (40 to 55 years of age) and can occur in mild, moderate, and severe forms. In the mildest form, there is diffuse, painless erythema of the gingiva. In the moderate to severe form, there are scattered red and gray areas involving the marginal and attached gingiva. The gingiva can usually be rubbed off with finger massage or blown off with an air syringe (Nikolsky's sign), leaving a bleeding surface. The papillae do not undergo necrosis; therefore, there is no interdental cratering. The patients complain of a burning sensation, thermal sensitivity, and pain when brushing the teeth. The mild form of this condition may be painless, but the severe form is extremely painful. Diagnosis is based on clinical findings and biopsy. Local treatment consists of gentle prophylaxis, plaque control, and elimination of all forms of local irritants. In the most severe cases, topical or systemic corticosteroids are used to supplement the local therapy. Topical hormones are often effective supplements to local therapy: for female patients, a cream containing 1.25 mg/g of conjugated estrogen, and for males, methyltestosterone ointment, 2 mg/g. Some therapists have successfully eliminated the condition by gingivectomy.

5. Infectious mononucleosis. This benign infectious disease is usually seen in children and young adults. The symptoms include a sudden

onset of fever, nausea, headache, vomiting, malaise, loss of appetite, swelling, and tenderness of the lymph nodes. The patient often complains first of a sore mouth and throat. Orally, there may be diffuse erythema of the mucosa and petechiae. The marginal gingiva and interdental papillae are swollen and inflamed, and bleed spontaneously or with gentle pressure. There is no ulceration or interdental crater formation, but secondary development of NUG affords a diagnostic challenge. Diagnosis is based on hematologic and immunologic findings.

6. Leukemia (Fig. 24-5). Oral manifestations occur with great frequency in patients with leukemia, particularly acute and subacute monocytic leukemia. Clinical changes may vary from diffuse cyanotic discoloration of the entire gingival mucosa to a tumorous gingival enlargement. The enlargement may be localized or generalized, diffuse or marginal, but in all cases it is associated with local irritants, such as plaque, calculus, faulty restorations, and trauma. The clinical signs of NUG are often superimposed on leukemic gingival enlargement. When there is a lack of response to local treatment of NUG, a complete blood count, urinalysis, and bone marrow studies are essential to rule out the presence of leukemia and other blood dyscrasias.

7. Agranulocytosis (malignant neutropenia). This condition is manifested orally as ulceration and necrosis of the gingiva, which resembles NUG. The ulcers are covered by a gray or gray-black membrane, but there is less inflammation associated with the lesions of agranulocytosis than NUG. Lesions are also observed in the oral mucosa, tonsils, and pharynx. The most common cause is a reaction to a wide variety of drugs. Diagnosis is based on blood studies and bone marrow biopsy.

8. Secondary syphilis (mucous patch). The oral lesions of syphilis are usually on the tongue, the gingiva, or the buccal mucosa. They are usually ovoid or irregularly shaped and are surrounded by an erythematous zone. The mucous patch rarely affects the marginal gingiva, and the overlying gray-white plaque is not detachable. The lesions are usually painless but are highly infectious. Diagnosis is made by positive results of serologic analysis and darkfield examination of an affected lymph node.

## Treatment of NUG

The therapist should attempt to:

1. Control the acute bacterial phase
2. Educate the patient in plaque control and the nature of the disease
3. Eliminate the predisposing factors, both local and systemic[12,13]

Early and vigorous local treatment during the acute phase will produce rapid and dramatic results in most cases. Antibiotics should be used only when systemic complications are evidenced.

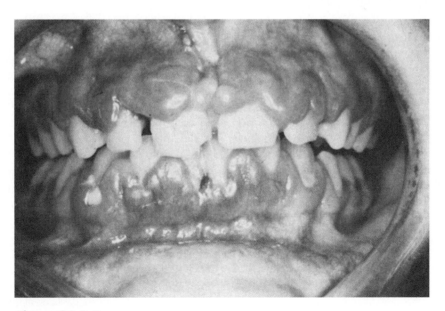

**Figure 24.5** ●

Drugs should never be considered a substitute for scaling and debridement for the following reasons:

1. Patients treated with antibiotics alone may come to believe that drugs, not plaque control, are the solution.
2. Antibiotics may mask underlying systemic diseases.

The basic steps in treatment follow.

## First Visit

1. Remove as much calculus, plaque, and debris as possible, as soon as possible, and as gently as possible. Ultrasonic or sonic instrumentation are the methods of choice because they provide irrigation and debridement.
2. Instruct the patient in plaque control. Begin patient education and motivation. Have the patient hold the soft toothbrush under warm water to soften the bristles further and then instruct in the proper use of the brush. Be sure to advise the patient to discard the old toothbrush and to use a new brush.
3. Antibiotics may be administered systemically if there is evidence of elevated temperature, lymphadenopathy, and general malaise. Most cases do not require antibiotics. Mild analgesics may be prescribed for pain.
4. Instruct the patient in specific home-care procedures. It is advisable to give the patient a mimeographed sheet of specific instructions to be followed at home.

## Recommended Home-Care Instructions for NUG Patients

1. Rinse the mouth vigorously with warm saline solution (1 teaspoon of table salt dissolved in one 8-oz glass of warm water) every 2 hours.
2. Follow a soft, bland diet of milk, eggnog, broth, and so forth. Dietary supplements (e.g., Boost, Ensure, Carnation Instant Breakfasts) are especially useful during this period.
3. Drink eight glasses of water every day.
4. Avoid foods that are hard, fried, coarse, spicy, or starchy.
5. Eliminate or reduce smoking and drinking of alcoholic beverages.
6. Rest as much as possible.
7. After eating, rinse the mouth with the warm saline solution.
8. Brush the teeth in the manner prescribed.
9. Return to the dental office after 24 hours.

## Second Visit

1. Check the oral hygiene and review plaque control procedures.

2. Continue the removal of calculus, plaque, and debris.
3. Polish the teeth.
4. Have the patient return after 24 to 48 hours.

## Third Visit

1. Check the oral hygiene and review plaque control procedures, if indicated.
2. Continue the elimination of all irritants, which includes all calculus, overhanging margins, and open contacts.
3. If the tissues have not responded dramatically by the third visit (48 to 72 hours), evaluate for systemic factors (leukemia, infectious mononucleosis, HIV or AIDS, and so forth). Refer for medical consultation, if necessary.
4. If improvement is apparent, make an appointment for reevaluation in 7 to 10 days; otherwise continue to see the patient every 24 to 48 hours.

## Fourth Visit

1. Check plaque control.
2. Check for calculus and other irritants. Remove if present.
3. Evaluate for further periodontal treatment.

NUG responds rapidly and dramatically to local therapy and effective plaque control. As a result, some patients and clinicians become somewhat complacent about the severity of the disease. It is important to remember, and to caution the patient accordingly, that unless the treatment is continued to completion, NUG is likely to recur. Likewise, uncontrolled NUG can result in localized osteonecrosis and extensive soft tissue destruction. Ludwig's angina has been observed in NUG cases in patients with infectious mononucleosis, acute leukemia, uncontrolled diabetes, and HIV. For this reason, if there has not been a dramatic response to local treatment of NUG by 72 hours, the patient should be referred for medical consultation.

# HYPERSENSITIVITY

Hypersensitivity is often a management problem for both the patient and the dentist. This is true despite the wide variety of medicaments and desensitizing paraphernalia available.

## Etiology

Hypersensitivity of exposed dentin can occur when dentinal tubules are exposed either by caries, fracture, periodontal disease, or periodontal instrumentation.[14] Trauma from occlusion may also be a cause of hypersensitivity. Under such circumstances, thermal stimuli (hot or cold foods) and tactile stimuli (toothbrushes and dental instruments) can excite a painful response. It is most discouraging to the patient, and futile for the dentist, to insist on vigorous plaque control when such procedures are painful.

## Treatment

Hypersensitivity can be controlled by eliminating the etiologic factors and by using desensitizing agents.[15] There are several patient-applied and dentist-applied preparations, all of which have some degree of success. One of the first treatments to be considered, especially after surgical procedures, should be occlusal adjustment. Even a slightly heavy occlusal contact can make a tooth or teeth in a recently treated area very sensitive. Refinement of the occlusal contacts often renders immediate relief.

Patient-applied commercial products can be very effective. Strontium chloride– and potassium nitrate–containing toothpastes may be used as medicaments, applied for 1 to 2 minutes after regular plaque control procedures. Relief should be achieved within 1 week.

Dentist-applied medicaments include ophthalmic suspensions of prednisolone acetate, sodium fluoride solution, stannous fluoride gels, fluoride varnish, sodium fluoride–glycerin–kaolin paste, and dibasic calcium phosphate. Each of these is applied after the sensitive area is polished with a suitable polishing agent. The medicament is then applied with a cotton pledget or Porte polisher. Several applications may be needed to achieve complete relief. Local anesthesia may be required before applying the medicaments. Dentine-bonding agents can be used in areas that are accessible. Refractory cases may require root canal therapy if the tooth is to be retained. Recently, lasers have been used with some success.

## PERIODONTAL AND ENDODONTIC PROBLEMS

### Diagnosis and Treatment

It is sometimes necessary to differentiate between a periodontal and periapical abscess. A nonvital pulp is usually indicative of a periapical abscess, and the tooth should be either treated endodontically or extracted. A clinically responsive vital pulp is not always assurance that the problem is still not pulpal. Radiography is of some assistance in differential diagnosis, but clinical findings, such

as extensive caries, tooth vitality testing, pocket formation, and continuity between the abscess and the gingival margin are of greater practical significance.

Various investigators have confirmed pulpal pathosis and infection in periodontally involved teeth. Thus, the probability exists that periodontitis can result in death of the pulp. It has also been demonstrated that because of pulpal disease, tissue destruction may proceed from the apical region toward the gingival margin. This process is termed retrograde periodontitis, to differentiate it from periodontitis, in which the disease spreads from the gingival margin to the apex of the tooth. Whether the periodontal pocket is a result of retrograde or marginal periodontitis or a combination of both is academic. In all cases, treatment should consist of either combined endodontic-periodontal therapy or extraction of the tooth. In cases in which the tooth is retained, endodontic therapy must be completed first.[16]

## CRACKED TOOTH SYNDROME

The diagnosis of fractured teeth can be very difficult. It is not unusual for the condition to be undiagnosed for months or years. Many classification systems have been devised during the years. The system presented here attempts to speak to the prognosis and treatment of fractures (Table 24-1). The most common fractures are incomplete crown root fractures and fractures of the root associated with prior endodontic therapy.[17–19]

### Diagnosis

Pain is a characteristic of fractured teeth. They are particularly sensitive to mastication and chewing. If the pulp is involved, the tooth will exhibit the signs and symptoms of acute or chronic pulpitis. A variety of diagnostic tools, such as the Tooth Sleuth, a rubber wheel, or a piece of a wooden tongue blade, enable the clinician to determine whether a particular cusp is sensitive to chewing forces and, therefore, possibly fractured.

Radiographs provide inconsistent results. Many, if not most, incomplete fractures cannot be visualized with radiographs. Complete fractures are more likely to be seen. Fiberoptic transillumination is also a useful diagnostic aid. Light will not cross a fracture line. If a fiberoptic light is shined on a tooth, a sharp distinction in illumination may indicate a fracture. Transillumination is less useful if a large restoration is present.

In many cases, periodontal probing is very helpful for the diagnosis of root fractures. A deep,

## TABLE 24.1

### Classification of Dental Fractures

| Classification | Prognosis | Treatment |
| --- | --- | --- |
| Crown—incomplete fracture | Fair to good | Possible endodontics, crown-lengthening surgery, and cast restoration |
| Crown—complete fracture | Fair to good | Possible endodontics, crown-lengthening surgery, and cast restoration |
| Root—incomplete fracture | Poor to hopeless | In some cases in which the fracture is limited to the coronal portion of the root, crown lengthening can be done, and a crown placed to splint the fracture |
| Root—complete fracture | Hopeless | Extraction |
| Tooth—incomplete fracture | Poor to hopeless | In some cases in which the fracture is limited to the coronal portion of the root, crown lengthening can be done, and a crown placed to splint the fracture |
| Tooth—complete fracture | Hopeless | Extraction |

narrow pocket is often a sign of a root fracture. This is especially true in a mouth that is otherwise periodontally healthy. In such a case, a deep, narrow pocket is almost always indicative of a fractured root or a periodontal or endodontic lesion. If there is no restoration in the tooth, and no history of trauma, the diagnosis is almost certainly a fractured tooth.

## REFERENCES

1. Gilbert GN, Moellering RC, Eliopoulos GM, Sande MA. The Sanford Guide to Antimicrobial Therapy, 35 ed. Hyde Park, VT: Antimicrobial Therapy, Inc, 2005:30.
2. Walker CB, Karpinia K, Baehni P. Chemotherapeutics: antibiotics and other antimicrobials. Periodontol 2000. 2004;36:146–165.
3. Gilbert GN, Moellering RC, Eliopoulos GM, Sande MA. The Sanford Guide to Antimicrobial Therapy, 35 ed. Hyde Park, VT: Antimicrobial Therapy, Inc, 2005:65.
4. Nitzan DW, Tal O, Sela MN, Shteyer A. Pericoronitis: a reappraisal of its clinical and microbiologic aspects. J Oral Maxillofac Surg 1985;43: 510–516.
5. Nabers JM. Treatment of the symptomatic periodontal lesions. Dent Clin North Am 1969;13: 169–180.
6. Herrera D, Roldan S, Gonzalez I, Sanz M. The periodontal abscess (I). Clinical and microbiological findings. J Clin Periodontol 2000;27:387–394.
7. Herrera D, Roldan S, Sanz M. The periodontal abscess: a review. J Clin Periodontol 2000;27: 377–386.
8. Novak MJ. Necrotizing ulcerative periodontitis. Ann Periodontol 1999;4:74–78.
9. Corbet EF. Diagnosis of acute periodontal lesions. Periodontol 2000 2004;34:204–216.
10. Albandar JM, Tinoco EMB. Epidemiology of periodontal diseases in children and young persons. Periodontol 2000 2002;29:153–176.
11. Ramfjord SP, Kerr DA, Ash MM. World Workshop in Periodontics. Ann Arbor, MI: University of Michigan Press, 1966:74–75.
12. Rowland RW. Necrotizing ulcerative gingivitis. Ann Periodontol 1999;4:65–73.
13. Johnson BD, Engel D. Acute necrotizing ulcerative gingivitis. A review of diagnosis, etiology and treatment. J Periodontol 1986;57:141–150.
14. Tavss EA, Fisher SW, Campbell S, Bonta Y, Darcy-Siegel J, Blackwell BL, Volpe AR, Miller SE. The scientific rationale and development of an optimized dentifrice for the treatment of dentin hypersensitivity. Am J Dent 2004;17:61–70.
15. Swift EJ Jr. Causes, prevention, and treatment of dentin hypersensitivity. Compend Contin Educ Dent 2004;25:95–106.
16. Rotstein I, Simon JH. Diagnosis, prognosis and decision-making in the treatment of combined periodontal-endodontic lesions. Periodontol 2000 2004; 34:165–203.
17. Gher ME Jr, Dunlap RM, Anderson MH, Kuhl LV. Clinical survey of fractured teeth. J Am Dent Assoc 1987;114:174–177.
18. Geurtsen W. The cracked-tooth syndrome: clinical features and case reports. Int J Periodontics Restorative Dent 1992;12:395–405.
19. Eakle WS, Maxwell EH, Braly BV. Fractures of posterior teeth in adults. J Am Dent Assoc 1986; 112:215–218.

## CHAPTER 24
## REVIEW QUESTIONS

1. Rectal temperatures generally measure less than oral temperatures, whereas, axillary temperatures are higher.
   a. True
   b. False

2. The first-line antibiotics of choice for oral infections in adult and pediatric patients, respectively, are:
   a. Augmentin and clindamycin
   b. Cefotetan and Augmentin
   c. Amoxicillin for both
   d. Amoxicillin and cefuroxime

3. The initial treatment of choice for a pericoronal infection would be to extract the underlying tooth involved.
   a. True
   b. False

4. Which statement best describes the management and healing of a periodontal abscess?
   a. An initial "I and D" (incision and drainage) of any fluctuant mass, prescribing systemic antibiotics with extraction at a later date
   b. Establish drainage via the "pocket" area first, with potential periodontal surgery at a later date
   c. Generally, one can readily determine the eventual prognosis of a tooth involved with a periodontal abscess on acute presentation
   d. The healing response in the second stage is generally compromised, given the early onset of the acute phase

5. The most pathognomonic finding with NUG (necrotizing ulcerative gingivitis ) is:
   a. Fetid odor
   b. Spontaneous bleeding
   c. Pain
   d. Ulcerative and cratered interdental papillae

6. Choose the best match for the therapeutic treatment with the oral condition.
   (1) Primary acute herpetic gingivostomatitis
   (2) Recurrent aphthous stomatitis (canker sore)
   (3) Desquamative gingivitis
   (4) Acute gingivitis
       a. Oral suspension of tetracycline
       b. Topical corticosteroids
       c. Debridement
       d. Dyclonine HCl

7. When treating NUG, if there has not been a dramatic improvement in presentation after _____, the patient should be referred for additional medical evaluation to rule out concurrent systemic disease.
   a. 24 hours
   b. 72 hours
   c. 3 days
   d. 7 days

8. Dentinal hypersensitivity immediately after periodontal surgery often has an occlusal component as an etiology.
   a. True
   b. False

9. What combination of prognoses is best associated with two different presentations: a complete and an incomplete root fracture?
   a. Poor and fair
   b. Hopeless and fair
   c. Both are hopeless
   d. Hopeless and poor

10. In determining the difference between a periodontal and endodontic abscess, which clinical finding would be most helpful in differentiating the two?
    a. Radiographic presentation
    b. Vital tooth
    c. Probing depths
    d. Pain

# Mucocutaneous Diseases of the Periodontium

Terry Rees

The tissues of the oral cavity are susceptible to a number of autoimmune or immunologically mediated diseases that affect skin and mucous membranes. Several of these disorders may affect the periodontal soft tissues as part of their overall oral manifestations. The conditions often present similar clinical features, and careful diagnosis is required. The following conditions will be discussed:

Lichen planus
Chronic ulcerative stomatitis
Mucous membrane pemphigoid
Pemphigus vulgaris
Lupus erythematosus
Graft-versus-host disease
Erythema multiforme

## LICHEN PLANUS

Lichen planus (LP) is a chronic inflammatory condition of unknown etiology. It affects from 1 to 2% of the population, and lesions may occur on skin or oral mucosa alone or in combination. A relationship with emotional and environmental stress has been suggested, but study results are inconclusive to date. A vulvovaginal-gingival syndrome has been described, and women diagnosed with oral LP should probably be referred for gynecologic examination.[1] Skin lesions usually manifest as violaceous, pruritic papules that are generally transient in nature, disappearing spontaneously within 1 to 2 years of onset. In contrast, oral lesions may persist for many years and undergo transition in their clinical appearance. Lesions are more common in women, and they generally affect individuals older than 50 years of age.[2]

Oral lesions may manifest as asymptomatic papular, reticular, or plaquelike white lesions, but they also occur in painful atrophic, ulcerative, or bullous forms. Reticular lesions occur most frequently, whereas bullous lesions are the least common (Fig. 25-1). For the purpose of this discussion, the atrophic, ulcerative, and bullous forms will be grouped collectively under the term *erosive lichen planus*.

Lichen planus can affect any surface of the oral cavity, although buccal mucosal lesions are most common. Erosive lesions, however, may frequently affect the gingiva and give the clinical appearance of desquamative gingivitis (sloughing of the gingival tissue surface) (Fig. 25-2). Histologic examination of LP reveals thickening of the epithelium (acanthosis with hyperorthokeratosis), a sawtoothed configuration of epithelial rete ridges, and liquefaction degeneration of the epithelial basal cell layer. The degeneration of the epithelial basal cells accounts for the tendency of the surface lesional tissue to slough when traumatized. Underlying connective tissue features a dense band of lymphocytic inflammatory cells immediately subjacent to the basement membrane. This type of infiltration may occur, however, in other mucocutaneous diseases including epithelial dysplasia and malignancy. If dysplastic changes are found, these areas should be carefully monitored and biopsied again in event of any significant changes in appearance.[3] Direct immunofluorescence (DIF) of a portion of the biopsy specimen may help establish the diagnosis by identifying the presence of fibrinogen in a linear pattern in the basal membrane zone or the presence of immunopositive cytoid bodies in underlying connective tissues. These features may also be found in other mucocutaneous diseases, thus positive DIF findings are considered supportive but not diagnostic for LP.[4]

A number of papers have suggested a possible relationship between oral LP and chronic hepatitis, especially that induced by the hepatitis C virus.[5] Some data suggest, however, that this relationship may be induced by a lichenoid reaction to interferon and other drugs used in the treatment of chronic hepatitis. In general, drug-induced lichenoid reactions will manifest with clinical, histologic, and immunofluorescence features consistent with idiopathic LP. These reactions are reasonably common in association with antimalarial drugs, antihypertensive medications, and nonsteroidal anti-inflammatory agents. In recent years, several studies and case reports have described an association between dental restorations, especially silver amalgam, and localized lichenoid reactions in tissue directly contacting the restoration to which the patient is hypersensitive (Fig. 25-3).[6,7] There are also reports of contact lichenoid reactions to flavoring agents such as cinnamic aldehyde that are used in many toothpastes, mouth rinses, soft drinks, candies, and chewing gums.[8]

Several studies and case reports indicate that a relationship may exist between the presence of oral LP and the development of oral squamous cell carcinoma. This remains a contentious issue, however, because some early dysplastic lesions may present with lichenoid features, creating the impression of malignant transformation from preexisting LP. A persuasive number of studies do suggest a weak association between the two conditions, and patients diagnosed with LP should be carefully monitored to ensure that any malignant changes are detected and treated early in the disease process. The clinician should be especially observant of plaquelike and erosive LP, as these types of lesions appear to create the greatest risk.[9]

The painless forms of LP usually do not require treatment. Proper management of erosive LP requires a careful diagnosis, elimination of drugs or other agents possibly causing a lichenoid reaction, control of local irritants, and application of topical or systemic corticosteroid therapy. Recently, a nonsteroidal drug, topical tacrolimus, has been used with significant success in management of oral LP.[10,11] Other therapies have been reported as sometimes successful, but not with the consistency of corticosteroids and topical tacrolimus. At present, therapeutic goals are directed toward elimination of erosive lesions and control of the painless forms of the disease. Lesions tend to recur, and long-term patient recall is necessary for this reason and to monitor affected patients for any tissue changes suggestive of possible malignant transformation.[12,13]

# CHRONIC ULCERATIVE STOMATITIS

Chronic ulcerative stomatitis (CUS) is a newly described autoimmune disease of the oral mucosa that may induce desquamative gingivitis, which closely resembles erosive lichen planus or oral lupus erythematosus in its clinical and histologic manifestations (Fig. 25-4). Diagnosis is generally based on specific direct and indirect immunofluorescence tests. CUS should be suspected in patients who fail to respond to routine therapy for lichen planus, and such patients should be referred to a dermatologist or oral medicine expert for diagnostic confirmation and treatment. Treatment may include topical corticosteroids, systemic corticosteroids, or antimalarial agents.[14,15]

# MUCOUS MEMBRANE PEMPHIGOID (CICATRICIAL PEMPHIGOID)

Mucous membrane pemphigoid (cicatricial pemphigoid [CP], benign mucous membrane pemphigoid) is a distinct chronic vesiculobullous disorder of the elderly that usually affects mucous membranes. The condition is autoimmune in origin, and oral lesions are almost invariably present. On occasion, concomitant lesions may affect the conjunctiva of the eye, the skin, genitalia, rectum, nares, larynx, or esophagus. Although oral lesions rarely heal with scarring, conjunctival scarring (symblepharon) can lead to loss of vision. For this reason, early ophthalmologic evaluation is an essential component in management of this disease.[2]

Lesions may occur on any mouth tissues. The gingiva is the most common target site, with involvement in approximately 97% of reported oral cases. Gingival lesions often feature blistering and loss of the epithelial surface in response to trauma (Nikolsky's sign). This leaves raw, painful erythematous gingival surfaces (Fig. 25-5). Blistering and ulceration may affect other mucosal tissues as well.[16,17]

Histologic examination of mucous membrane pemphigoid (MMP) reveals a separation of the surface epithelium from underlying connective tissue by a split just beneath the epithelial basal cell layer. Direct immunofluorescence reveals the presence of immunoglobin G (IgG) and complement in a linear pattern at the basal membrane zone of the tissue.[18]

Treatment depends on the severity and responsiveness of the oral lesions. Topical or intralesional corticosteroids should be applied, but systemic intervention is often necessary. Corticosteroids are most commonly used for systemic therapy, but dapsone has also been used with some success.

Meticulous oral hygiene is very important in managing oral MMP, but patients often have difficulty with oral physiotherapy because of gingival discomfort. Frequent, gentle debridement and scaling is often necessary to help promote patient comfort. The dentist is the health-care provider best qualified to evaluate progress in management of the oral condition.[19,20]

Bullous pemphigoid is a related condition that usually affects skin as the primary site, although oral mucosal lesions may occur. Oral lesions are very similar in appearance to CP clinically, histologically, and by direct immunofluorescence. Diagnosis is usually based on skin manifestations and by the presence of circulating immunoglobulins (indirect immunofluorescence) in approximately 70% of affected patients. Systemic therapy is usually required.[21]

## PEMPHIGUS VULGARIS

The term *pemphigus* refers to a group of autoimmune vesiculobullous diseases that affect mucosa and skin. Pemphigus vulgaris (PV) is the most common and severe form of the disorder. It can occur at any age, but it is more common in adults between the fourth and sixth decades. Skin lesions manifest as large bullae that rupture and leave eroded, weeping wounds, which may significantly alter the patient's fluid and electrolyte balance, and which may become secondarily infected. Pemphigus vulgaris is fatal in from 5 to 15% of affected individuals.[22]

Oral lesions are very common, and they often precede skin manifestations. Early diagnosis and treatment of oral lesions may enable afflicted patients to avoid the more serious effects of the disease. Oral lesions are similar to those occurring on the skin. Blisters develop and burst quickly, leaving painful eroded areas with irregular borders (Fig. 25-6). Gingival desquamative lesions are common and on occasion may be the only manifestation of the disease (Fig. 25-7).[23]

Histologic examination of PV reveals separation of the cells of the epithelium (acantholysis) and blistering within the epithelium above the basal cell layer. Direct immunofluorescence reveals a distinct pattern of IgG and complement located between the cells of the epithelium. In this and other autoimmune mucocutaneous diseases, immunofluorescence findings may be positive even in clinically normal mucosa.

Systemic corticosteroids are frequently used in therapy for PV although favorable results have also been reported with a variety of other immunosuppressive agents. Again, maintenance of

meticulous oral hygiene is important for patient comfort.[24,25]

Pemphigus vulgaris-like lesions have been associated with medications including captopril and penicillamine, and, on occasion, an association between PV and underlying malignancy has been identified. Paraneoplastic pemphigus lesions may be present exclusively in the oral cavity owing to the presence of a variety of underlying benign or malignant neoplasms (Fig. 25-8).[26]

## LUPUS ERYTHEMATOSUS

Lupus erythematosus (LE) is an autoimmune disease that may involve skin, mucosa, and multiple body systems. It occurs more commonly in women and blacks. The discoid form of the disease exclusively involves skin and mucosa. Mouth lesions are common. In systemic LE, various organ systems may be involved, and oral lesions are present in 25 to 40% of affected individuals. Typical oral lesions in either form of LE are characterized by a central erythematous erosion or ulceration surrounded by radiating keratotic striae (Fig. 25-9). The gingiva may appear erythematous, and LE can easily be clinically misdiagnosed as one of the desquamative diseases described above (Fig. 25-10).[27]

Diagnosis is based on clinical, histologic, and immunologic data. Microscopic features include hyperkeratosis, atrophy of rete ridges, and liquefaction degeneration of the basal layer of epithelium. A bandlike lymphocytic inflammatory infiltrate is evident in superficial connective tissue. These features are similar in some respects to lichen planus, and an LP–LE overlap condition has been described in which exact diagnosis is quite difficult. Direct immunofluorescence discloses granular deposits of IgG, complement, and fibrinogen in the basement membrane zone, thus displaying features that might be confused with cicatricial pemphigoid.[28]

Because of the similarities in the oral features of lupus erythematosus, lichen planus, and mucous membrane pemphigoid, treatment must occasionally be empiric. Oral and skin LE may respond to topical or systemic corticosteroids, but results are unpredictable. Antimalarial drugs sometimes yield satisfactory therapeutic results, as do immunosuppressive or cytotoxic drugs.[29]

## GRAFT-VERSUS-HOST DISEASE

As many as 70 to 80% of individuals receiving bone marrow transplants may experience oral complications associated with an effort by the engrafted marrow to reject its new host. Other tissues such as the liver, gastrointestinal tract, and skin may be involved, and the condition may result in considerable morbidity and even mortality. In the oral cavity, graft-versus-host disease (GVHD) often mimics lichenoid lesions or oral lupus erythematosus with or without significant ulcerations. Overall treatment for GVHD rests with the medical team that is managing the patient, but the dentist may be asked to participate in controlling the oral lesions. Oral therapy includes elimination of local irritants and use of topical corticosteroids, topical cyclosporine, or other anti-inflammatory drugs. Chlorhexidine gluconate mouth rinses may be of great benefit in assisting the patient in maintenance of dental and periodontal health.[29,30]

## ERYTHEMA MULTIFORME

Erythema multiforme (EM) is an acute, inflammatory, mucocutaneous disorder that may manifest with distinct, so-called target lesions of skin, with or without mucosal involvement. A target skin lesion appears as a central dusky-red zone surrounded by a raised, circumferential, erythematous zone. The oral cavity may be involved, and dentists often encounter patients with oral lesions in the absence of skin manifestations. Mouth lesions appear as bullae that burst rapidly and leave erythematous erosions and ulcerations that develop a grayish pseudomembrane, creating a "parboiled" appearance. Hemorrhagic crusting of the lips is very common. In the major form of EM (Stevens-Johnson syndrome), lesions may also occur on the genitalia and conjunctiva, and multiorgan involvement may be present.[31]

The condition is believed to represent a hypersensitivity reaction to an antigen that may or may not be identifiable. Sulfonamide drugs have been implicated, as have many additional drugs, including antibiotics and anticoagulants. Occasionally EM is preceded by bacterial or viral infections, and recent outbreaks of herpes simplex virus lesions have been described preceding the development of EM.

Clinically, EM patients may experience prodromal symptoms such as fever, headache, and general malaise. Once lesions begin to occur, they may take 10 days to several months to fully develop. Spontaneous remission may occur 2 to 3 weeks after onset, but resolution may also take many months.

The histopathologic and immunofluorescence features of EM are not specific, and diagnosis is often based on clinical features. Erythema multiforme can be differentiated from the other bullous diseases by its acute onset, by the presence of target skin lesions, and, occasionally, by the presence of slight fever. When lesions are confined to the oral cavity, however, the clinical features may be very similar to those encountered in primary herpetic gingivostomatitis (Fig. 25-11). Once the diagnosis is established, treatment usually includes administration of systemic corticosteroids and elimination of any drug associated with disease onset.[32]

## SUMMARY

Mucocutaneous diseases are relatively uncommon, yet they occur with sufficient frequency to suggest that all dentists and dental hygienists will encounter them in clinical practice. Many of these diseases produce gingival and other soft tissue lesions that require careful differential diagnosis and knowledgeable management. Primary management responsibility may rest in the hands of a physician or an oral medicine specialist, but all dental healthcare providers share in the responsibility for successful management of these troublesome disorders.

## REFERENCES

1. Eisen D. The evaluation of cutaneous, genital, scalp, nail, esophageal, and ocular involvement in patients with oral lichen planus. Oral Surg Oral Med Oral Pathol Oral Radiol Endod 1999;88:431–436.
2. Plemons JM. Position paper of the American Academy of Periodontology. Vesiculobullous diseases of the oral cavity. J Periodontol 2003;74:1545–1556.
3. Lozada-Nur F. Oral lichen planus and oral cancer: is there enough epidemiologic evidence. Oral Surg Oral Med Oral Pathol Oral Radiol Endod 2000;89:265–266.
4. Silverman S Jr, Eversole LR. Immunopathologic mucosal lesions. In: Silverman S Jr, Eversole LR, Truelove EL, eds. Essentials of Oral Medicine. Hamilton, Ontario: BC Decker Inc, 2001:206–217.
5. Carrozzo M, Gandolfo, S, Carbone M, Colombatto P, Broccoletti R, Garzino-Demo P, Ghisetti V. Hepatitis C virus infection in Italian patients with oral lichen plans: a prospective case-control study. J Oral Pathol Med 1996;25:527–533.
6. Issa Y, Brunton PA, Glenny AM, Duxbury AJ. Healing of oral lichenoid lesions after replacing amalgam restorations: a systematic review. Oral Surg Oral Med Oral Pathol Oral Radiol Endod 2004;98:553–565.
7. Laeijendecker R, Dekker SK, Burger PM, Mulder PG, Van Joost T, Neumann MH. Oral lichen planus and allergy to dental amalgam restorations. Arch Dermatol 2004;140:1434–1438.
8. Clayton R, Orton D. Contact allergy to spearmint oil in a patient with oral lichen planus. Contact Dermatitis 2004;51:314–315.
9. Silverman S Jr. Oral lichen planus: a potentially premalignant lesion. J Oral Maxillofac Surg 2000;58:1286–1288.

10. Byrd JA, Davis MD, Bruce AJ, Drage LA, Rogers RS 3rd. Response of oral lichen planus to topical tacrolimus in 37 patients. Arch Dermatol 2004;140: 1508–1512.

11. Lener EV, Brieva J, Schachter M, West LE, West DP, el-Azhary RA. Successful treatment of erosive lichen planus with topical tacrolimus. Arch Dermatol 2001;137:419–422.

12. Chan ES, Thornhill M, Azkrzewska J. Interventions for treating oral lichen planus. Cochrane Database Syst Rev 2000;(2):CD001168.

13. Mollaoglu N. Oral lichen planus: a review. Br J Oral Maxillofac Surg 2000;28:210–215.

14. Lorenzana ER, Rees TD, Glass M, Detweiler JF. Chronic ulcerative stomatitis: a case report. J Periodontol 2000;71:104–111.

15. Solomon LW, Aguirre A, Neiders M, Costales-Spindler A, Jividen GJ Jr, Zwick MG, Kumar V. Chronic ulcerative stomatitis: clinical, histopathologic, and immunopathologic findings. Oral Surg Oral Med Oral Pathol Oral Radiol Endod 2003;96: 718–726.

16. Alkan A, Gunhan O, Alkan A, Otan F. A clinical study of oral mucous membrane pemphigoid. J Int Med Res 2003;31:340–344.

17. Scully C, Carrozzo M, Gandolfo S, Puiatti P, Monteil R. Update on mucous membrane pemphigoid. Oral Surg Oral Med Oral Pathol Oral Radiol Endod 1999;88:56–68.

18. Cheng YS, Rees TD, Wright JM, Plemons JM. Childhood oral pemphigoid: a case report and review of the literature. J Oral Pathol Med 2001;30: 372–377.

19. Damoulis PD, Gagari E. Combined treatment of periodontal disease and benign mucous membrane pemphigoid. Case report with 8 years maintenance. J Periodontol 2000;71:1620–1629.

20. Lamey PJ, Rees TD, Binnie WH, Rankin KV. Mucous membrane pemphigoid. Treatment experience at two institutions. Oral Surg Oral Med Oral Pathol 1992;74:50–53.

21. Holmstrup P. Non-plaque induced gingival lesions. Ann Periodontol 1999;4:20–31.

22. Ettlin DA. Pemphigus. Dent Clin North Am 2005;49:107–125, viii–ix.

23. Sirois D, Leigh JE, Sollecito TP. Oral pemphigus vulgaris preceding cutaneous lesions: recognition and diagnosis. J Am Dent Assoc 2000;131: 1156–1160.

24. Lamey PJ, Rees TD, Binnie WH, Wright JM, Rankin KV, Simpson NB. Oral presentation of pemphigus vulgaris and its response to systemic steroid therapy. Oral Surg Oral Med Oral Pathol 1992;74:54–57.

25. Mignogna MD, Lo Muzio L, Mignogna RE, Carone R, Ruoppo E, Bucci E. Oral pemphigus: long term behavior and clinical response to treatment with deflazacort in sixteen cases. J Oral Pathol Med 2002;29: 145–152.

26. Kaplan I, Hodak E, Ackerman L, Mimouni D, Anhalt GJ, Calderon S. Neoplasms associated with paraneoplastic pemphigus: a review with emphasis on non-hematologic malignancy and oral mucosa manifestations. Oral Oncol 2004;40:553–562.

27. Brennan MT, Valerin MA, Napenas JJ, Lockhart PB. Oral manifestations of patients with lupus erythematosus. Dent Clin North Am 2005;49:127–141.

28. Gonzales TS, Coleman GC. Periodontal manifestations of collagen vascular disorders. Periodontol 2000 1999;21:94–105.

29. Majorana A, Schubert MM, Porta F, Ugazio AG, Sapelli PL. Oral complications of pediatric hematopoietic cell transplantation: diagnosis and management. Support Care Cancer 2000;8: 353–365.

30. Nicolatou-Galitis O, Kitra V, Van Vliet-Constantinidou C, Peristeri J, Goussetis E, Petropoulos D, Grafakos S. The oral manifestations of chronic graft-versus-host disease (cGVHD) in paediatric allogeneic bone marrow transplant. J Oral Pathol Med 2001;30:148–153.

31. Ayangeo L, Rogers RS 3rd. Oral manifestations of erythema multiforme. Dermatol Clin 2003;21:195–205.

32. Williams PM, Conklin RJ. Erythema multiforme: a review and contrast from Stevens-Johnson syndrome/toxic epidermal necrolysis. Dent Clin North Am 2005;49:67–76, viii.

## CHAPTER 25
## REVIEW QUESTIONS

1. Which of the following statements is true regarding oral lichen planus?
   a. Skin lichen planus lesions persist longer than oral lesions.
   b. Women with gingival lichen planus should be evaluated for possible coexistent vulvo-vaginal lichen planus.
   c. Reticular oral lichen planus is the least common form of the disease.
   d. Positive findings on direct immunofluorescence evaluation of tissue biopsies are diagnostic for oral lichen planus.

2. Drug-induced oral lichenoid lesions may:
   a. Differ markedly on clinical examination from idiopathic oral lichen planus
   b. Show similar histologic and immunofluorescence features
   c. Be caused by hepatitis C infection
   d. Only occur when skin lesions are also present

3. What forms of oral lichen planus have most often been associated with hidden or developing malignant changes?
   a. Reticular and papular
   b. Reticular and plaquelike
   c. Papular and erosive
   d. Plaquelike and erosive

4. Chronic ulcerative stomatitis is a newly identified disease that may be mistaken for:
   a. Erosive lichen planus
   b. Mucous membrane pemphigoid
   c. Pemphigus vulgaris
   d. Erythema multiforme

5. Which of the following statements is true regarding mucous membrane pemphigoid (MMP)?
   a. Occurs most often in teenagers and young adults
   b. Only affects the oral cavity
   c. Primarily affects the gingiva
   d. Infection is the primary etiologic factor

6. Histologic examination of MMP reveals:
   a. A split between epithelial cells
   b. Liquefaction degeneration of the basal epithelial cells
   c. An intense lymphocytic inflammatory infiltrate
   d. A split between the epithelial basal cell layer and the connective tissue

7. Which of the following statements is false regarding pemphigus vulgaris (PV)?
   a. It is the most common of a group of similar diseases.
   b. It usually affects adults past the age of 50.
   c. It may be life-threatening.
   d. It only occurs in the oral cavity after severe skin lesions are present.

8. Histologic examination of PV reveals:
   a. Cell separation and blistering within the epithelium
   b. Liquefaction degeneration of the basal epithelial cells
   c. An intense lymphocytic inflammatory infiltrate
   d. A split between the epithelial basal cell layer and the connective tissue

9. Which of the following statements is false regarding lupus erythematosus (LE)?
   a. It occurs more often in women and blacks.
   b. The discoid form may be localized on skin or in the mouth.
   c. The systemic form is usually associated with ulcerated oral lesions.
   d. Clinically it may appear similar to desquamative gingivitis.

10. Which of the following statements is false regarding graft-versus-host disease (GVHD)?
    a. It represents an effort by the host to reject engrafted bone marrow.
    b. It affects more than half of individuals who receive bone marrow transplants.
    c. Oral lesions may mimic lichen planus or lupus erythematosus.
    d. The dentist should not be the primary care provider for the condition.

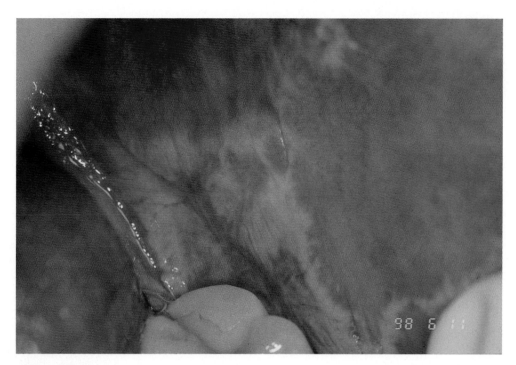

*Figure 25.1* ●

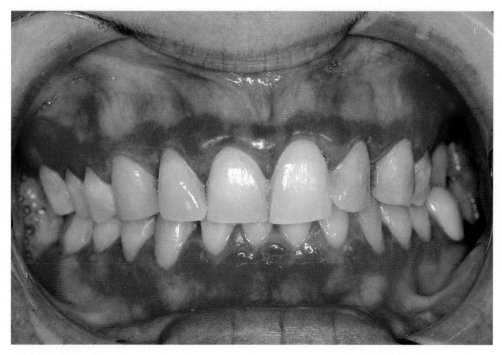

*Figure 25.2* ●

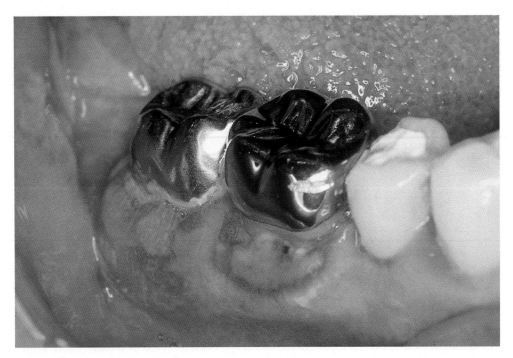

*Figure 25.3a* ●

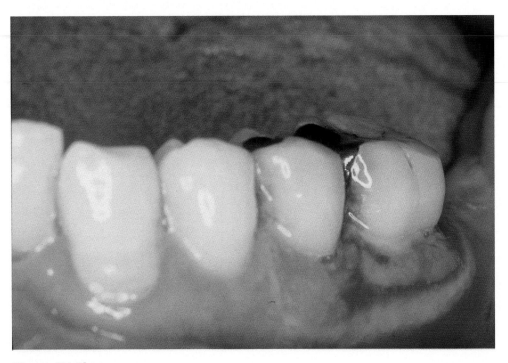

*Figure 25.3b* ●

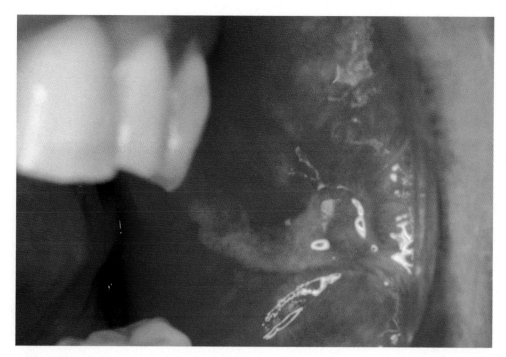

*Figure 25.4a* ●

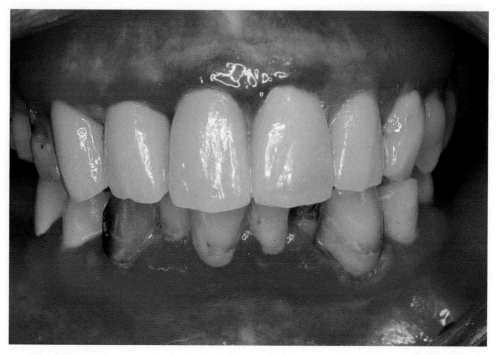

*Figure 25.4b* ●

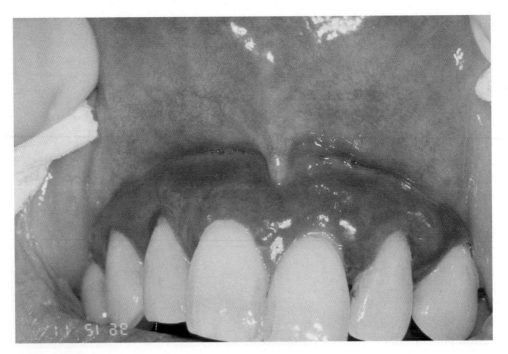

Figure 25.5 ●

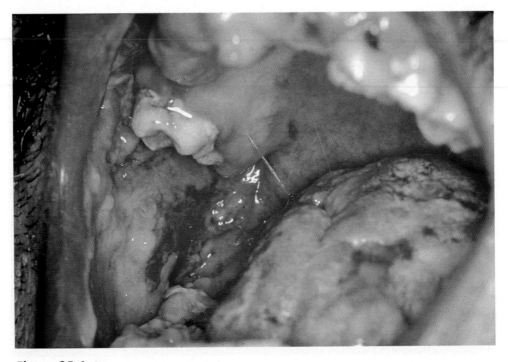

Figure 25.6 ●

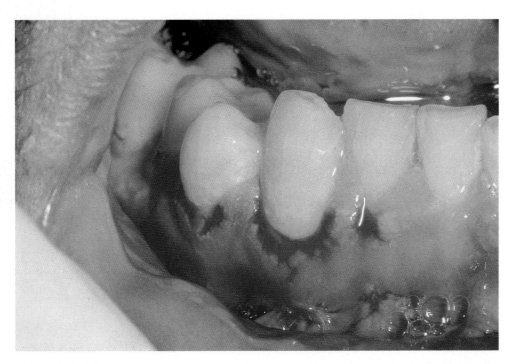

*Figure 25.7* ●

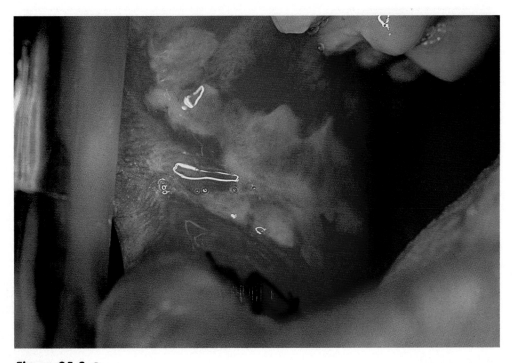

*Figure 25.8* ●

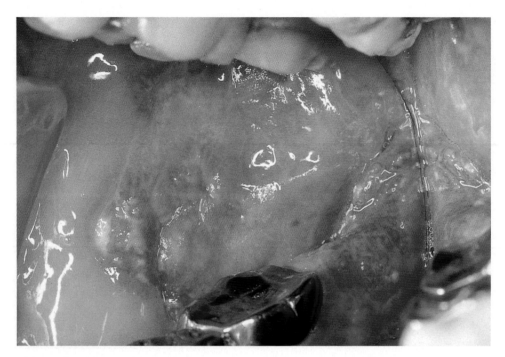

*Figure 25.9* ●

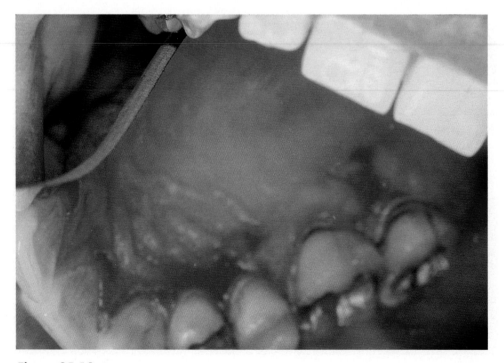

*Figure 25.10* ●

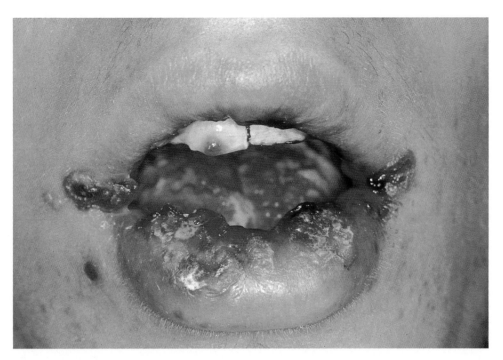

*Figure 25.11a* ●

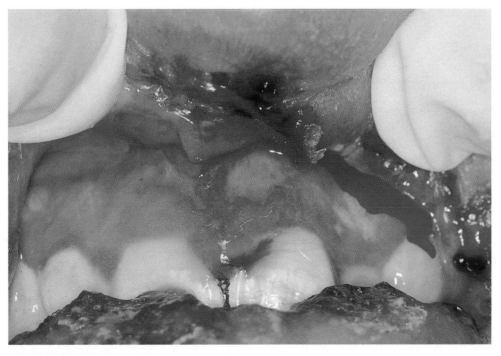

*Figure 25.11b* ●

# Answers to Review Questions

## CHAPTER 1
**REVIEW QUESTIONS**

1. b
2. d
3. e
4. b
5. b
6. b
7. c
8. a
9. b
10. c

## CHAPTER 2
**REVIEW QUESTIONS**

1. a
2. d
3. a
4. d
5. a
6. a
7. c
8. a
9. b
10. a

## CHAPTER 3
**REVIEW QUESTIONS**

1. a
2. b
3. b
4. d
5. c
6. a
7. d
8. d

9. b
10. b

## CHAPTER 4
**REVIEW QUESTIONS**

1. a
2. b
3. a
4. d
5. a
6. a
7. a
8. a
9. d
10. a

## CHAPTER 5
**REVIEW QUESTIONS**

1. a
2. a
3. d
4. b
5. c
6. b
7. b
8. b
9. a
10. c

## CHAPTER 6
**REVIEW QUESTIONS**

1. a
2. a
3. d
4. a
5. c

6. a
7. a
8. c
9. b
10. a

6. a
7. b
8. a
9. c
10. b

## CHAPTER 7
**REVIEW QUESTIONS**

1. c
2. b
3. c
4. d
5. a
6. d
7. c
8. e
9. b
10. a

## CHAPTER 11
**REVIEW QUESTIONS**

1. b
2. answers may vary
3. e
4. b
5. a
6. c
7. b
8. d
9. a
10. d

## CHAPTER 8
**REVIEW QUESTIONS**

1. b
2. c
3. a
4. c
5. a
6. d
7. d
8. c
9. d
10. c

## CHAPTER 12
**REVIEW QUESTIONS**

1. a
2. b
3. c
4. d
5. c
6. b
7. a
8. a
9. c
10. c

## CHAPTER 9
**REVIEW QUESTIONS**

1. a
2. c
3. b
4. a
5. c
6. c
7. b
8. d
9. c
10. a

## CHAPTER 13
**REVIEW QUESTIONS**

1. a
2. c
3. b
4. d
5. d
6. b
7. b
8. a
9. b
10. a

## CHAPTER 10
**REVIEW QUESTIONS**

1. d
2. a
3. f
4. c
5. d

## CHAPTER 14
**REVIEW QUESTIONS**

1. c
2. b
3. a
4. d
5. c

6. d
7. a
8. c
9. b
10. d

## CHAPTER 15
### REVIEW QUESTIONS

1. a
2. d
3. d
4. d
5. c
6. a
7. b
8. c
9. a
10. d
11. c

## CHAPTER 16
### REVIEW QUESTIONS

1. a
2. c
3. a
4. b
5. d
6. b
7. b
8. a
9. a
10. c

## CHAPTER 17
### REVIEW QUESTIONS

1. c
2. a
3. d
4. c
5. c
6. d
7. a
8. a
9. b
10. a

## CHAPTER 18
### REVIEW QUESTIONS

1. c
2. d
3. c
4. b
5. b

6. b
7. b
8. c
9. c
10. c
11. b
12. b
13. b
14. c
15. b
16. e

## CHAPTER 19
### REVIEW QUESTIONS

1. b
2. a
3. c
4. b
5. d
6. b
7. d
8. b
9. a
10. b

## CHAPTER 20
### REVIEW QUESTIONS

1. c
2. c
3. b
4. c
5. a
6. d
7. c
8. a
9. c
10. a

## CHAPTER 21
### REVIEW QUESTIONS

1. a
2. b
3. a
4. a
5. d
6. c
7. c
8. c
9. c
10. d
11. a
12. a
13. b

CHAPTER 22
## REVIEW QUESTIONS

1. c
2. b
3. c
4. b
5. b
6. b
7. b
8. c
9. d
10. b

CHAPTER 23
## REVIEW QUESTIONS

1. a
2. b
3. d
4. c
5. b
6. c
7. d
8. b
9. c
10. a

CHAPTER 24
## REVIEW QUESTIONS

1. b
2. d
3. b
4. b
5. d
6. (1) d; (2) a; (3) b; (4) c
7. b
8. a
9. d
10. c

CHAPTER 25
## REVIEW QUESTIONS

1. b
2. b
3. d
4. a
5. c
6. d
7. d
8. a
9. c
10. a

# Index

Page numbers followed by a t indicate table; those followed by an f indicate figure.